T0259570

Anemia

Editor

THOMAS G. DELOUGHERY

MEDICAL CLINICS
OF NORTH AMERICA

www.medical.theclinics.com

Consulting Editor
BIMAL H. ASHAR

March 2017 • Volume 101 • Number 2

ELSEVIER

1600 John F. Kennedy Boulevard • Suite 1800 • Philadelphia, Pennsylvania, 19103-2899

http://www.theclinics.com

MEDICAL CLINICS OF NORTH AMERICA Volume 101, Number 2
March 2017 ISSN 0025-7125, ISBN-13: 978-0-323-50980-0

Editor: Jessica McCool
Developmental Editor: Alison Swety

Medical Clinics of North America (ISSN 0025-7125) is published bimonthly by Elsevier Inc., 360 Park Avenue South, New York, NY 10010-1710. Months of publication are January, March, May, July, September, and November. Business and editorial offices: 1600 John F. Kennedy Boulevard, Suite 1800, Philadelphia, PA 19103-2899. Periodicals postage paid at New York, NY, and additional mailing offices. Subscription prices are USD $268.00 per year (US individuals), $563.00 per year (US institutions), $100.00 per year (US Students), $330.00 per year (Canadian individuals), $731.00 per year (Canadian institutions), $200.00 per year (Canadian and foreign students), $402.00 per year (foreign individuals), and $731.00 per year (foreign institutions). To receive student/resident rate, orders must be accompanied by name of affiliated institution, date of term, and the signature of program/residency coordinator on institution letterhead. Orders will be billed at individual rate until proof of status is received. Foreign air speed delivery is included in all Clinics' subscription prices. All prices are subject to change without notice. **POSTMASTER:** Send address changes to *Medical Clinics of North America*, Elsevier Health Sciences Division, Subscription Customer Service, 3251 Riverport Lane, Maryland Heights, MO 63043. **Customer Service: Telephone: 1-800-654-2452** (U.S. and Canada); **1-314-447-8871** (outside U.S. and Canada). **Fax: 314-447-8029. E-mail: journalscustomerserviceusa@elsevier.com** (for print support); **journalsonlinesupport-usa@elsevier.com** (for online support).

Reprints. For copies of 100 or more of articles in this publication, please contact the Commercial Reprints Department, Elsevier Inc., 360 Park Avenue South, New York, NY 10010-1710. Tel.: 212-633-3874; Fax: 212-633-3820; E-mail: reprints@elsevier.com.

Medical Clinics of North America is also published in Spanish by McGraw-Hill Interamericana Editores S. A., P.O. Box 5-237, 06500 Mexico, D.F., Mexico.

Medical Clinics of North America is covered in *MEDLINE/PubMed (Index Medicus), Current Contents, ASCA, Excerpta Medica, Science Citation Index,* and *ISI/BIOMED.*

PROGRAM OBJECTIVE
The goal of the *Medical Clinics of North America* is to keep practicing physicians up to date with current clinical practice by providing timely articles reviewing the state of the art in patient care.

TARGET AUDIENCE
All practicing physicians and other healthcare professionals.

LEARNING OBJECTIVES
Upon completion of this activity, participants will be able to:
1. Review the presentation and diagnosis various types of anemia including iron deficiency anema, anemia of inflammation, and congenital haemolytic anemia, among others.
2. Discuss the evaluation and treatment of various types of anemia.
3. Recognize unusual presentations of anemia.

ACCREDITATION
The Elsevier Office of Continuing Medical Education (EOCME) is accredited by the Accreditation Council for Continuing Medical Education (ACCME) to provide continuing medical education for physicians.

The EOCME designates this enduring material for a maximum of 15 *AMA PRA Category 1 Credit*(s)™. Physicians should claim only the credit commensurate with the extent of their participation in the activity.

All other health care professionals requesting continuing education credit for this enduring material will be issued a certificate of participation.

DISCLOSURE OF CONFLICTS OF INTEREST
The EOCME assesses conflict of interest with its instructors, faculty, planners, and other individuals who are in a position to control the content of CME activities. All relevant conflicts of interest that are identified are thoroughly vetted by EOCME for fair balance, scientific objectivity, and patient care recommendations. EOCME is committed to providing its learners with CME activities that promote improvements or quality in healthcare and not a specific proprietary business or a commercial interest.

The planning committee, staff, authors and editors listed below have identified no financial relationships or relationships to products or devices they or their spouse/life partner have with commercial interest related to the content of this CME activity:
Bimal H. Ashar, MD, MBA, FACP; Sharl Azar, MD; Michael J. Cascio, MD; Kim-Hien T. Dao, DO, PhD; Ananya Datta Mitra, MD; Molly Maddock Daughety, MD; Thomas G. DeLoughery, MD, MACP, FAWM; Anjali Fortna; Paula G. Fraenkel, MD; Lawrence Tim Goodnough, MD; Ralph Green, MD, PhD; Kristina Haley, DO, MCR; Howard A. Liebman, MA, MD; Jessica McCool; Premkumar Nandhakumar; Anil K. Panigrahi, MD, PhD; Joseph J. Shatzel, MD; Jason A. Taylor, MD, PhD; Ilene C. Weitz, MS, MD; Amy Williams; Trisha E. Wong, MD, MS.

UNAPPROVED/OFF-LABEL USE DISCLOSURE
The EOCME requires CME faculty to disclose to the participants:
1. When products or procedures being discussed are off-label, unlabelled, experimental, and/or investigational (not US Food and Drug Administration [FDA] approved); and
2. Any limitations on the information presented, such as data that are preliminary or that represent ongoing research, interim analyses, and/or unsupported opinions. Faculty may discuss information about pharmaceutical agents that is outside of FDA-approved labelling. This information is intended solely for CME and is not intended to promote off-label use of these medications. If you have any questions, contact the medical affairs department of the manufacturer for the most recent prescribing information.

TO ENROLL
To enroll in the *Medical Clinics of North America* Continuing Medical Education program, call customer service at 1-800-654-2452 or sign up online at http://www.theclinics.com/home/cme. The CME program is available to subscribers for an additional annual fee of USD $295.

METHOD OF PARTICIPATION
In order to claim credit, participants must complete the following:
1. Complete enrolment as indicated above.
2. Read the activity.

3. Complete the CME Test and Evaluation. Participants must achieve a score of 70% on the test. All CME Tests and Evaluations must be completed online.

CME INQUIRIES/SPECIAL NEEDS

For all CME inquiries or special needs, please contact elsevierCME@elsevier.com.

MEDICAL CLINICS OF NORTH AMERICA

THE CLINICS ARE AVAILABLE ONLINE!
Access your subscription at:
www.theclinics.com

Contributors

CONSULTING EDITOR

BIMAL H. ASHAR, MD, MBA, FACP
Associate Professor of Medicine, Division of General Internal Medicine, Johns Hopkins University School of Medicine, Baltimore, Maryland

EDITOR

THOMAS G. DeLOUGHERY, MD, MACP, FAWM
Professor of Medicine, Pathology, and Pediatrics, Division of Hematology/Medical Oncology, Department of Medicine, Knight Cancer Institute, Oregon Health and Science University, Portland, Oregon

AUTHORS

SHARL AZAR, MD
Fellow, Division of Hematology and Medical Oncology, Department of Medicine, Oregon Health and Science University, Portland, Oregon

MICHAEL J. CASCIO, MD
Assistant Professor, Department of Pathology, Oregon Health and Science University, Portland, Oregon

KIM-HIEN T. DAO, DO, PhD
Hematology and Medical Oncology, Knight Cancer Institute, Oregon Health and Science University, Portland, Oregon

ANANYA DATTA MITRA, MD
Resident, Department of Pathology and Laboratory Medicine, UC Davis Medical Center, University of California Davis Health System, Sacramento, California

MOLLY MADDOCK DAUGHETY, MD
Division of Hematology/Medical Oncology, Department of Medicine, Division of Laboratory Medicine, Department of Pathology, Oregon Health and Science University, Portland, Oregon

THOMAS G. DeLOUGHERY, MD, MACP, FAWM
Professor of Medicine, Pathology, and Pediatrics, Division of Hematology/Medical Oncology, Department of Medicine, Knight Cancer Institute, Oregon Health and Science University, Portland, Oregon

PAULA G. FRAENKEL, MD
Assistant Professor, Department of Medicine, Harvard Medical School, Division of Hematology/Oncology, Cancer Research Institute, Beth Israel Deaconess Medical Center, Boston, Massachusetts

LAWRENCE TIM GOODNOUGH, MD
Professor, Departments of Pathology and Medicine, Stanford University, Stanford, California

RALPH GREEN, MD, PhD
Distinguished Professor, Department of Pathology and Laboratory Medicine, UC Davis Medical Center, University of California Davis Health System, Sacramento, California

KRISTINA HALEY, DO, MCR
Division of Pediatric Hematology/Oncology, Department of Pediatrics, Oregon Health and Science University, Portland, Oregon

HOWARD A. LIEBMAN, MA, MD
Professor of Medicine and Pathology, Jane Anne Nohl Division of Hematology, Department of Medicine, Keck School of Medicine, University of Southern California, Los Angeles, California

ANIL K. PANIGRAHI, MD, PhD
Clinical Instructor, Departments of Pathology and Anesthesiology, Stanford University, Stanford, California

JOSEPH J. SHATZEL, MD
Fellow, Division of Hematology and Medical Oncology, Knight Cancer Institute, Oregon Health and Science University, Portland, Oregon

JASON A. TAYLOR, MD, PhD
Associate Professor, Division of Hematology and Medical Oncology, Portland VA Medical Center, Knight Cancer Institute, Associate Director, The Hemophilia Center, Oregon Health and Science University, Portland, Oregon

ILENE C. WEITZ, MS, MD
Associate Clinical Professor of Medicine, Jane Anne Nohl Division of Hematology, Department of Medicine, Keck School of Medicine, University of Southern California, Los Angeles, California

TRISHA E. WONG, MD, MS
Assistant Professor, Divison of Hematology/Oncology, Department of Pediatrics, Division of Transfusion Services, Department of Pathology, Oregon Health and Science University, Portland, Oregon

Contents

Anemia is among the most common medical problems and clinical and laboratory evaluation need to be approached logically. The complete blood count with red cell indices offers clues to diagnosis. Many anemias have characteristic red cell morphology. The reticulocyte count serves as a useful screen for hemolysis or blood loss. Testing for specific causes of the anemia is performed. Occasionally, examination of the bone marrow is required for diagnosis. Molecular testing is increasingly being use to aid the diagnostic process. This article reviews diagnostic tests for anemia and suggests a rational approach to determining the etiology of a patient's anemia.

Impaired iron homeostasis and the suppressive effects of proinflammatory cytokines on erythropoiesis, together with alterations of the erythrocyte membrane that impair its survival, cause anemia of inflammation. Recent epidemiologic studies have connected inflammatory anemia with critical illness, obesity, aging, kidney failure, cancer, chronic infection, and auto-immune disease. The proinflammatory cytokine, interleukin-6, the iron regulatory hormone, hepcidin, and the iron exporter, ferroportin, interact to cause iron sequestration in the setting of inflammation. Although severe anemia is associated with adverse outcomes in critical illness, experimental models suggest that iron sequestration is part of a natural defense against pathogens.

Vitamin B_{12} and folate deficiencies are major causes of megaloblastic anemia. Causes of B_{12} deficiency include pernicious anemia, gastric surgery, intestinal disorders, dietary deficiency, and inherited disorders of B_{12} transport or absorption. The prevalence of folate deficiency has decreased because of folate fortification, but deficiency still occurs from malabsorption and increased demand. Other causes include drugs and inborn metabolic errors. Clinical features of megaloblastic anemia include anemia, cytopenias, jaundice, and megaloblastic marrow morphology. Neurologic symptoms occur in B_{12} deficiency, but not in folate deficiency. Management includes identifying any deficiency, establishing its cause, and replenishing B_{12} or folate parenterally or orally.

Iron deficiency is one of the most common causes of anemia. The 2 main etiologies of iron deficiency are blood loss due to menstrual periods and blood loss due to gastrointestinal bleeding. Beyond anemia, lack of iron has protean manifestations, including fatigue, hair loss, and restless legs. The most efficient test for the diagnosis of iron deficiency is the serum ferritin. Iron replacement can be done orally, or in patients in whom oral iron is not effective or contraindicated, with intravenous iron.

Myelodysplastic syndrome (MDS) is a heterogeneous, clonal stem cell disorder of the blood and marrow typically diagnosed based on the presence of persistent cytopenia(s), dysplastic cells, and genetic markers. Common issues that arise in the clinical management include difficulty confirming MDS diagnosis, lack of a standard approach with novel agents in MDS, and few prospective long-term, randomized controlled MDS clinical studies to guide allogeneic blood and marrow transplant. With the recent genetic characterization of MDS, certain aspects of these issues will be better addressed by integrating genetic data into clinical study design and clinical practice.

Autoimmune hemolytic anemia is an acquired autoimmune disorder resulting in the production of antibodies directed against red blood cell antigens causing shortened erythrocyte survival. The disorders can present as a primary disorder (idiopathic) or secondary to other autoimmune disorders, malignancies, or infections. Treatment involves immune modulation with corticosteroids and other agents.

Red blood cell (RBC) destruction can be secondary to intrinsic disorders of the RBC or to extrinsic causes. In the congenital hemolytic anemias, intrinsic RBC enzyme, RBC membrane, and hemoglobin disorders result in hemolysis. The typical clinical presentation is a patient with pallor, anemia, jaundice, and often splenomegaly. The laboratory features include anemia, hyperbilirubinemia, and reticulocytosis. For some congenital hemolytic anemias, splenectomy is curative. However, in other diseases, avoidance of drugs and toxins is the best therapy. Supportive care with transfusions are also mainstays of therapy. Chronic hemolysis often results in the formation of gallstones, and cholecystectomy is often indicated.

Sickle cell disease (SCD) is an inherited monogenic disease characterized by misshapen red blood cells that causes vaso-occlusive disease, vasculopathy, and systemic inflammation. Approximately 300,000 infants are born per year with SCD globally. Acute, chronic, and acute-on-chronic complications contribute to end-organ damage and adversely affect quantity and quality of life. Hematopoietic stem cell transplantation is the only cure available today, but is not feasible for the vast majority of people suffering from SCD. Fortunately, new therapies are in late clinical trials and more are in the pipeline, offering hope for this unfortunate disease, which has increasing global burden.

Thrombotic thrombocytopenia purpura (TTP) and the hemolytic uremic syndrome (HUS) are rare thrombotic microangiopathies that can be rapidly fatal. Although the acquired versions of TTP and HUS are generally highest on this broad differential, multiple rarer entities can produce a clinical picture similar to TTP/HUS, including microangiopathic hemolysis, renal failure, and neurologic compromise. More recent analysis has discovered a host of genetic factors that can produce microangiopathic hemolytic syndromes. This article discusses the current understanding of thrombotic microangiopathy and outlines the pathophysiology and causative agents associated with each distinct syndrome as well as the most accepted treatments.

Many processes lead to anemia. This review covers anemias that are less commonly encountered in the United States. These anemias include hemoglobin defects like thalassemia, bone marrow failure syndromes like aplastic anemia and pure red cell aplasia, and hemolytic processes such as paroxysmal nocturnal hemoglobinuria. The pathogenesis, diagnostic workup, and treatment of these rare anemias are reviewed.

Transfusion of red blood cells (RBCs) is a balance between providing benefit for patients while avoiding risks of transfusion. Randomized, controlled trials of restrictive RBC transfusion practices have shown equivalent patient outcomes compared with liberal transfusion practices, and meta-analyses have shown improved in-hospital mortality, reduced cardiac events, and reduced bacterial infections. This body of level 1 evidence has led to substantial, improved blood utilization and reduction of inappropriate blood transfusions with implementation of clinical decision support via electronic medical records, along with accompanying educational initiatives.

Foreword

This Is Not an Anemic Issue

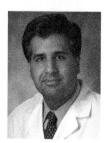

Bimal H. Ashar, MD, MBA, FACP
Consulting Editor

In a recent article (*Perspectives in Biology and Medicine* 2015,58:419-43), physician and medical historian John G. Sotos suggests that former first lady Mary Todd Lincoln suffered from pernicious anemia. In the years following her husband's assassination, Mrs Lincoln was noted to become socially isolated and mentally unstable. Those around her labeled her as hypochondriacal. Dr Sotos goes on to describe how the former first lady manifested a number of signs and symptoms over 3 decades that "...included sore mouth, pallor, paresthesias, the Lhermitte symptom, fever, headaches, fatigue, resting tachycardia, edema, episodic weight loss, progressive weakness, ataxia, and visual impairment." He concluded that these were all consistent with undiagnosed vitamin B12 deficiency due to chronic multisystem pernicious anemia.

One hundred thirty-five years after the death of Mrs Lincoln, significant advances have been made in the diagnosis of anemia. The World Health Organization estimates that anemia afflicts 1.6 billion people worldwide (about one-fourth of the world's population). Its widespread prevalence has led to it becoming an adjective in the nonmedical English lexicon, meaning feeble, weak, or bland. Yet, anemia is still frequently underrecognized and untreated. It is also seen as a poor prognostic indicator for many diseases.

In this issue of *Medical Clinics of North America*, Dr DeLoughery and colleagues provide an extensive overview of common and uncommon causes of anemia. I hope that

Med Clin N Am 101 (2017) xiii–xiv
http://dx.doi.org/10.1016/j.mcna.2016.12.002
0025-7125/17/© 2016 Published by Elsevier Inc.

this overview will serve as a thorough reference for practicing clinicians, assisting them in diagnosing and managing this pervasive condition.

Bimal H. Ashar, MD, MBA, FACP
Division of General Internal Medicine
Johns Hopkins University School of Medicine
601 North Caroline Street
#7143
Baltimore, MD 21287, USA

E-mail address:
Bashar1@jhmi.edu

Preface

Anemia: Things Have Changed!

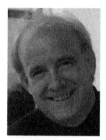

Thomas G. DeLoughery, MD, MACP, FAWM
Editor

Anemia is one of the most common diagnoses patients present with and also can complicate the course of many illnesses. In the last few years, there has been an explosion of new information about pathogenesis, diagnosis, and treatment of anemia. This issue of the *Medical Clinics of North America* has a team of experts to provide state-of-the-art reviews of a wide array of topics related to anemia to bring the reader up-to-date on this exciting area of Hematology.

Dr Cascio provides an overview of tests both old and new for anemia, ranging from the time-honored review of the blood smear to the role of molecular diagnostics. Dr Fraenkel reviews the pathogenesis of the anemia of inflammations, its role in many disease states, and possibilities for treatment.

Then, nutritional anemias take the stage. Drs Green and Datta Mitra thoroughly review all aspects of megaloblastic anemia, focusing on vitamin B12 and folate deficiency but also reviewing rarer causes. Then, I discuss iron deficiency and review the data of the harmful effects of nonanemic iron deficiency and treatment options.

Dr Dao uses a case-based approach to make comprehensible issues in diagnosis and treatment of myelodysplastic syndromes. The many forms of autoimmune hemolytic anemia are discussed by Drs Liebman and Weitz, focusing on aspects of pathogenesis, presentation, testing, and treatment. Congenital hemolytic anemia is the focus of Dr Haley's article, where she reviews the protean manifestations of these anemias, the clues to diagnosis, and some of the most common hemolytic anemias.

Drs Azar and Wong review sickle cell anemia with a discussion on new trends in treatment for this disabling disease. Drs Shatzel and Taylor review the range of thrombotic microangiopathies, ranging from thrombotic thrombocytopenic purpura to rare causes of hemolytic uremic syndromes and the new treatment options for these conditions. Then, discussions of anemia come to a close with Dr Daughety reviewing less common anemias.

Finally, Drs Goodnough and Panigrahi review red cell transfusions therapy and provide an overview of the crucial clinic trials that have recently helped define appropriate use of this commonly given therapy.

Med Clin N Am 101 (2017) xv–xvi
http://dx.doi.org/10.1016/j.mcna.2016.12.001
0025-7125/17/© 2016 Published by Elsevier Inc.

medical.theclinics.com

I am proud of the talent that took time to write these state-of-the-art reviews for this issue of *Medical Clinics of North America*, and I hope the readers of these articles find them both enlightening and helpful in their care for patients.

Thomas G. DeLoughery, MD, MACP, FAWM
Division of Hematology/Medical Oncology
Department of Medicine
Knight Cancer Institute
Oregon Health and Science University
MC L586
3181 Southwest Sam Jackson Park Road
Portland, OR 97239, USA

E-mail address:
delought@ohsu.edu

Anemia
Evaluation and Diagnostic Tests

Michael J. Cascio, MD[a], Thomas G. DeLoughery, MD, MACP, FAWM[b,c],*

KEYWORDS

- Red cell indices • Schistocytes • Microcytic • Macrocytic • Cytogenetics • Anemia
- Diagnostic testing

KEY POINTS

- Both the red cell indices and blood smear can offer clues to diagnosis and help to guide laboratory testing.
- Classification of anemia by either size of the red cell or mechanism (decreased production or increased loss) can narrow down the differential diagnosis.
- New molecular technologies may offer improved diagnostic sensitivity and specificity.

ANEMIA: DEFINITION

Although anemia is common, the exact cutoff to establish a diagnosis can be elusive. The standard definition is population-based and varies by gender and race. Current hemoglobin cutoff recommendations range from 13 to 14.2 g/dL in men and 11.6 to 12.3 g/dL in women.[1] Data from large population studies suggests that hemoglobin levels for African Americans tend to be 0.8 to 0.7 g/dL lower, perhaps owing to the high frequency of alpha-thalassemia in this population.[2] Another important factor is the trend of hemoglobin. For example, a patient with previous hemoglobin values at the higher end of the normal range, who now presents with a hemoglobin concentration at the lower end of the normal range, can now be considered anemic.

SYMPTOMS AND SIGNS OF ANEMIA

In general, the signs and symptoms of anemia are unreliable in predicting the degree of anemia. Several factors determine the symptomatology of anemia, with time of

The authors report no conflict of interest.
a Department of Pathology, Oregon Health and Science University, 3181 SW Sam Jackson Park Road, MC L-471, Portland, OR, 97239, USA; b Division of Hematology/Medical Oncology, Department of Medicine, Knight Cancer Institute, Oregon Health and Science University, MC L586, 3181 Southwest Sam Jackson Park Road, Portland, OR 97239, USA; c Division of Laboratory Medicine, Department of Pathology, Oregon Health and Science University, Hematology L586, 3181 Southwest Sam Jackson Park Road, Portland, OR 97201-3098, USA
* Corresponding author. Division of Hematology/Medical Oncology, Department of Medicine, Knight Cancer Institute, Oregon Health and Science University, MC L586, 3181 Southwest Sam Jackson Park Road, Portland, OR 97239, USA.
E-mail address: delought@ohsu.edu

Med Clin N Am 101 (2017) 263–284
http://dx.doi.org/10.1016/j.mcna.2016.09.003
0025-7125/17/© 2016 Elsevier Inc. All rights reserved.

onset and overall baseline health of the patient being the most important. Patients who gradually develop anemia over a period of months can tolerate lower hemoglobin owing to the use of compensatory mechanisms. An example would be a patient with sickle cell disease who can tolerate a chronic hemoglobin concentration of 7 g/dL. Because blood delivers oxygen, many of the signs are related to lack of oxygen delivery, chiefly, fatigue and shortness of breath. On physical examination, anemia is manifested by paleness of the mucous membranes and resting tachycardia. One should look for other physical examination clues to a possible source of anemia, such as splenomegaly, guaiac-positive stools, or oral telangiectasia.

COMPENSATION FOR ANEMIA

There are 3 physiologic compensatory mechanisms for anemia. The first is by increasing cardiac output. Because oxygen delivery is cardiac output times hemoglobin, patients with decreased hemoglobin can maintain the same level of oxygen delivery by increasing cardiac output. Therefore, patients with limited cardiac reserve (heart failure, coronary artery disease) will have symptoms at higher hemoglobin concentrations than those with normal cardiac function. Increasing plasma volume is the second compensatory mechanism. This allows the remaining red cells to move around more efficiently owing to decreased viscosity. The increased plasma volume also increases cardiac output and helps to maintain blood pressure. Finally, red cell 2,3-diphosphoglycerate increases, which decreases oxygen affinity for hemoglobin. This results in more oxygen delivery to tissues. The high ambient oxygen tension in the alveoli leads to full oxygenation of hemoglobin despite its decreased oxygen affinity, but at the tissue level this results in more delivery of oxygen.

CLASSIFICATION

There are 2 classification systems for anemia (**Box 1**). The first is based on Wintrobe observations that red cell size can differentiate potential etiologies of anemia. This led to the concepts of "microcytic," "normocytic," and "macrocytic" anemia.[3] Microcytic anemias are those with a mean corpuscular volume (MCV) less than normal (<80 fL). Microcytic anemias reflect defects in hemoglobin synthesis. Lack of iron, either owing to deficiency or sequestration (anemia of inflammation), thalassemia, or sideroblastic anemias (defect of heme synthesis) all can lead to microcytosis.

There are 2 general etiologies of macrocytic anemias (MCV > 100 fL)[4]—red cell membrane defects and DNA synthesis defects. Red cell membrane defects can occur in the setting of liver disease or hypothyroidism. Macrocytic red blood cells (RBCs) in this setting tend to be round on review of the peripheral smear. In contrast, defects in DNA synthesis (such as those seen with megaloblastic anemia or chemotherapy) show a prominent oval macrocytosis. One of the most common causes of macrocytic anemia is the presence of a reticulocytosis. The average size of the reticulocyte (160 fL) can yield an high MCV in the setting of hemolysis.

The difficulty in using red cell size as a means of distinguishing potential etiologies for anemia is that, in many cases, the red cells demonstrate a normal size ("normocytic anemia," MCV 80–100 fL). This may occur during early stages of a process (such as iron deficiency) or when multiple processes occur simultaneously (concurrent iron deficiency and liver disease) and lead to a red cell size within the normal range.

The other classification schema uses the underlying mechanism of anemia (increase in RBC loss or decrease in RBC production). The first branch point is if red cell

> **Box 1**
> **Classification of anemia**
>
> *Size*
>
> - Microcytic
>   - Iron deficiency
>   - Thalassemia
>   - Sideroblastic anemia
>   - Anemia of inflammation
> - Macrocytic
>   - Round
>   - Aplastic anemia
>   - Hypothyroidism
>   - Liver disease
>   - Renal disease
>   - Reticulocytosis
>   - Thyroid disease
>   - Oval
>   - Vitamin B_{12} and folate deficiency
>   - Chemotherapy
>   - Myelodysplastic syndrome
> - Normocytic
>   - Anemia of inflammation
>   - Acute onset hemolysis or blood loss
>   - Renal disease
>
> *Mechanism*
>
> - Increased loss
>   - Hemorrhage
>   - Hemolysis (immune, microangiopathic, intrinsic red blood cell defects)
> - Decreased production
>   - Stem cell (myelodysplastic syndrome, acute leukemia)
>   - Nutritional (iron, vitamin B_{12}, folate, copper)
>   - Toxin/drug
>   - Lack of growth factors (renal disease, anemia of chronic disease)
>   - Myelophthisic process (metastatic cancer, infection, fibrosis)

production is increased or decreased as determined by the reticulocyte count. If increased, then hemolysis and blood loss are primary considerations. If red cell production seems to be decreased, then basic causes of impaired marrow production should be considered:

- Nutritional: iron, vitamin B_{12}, folate, copper deficiency
- Marrow failure: aplastic anemia, pure red cell aplasia, myelodysplasia, leukemia
- Lack of growth factors: lack of erythropoietin (EPO) owing to chronic renal disease
- Myelophthisic process: cancer, infection

DIAGNOSTIC TESTS

Diagnostic testing should focus on (1) determining whether an anemia is present and (2) identifying the underlying etiology. Basic assays (complete blood count, reticulocyte count, and blood smear) will be reviewed first, with more specific assays covered elsewhere in this article.

Complete Blood Count

The complete blood count is probably one of the most widely performed tests in the world. The complete blood count was originally performed by manual methods, but currently there are 2 main forms of automated technology that are used. Each automated method directly measures the number of cells, the volume of individual cells, and the hemoglobin concentration.

The first automated method was devised by Wallace Coulter in the 1950s and relies on electrical impedance. When RBCs flow through an aperture in a current-conducting solution, the nonconducting RBCs induce a momentary alteration in current impedance between the sensing electrodes. Each impedance pulse correlates with an individual RBC passing through an aperture, whereas the magnitude of the impulse is directly proportional to cell size.

A newer method uses laser light scatter properties. In this assay, RBCs are hydrodynamically focused in a flow cell and a beam of laser light is applied. A photodetector then captures the light scatter emitted from each cell. The photodetector then converts this light scatter to electrical impulses, the number of which is proportional to the number of RBCs passing through the laser. Similar to the impedance method, the amplitude of the light scatter pulse is proportional to RBC size.

Hemoglobin concentration is determined by photospectometry after erythrocyte lysis. Although red cell number, size, and hemoglobin concentration are directly measured, the hematocrit is a calculated value, and can be less reliable when there is inaccuracy in the measurements of the other red cell indices.

Peripheral Blood Smear Assessment

The blood smear can offer valuable diagnostic clues to the etiology of anemia (**Table 1**). The clinician can request a formal blood smear review by the laboratory technologist or pathologist to assess red cell, white cell, and platelet morphology. When initiating such requests, it is important to convey relevant clinical and laboratory findings that may not be available to the pathologist.

Assessment of red cell size is an important part of the peripheral smear evaluation. Normocytic red cells are approximately the same size as the nucleus of a small resting lymphocyte (**Fig. 1**). Red cells that are larger than the lymphocyte nucleus are considered macrocytic and those that are smaller are microcytic. As noted, when a macrocytic anemia is present, it is important to distinguish round and oval macrocytosis owing to differing underlying etiologies.

Microcytosis may be seen in the setting of iron deficiency, hemoglobin H disease, thalassemia minor, sideroblastic anemias, and in some cases of anemia of chronic disease. When evaluating a microcytosis, assessment for hypochromia can be helpful in determining whether the changes may be owing to or in part reflect iron deficiency. In normal red cells, central pallor occupies approximately one-third of the RBC diameter. An increase in the central pallor is indicative of hypochromia, which generally occurs at hemoglobin concentrations less than 10 g/dL and the degree of which correlates with the severity of the anemia (**Figs. 2 and 3**). The differential diagnosis for microcytic hypochromic anemia includes thalassemia, iron deficiency, sideroblastic anemias, and anemia of chronic disease.

Anisocytosis and poikilocytosis refer to the variation of red cell size and shape, respectively. Although a mild increase in anisopoikilocytosis lacks diagnostic specificity, it is important to note whether the RBC abnormality observed is a high frequency or low frequency abnormality. High frequency abnormalities, as the name suggests, are RBC types that occur more often in normal blood films. Examples include

Table 1
RBC morphologic findings

RBC Finding	Mechanism	Clinical Setting
Coarse basophilic stippling	Remnant of ribosomes	Lead poisoning, marrow stress, thalassemia
Bite cells	Hemoglobin denaturation and removal by RES	Oxidative hemolytic anemia
Burr cells	Membrane alteration related to increased lipids, calcium	Artifact, liver disease, uremia, hyperlipidemia
Acanthocytes	Increased cholesterol in RBC membrane	Liver disease, abetalipoproteinemia, McLeod syndrome
Elliptocytes	RBC cytoskeletal defects	Heredity elliptocytosis, iron deficiency
Howell-Jolly bodies	RNA remnants	Splenectomy or functional hyposplenism
Nucleated red cells	Retention of nucleus	Splenectomy, marrow stress, myelopthisis
Schistocytes	Mechanical RBC damage	Microangiopathic hemolytic anemia
Reticulocytosis (shift cells)	High RNA content	Hemolysis, marrow stress
Spherocytosis	Loss of RBC membrane, cytoskeletal defect	Hereditary spherocytosis, autoimmune hemolytic anemia
Target cells	Excess RBC membrane cholesterol, decreased hemoglobin	Thalassemia, hemoglobin C and E disease, obstructive liver disease
Tear drop cells	Extension of RBC cytoplasm	Myelophthisis, fibrosis, extramedullary hematopoiesis

Abbreviations: RBC, red blood cells; RES, reticuloendothelial system.

acanthocytes, echinocytes, target cells, and ovalocytes. In contrast, low frequency abnormalities are rare or seldom seen in blood of healthy individuals. These include schistocytes, tear drop cells, and blister cells, among others. The severity of the poikilocytosis can be estimated based on the relative percent of each abnormal RBC type observed, which are commonly reported by the laboratory in a tiered grading scheme.

Schistocytes, or helmet cells, are red cell fragments that contain 2 or 3 pointed ends (**Fig. 4**). The presence of an increased number of schistocytes implies intravascular damage to red cells. The mechanism of schistocyte formation involves mechanical shearing of the red cell membrane by intravascular deposits, such as fibrin strands or platelet aggregates. Schistocytes can be increased in the setting of disseminated intravascular coagulation, thrombotic thrombocytopenia purpura, hypertension, preeclampsia, mechanical heart valves, and a ventricular assist device.

Spherocytes appear as round, slightly smaller red cells that lack central pallor and have a more deeply red appearance than other red cells. Spherocytes are formed through loss of red cell membrane; this converts the biconcave disk (most surface area for a given volume) to a sphere, which is the least amount of surface area. An increased number of spherocytes is seen in hereditary spherocytosis, hemolytic anemias mediated by immune mechanisms, and in microangiopathic hemolytic anemias (see **Fig. 4**).

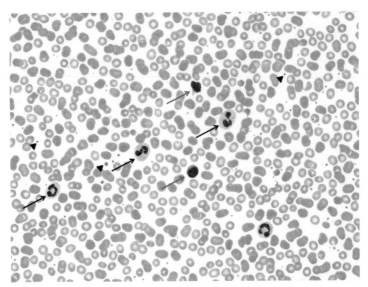

Fig. 1. Normal peripheral blood smear (original magnification, ×400). Red blood cells (RBCs) show a normal central pallor (less than one-third of the diameter of the RBC) and have a size that is roughly equal to the size of the nucleus of a small lymphocyte (*red arrows*). Normal neutrophils (*black arrows*) with segmented nuclei and pink cytoplasm are shown. Platelets with normal size and blue-purple alpha granules are easily identified in the background (*black arrowheads*).

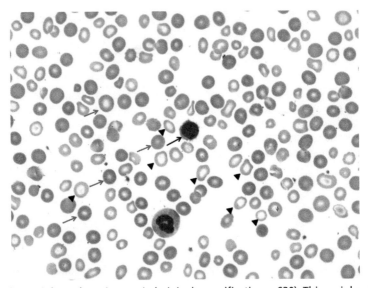

Fig. 2. Microcytic hypochromic anemia (original magnification, ×630). This peripheral blood film was from a patient with iron deficiency anemia. Note the "dimorphic" red cell populations. One population (*black arrowheads*) seems to be smaller than the nucleus of a small lymphocyte (*black arrow*) and shows an increase in central pallor. The second population shows a more normal size and lacks central pallor (less than one-third of the red blood cell diameter, *red arrows*).

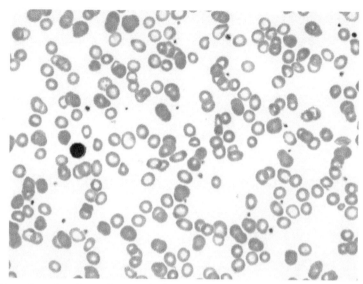

Fig. 3. Hypochromic microcytic anemia (original magnification, ×630). In contrast with **Fig. 2**, the red blood cells (RBCs) on this smear show a relatively uniform appearance, with "normal appearing" RBCs absent.

Elliptocytes (ovalocytes) are oval to elongated rodlike red cells. A uniform increase in elliptocytes is mainly seen in the setting of hereditary elliptocytosis, which is caused by abnormalities in red cell membrane or cytoskeletal proteins, alpha-spectrin (*SPTA1*), beta-spectrin (*SPTB*), or protein 4.1R[5] (**Fig. 5**). In iron deficiency, elliptocytes

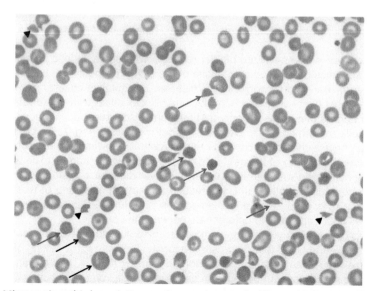

Fig. 4. Microangiopathic hemolytic anemias are characterized by an increase in spherocytes (*blue arrows*), schistocytes (*red arrows*), nonspecific red cell fragments (*black arrowheads*), and polychromatophilic cells (*black arrows*) (original magnification, ×630).

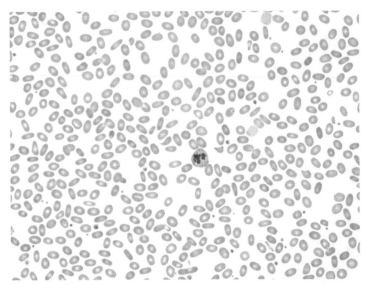

Fig. 5. Elliptocytes are increased in a variety of conditions. Here, a relatively uniform population of elliptocytes is noted incidentally on peripheral smear review during a bleeding diathesis work up. The patient had a positive family history of hereditary elliptocytosis (original magnification, ×400).

are microcytic and more elongate and are termed "pencil" cells. A dramatic increase in anisopoikilocytosis with hypochromic microcytes can help to support a diagnosis of iron deficiency. Ovalocytes can be seen in the setting of hereditary conditions such as southeast Asian ovalocytosis or in acquired cases, such as myelodysplastic syndrome (MDS). Southeast Asian ovalocytosis results from mutations in *SLC4A1* and occurs in a geographic distribution that parallels that of malaria endemic regions. The presence of this mutation confers resistance to *Plasmodium falciparum* and *Plasmodium vivax*.[5]

Drepanocytes (sickle cells) are bipolar red cells with characteristic points at each end (**Fig. 6**). These cells are characteristic of the sickling syndromes, such as Sickle cell disease or trait and hemoglobin SC disease. Quantitative assessment of sickle cells on peripheral smear review is of dubious clinical value, with no correlation between the degree of disease severity and the number of drepanocytes observed.

Target cells are formed owing to excess red cell membrane (**Fig. 7**). On blood smear review, they have a characteristic "bull's eye" appearance owing to hemoglobin occupying the central portion of the cell. Target cells occur when there is excess red cell membrane compared with hemoglobin level. In liver disease, target cell formation is owing to altered lipid metabolism, whereas in the setting of setting of thalassemia, the abnormality is owing to lack of hemoglobin production. Clinical findings, MCV, and red cell count can help to differentiate between the two.

Teardrop cells (dacrocytes) have an extended cytoplasmic projection resembling a tail. Increased numbers of tear drop cells are most often seen in the setting of marrow myelophthisis (such as metastatic carcinoma), marrow fibrosis, and extramedullary hematopoiesis, but also can be found in cases of severe iron deficiency.

Spur cells (acanthocytes) have a few, irregularly spaced and variably sized projections on their surface (**Fig. 8**). Additionally, the central pallor of the RBC is absent and the red cell has a "contracted" or dense appearance. Acanthocyte formation is related

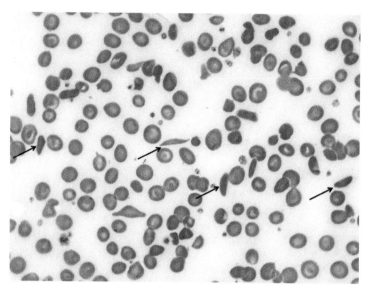

Fig. 6. Drepanocytes (sickle cells) are denoted by black arrows (original magnification, ×630).

to defects in the lipid or protein composition in the red cell membrane, most commonly seen in the setting of severe liver disease. Other less common causes include abeta-lipoproteinemia, malnutrition, McLeod phenotype (lack of Kx antigen), and neuroacan-thocytosis syndrome.

Burr cells (echinocytes) are red cells with short, evenly spaced, uniform projections and preserved central pallor (see **Fig. 8**). Probably the most common cause of Burr

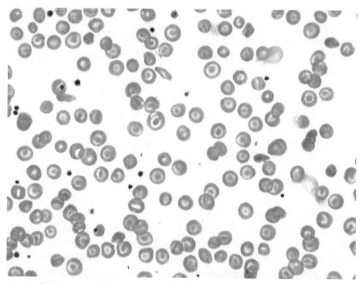

Fig. 7. Innumerable target cells are present in this patient with hemoglobin C disease (original magnification, ×630).

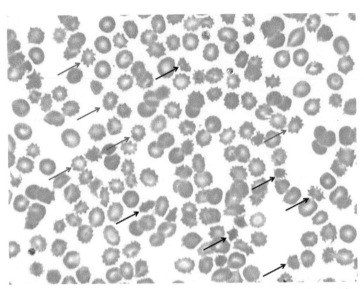

Fig. 8. Acanthocytes (*black arrows*) and Burr cells (*red arrows*) in a patient with end-stage liver disease owing to hepatitis C virus infection (original magnification, ×630). Note the irregularly spaced, "sharp" projections and loss of central of the acanthocyte versus the more "blunt" and regularly distributed projections and retained central pallor of the Burr cell.

cells is artifact related to prolonged storage before smear preparation. Pathologically, Burr cells are seen in end-stage kidney disease (uremia) and obstructive liver disease.

Bite cells (degmacytes) have semicircular defects in the edge of the red cell membrane that resembles a "bite." During oxidative stress, hemoglobin precipitates out of solution to form insoluble aggregates (Heinz bodies) that are then removed by the reticuloendothelial system of the spleen and liver. Bite cells and blister cells are seen in the setting of glucose-6-phosphate dehydrogenase deficiency and drug-induced oxidant hemolysis (**Fig. 9**).

When evaluating for a macrocytic anemia, the recognition of polychromatophilic red cells can be an important finding in determining the cause of red cell macrocytosis. Polychromatophilic cells are macrocytic, lack central pallor, and have a blue-gray appearance (**Fig. 10**). Their appearance is a function of their immaturity, with their distinctive color attributable to the presence of residual polyribosomes not found in mature RBCs. An increase in polychromatophilic cells is seen under conditions of marrow stress or hemolysis and can be a useful marker of a raised reticulocyte count. Identification of reticulocytes, and thus, the calculation of the reticulocyte count, requires special staining protocols with fluorescent or supravital dyes (ie, methylene blue).

Nucleated red cells (nRBCs) are not normally present in the peripheral blood (see **Fig. 10**). nRBCs can be seen in several situations and usually indicate the presence of severe hemolysis, hemoglobinopathies, a myelophthisic process, or severe physiologic stress. Because the spleen normally functions to remove nRBCs from the circulation, postsplenectomy patients will demonstrate an increased number of nRBCs in addition to significant anisopoikilocytosis and Howell-Jolly body formation.

Rouleaux is manifest in the thin part of the smear by the stacking of greater than 3 red cells, resembling a "stack of coins" (**Fig. 11**). This is an in vitro phenomenon related

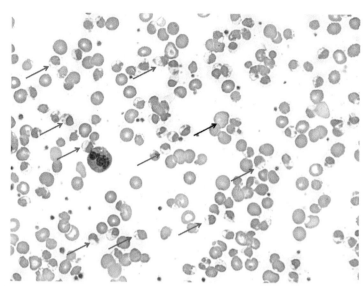

Fig. 9. Blister cells are seen in settings of drug or medication induced oxidative injury, usually in patients with glucose-6-phosphate-dehydrogenase deficiency. Note the presence of numerous "blister" cells (*red arrows*), as characterized by the puddling of hemoglobin at 1 aspect of the cell with the other aspect having a "cleared-out" look surrounded by a thin rim of red membrane (original magnification, ×600). A few polychromatophilic cells are present (*black arrow*).

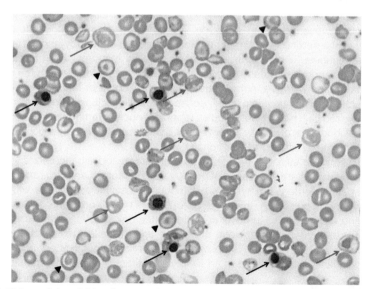

Fig. 10. This peripheral blood smear demonstrates numerous nucleated red blood cells (*black arrows*), polychromatophilic cells (*red arrows*), and target cells (*black arrowheads*; original magnification, ×630). The patient had beta thalassemia/hemoglobin E disease.

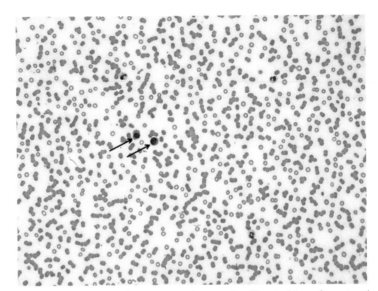

Fig. 11. Rouleaux is an in vitro phenomenon characterized by stacking of greater than 3 red blood cells and is mainly seen in the setting of increased serum protein levels, typically in patients with a severe infectious/inflammatory process or a monoclonal protein spike. This peripheral blood smear demonstrates an increase in Rouleaux formation in a patient with plasma cell myeloma (original magnification, ×50). Rare circulating plasma cells are identified (*black arrows*).

to an high protein concentration, which functions to disrupt the zeta potential on the red cell surface that normally causes the RBCs to repel one another. Rouleaux can occur in the setting of increased acute phase reactant proteins (ie, fibrinogen) in inflammatory states or in the presence of a monoclonal paraprotein.

Autoagglutination manifests as rounded aggregates or clumps of RBCs that form owing to the presence of an antibody. This in vitro phenomenon occurs most commonly in the setting of an immunoglobulin (Ig)M autoantibody and is referred to as "cold agglutinins." Although many cold agglutinins may not have clinical significance, from a laboratory perspective, their presence may interfere with the ability of the automated analyzer to accurately determine RBC count or MCV.

Howell-Jolly bodies are single small, dense basophilic inclusions located at the periphery of the red cell. Howell-Jolly bodies represent nuclear remnants (DNA). Because Howell-Jolly bodies are usually removed by the spleen, their presence indicates a hyposplenic state (anatomic or functional).

Coarse basophilic stippling manifests as punctate basophilic inclusions in the red cell. These inclusions are composed of precipitated ribosomes and RNA and are indicative of impaired hemoglobin synthesis. Although classically associated with lead or other heavy metal poisoning, in clinical practice it is more commonly seen in conditions with increased red cell turnover and altered hemoglobin synthesis, especially hemoglobinopathies, dyserythropoietic states, or any process that leads to marrow stress. Fine basophilic stippling is observed in polychromatophilic cells and is a clinically insignificant artifact related to an air-drying artifact of the peripheral smear.

Reticulocyte Count

The reticulocyte count is a measure of the production of new red cells by the marrow. Because the average lifespan of a red cell is 120 days, approximately 1% of red cells will be removed from the circulation each day. To maintain steady state, the marrow needs to constantly produce new RBCs. Reticulocytes are immature, nonnucleated RBCs that circulate in the peripheral blood for 1 day before losing their RNA and becoming mature RBCs.

The traditional method of measuring the reticulocyte count is a manual method that uses supravital stains (such as methylene blue) to highlight the reticulum (RNA) network of this immature red cell fraction. The technologist then enumerates the number of reticulocytes and expresses this value as a percent of total RBCs. The main difficulty with this test is that it depends on the hematocrit. Thus, a reticulocyte count of 1% in a patient with a hematocrit of 45 would "increase" to 2% if the hematocrit decreased to 22.5. Therefore, the raw number needs to be corrected for the hematocrit by multiplying the value by patient's hematocrit divided by 45 (corrected reticulocyte count = retic % [Hct%/45]). So, in the above example, the corrected reticulocyte count would be 2% times (22.5/45) equals 1%.

The number of reticulocytes can be measured directly by most automated analyzers by staining the remnant RNA with a fluorescent dye. This is known as the absolute reticulocyte count. Advantages of automated methods include improved turnaround time, measurement precision, and lack of need to adjust for hematocrit.

The usefulness of the reticulocyte count is in assessing the marrow response to anemia. If the reticulocyte count is elevated, then either blood loss or hemolysis is suggested. "Normal" reticulocyte counts are indicative of production causes of anemia. Very low reticulocyte counts (<0.1% or 10,000/µL) are seen in aplastic anemia or pure red cell aplasia.

RED CELL INDICES: OLD AND NEW

Originally, 3 of the red cell indices were derived or calculated (**Table 2**): (1) MCV, (2) mean corpuscular hemoglobin concentration (MCHC), and (3) mean corpuscular hemoglobin (MCH). On most new analyzers MCV, hemoglobin, and red cell count are directly measured and MCHC and MCH are calculated. Because the MCHC and MCH tend to trend with the MCV, these indices are rarely used anymore.

With more widespread use of new automated complete blood count analyzers, there are now a wider array of newer "indices" available.[6] With the ability to rapidly identify reticulocytes these machines can determine both reticulocyte MCV and reticulocyte MCHC, and from this derive an MCH (CHr/Ret-He). Most studies of these newer indices have been in patients receiving EPO who develop "functional" iron deficiency where the delivery of iron to the developing red cell cannot keep up with demand. The CHr/Ret-He falls with the onset of iron deficiency and is the first to increase with iron supplementation. However, the CHr/Ret-He also can be reduced in thalassemia; therefore, hemoglobinopathies should be excluded before it is used to assess iron status.

Table 2 RBC indices		
Index	**Normal Values**	**Comment**
MCV	80–100 fL	RBC size
Mean corpuscular hemoglobin concentration	33.8–34.2 m/dL	Increased in spherocytosis
Mean corpuscular hemoglobin	28.5–32.3 pg	Trends with MCV

Abbreviations: MCV, mean corpuscular volume; RBC, red blood cell.

BONE MARROW EXAMINATION

For some causes of anemia a bone marrow evaluation is required. A common issue that arises is determining when a bone marrow examination should be performed in the evaluation of anemia. In general, a bone marrow examination should be considered if:

- Circulating immature cells are identified on peripheral smear (blasts, etc);
- Severe pancytopenia (decreased numbers of all cell types);
- Very low reticulocyte counts (<0.1%);
- Circulating nucleated RBCs;
- Evidence of marrow infiltration (leukoerythroblastic blood picture);
- Evaluation of a monoclonal paraproteins; and
- Unexplained severe anemia, especially if there is suspicion of myelodysplasia.

The aspirate part of the procedure involves withdrawing the liquid marrow. From the aspirate, smears are made for morphologic review (**Fig. 12**) and material can be sent for flow cytometry, cytogenetics (karyotyping and fluorescence in situ hybridization studies), molecular diagnostics, and microbiologic studies. A core biopsy should also be obtained for accurate assessment of marrow cellularity (**Fig. 13**). The core biopsy also provides the opportunity to identify disease processes that may show patchy involvement of the marrow space, such as in the case of some lymphomas and granulomatous infectious/inflammatory infiltrates.

CYTOGENETICS AND MOLECULAR TESTS

Cytogenetic and molecular studies are a useful adjunct in the workup of a patient with unexplained anemia. To achieve optimal results, good quality aspirate material should

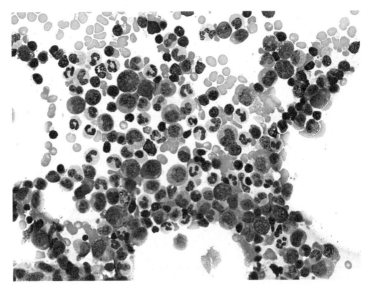

Fig. 12. Normal bone marrow aspirate (original magnification, ×400). This aspirate shows the presence of a mixture of maturing granulocytic and erythroid precursors. Well prepared aspirate smears with adequate spicules should be obtained when considering a diagnosis of myelodysplastic syndrome.

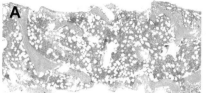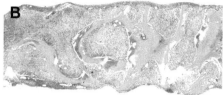

Fig. 13. (*A*) Normal bone marrow core biopsy (stain: hematoxylin and eosin; original magnification, ×25). The normal adult marrow shows a cellularity of 30% to 70%, which is estimated by comparing the proportion of cells to adipocytes. The core biopsy is important for determining marrow cellularity and the presence of any focal infiltrates such as granulomas, lymphoma, or metastatic cancer. (*B*) Bone marrow core biopsy demonstrating cellularity of greater than 95% in a patient with myelodysplastic syndrome (stain: hematoxylin and eosin; original magnification, ×25).

be obtained and with minimal peripheral blood hemodilution. Additionally, the treating clinician should communicate diagnostic considerations to the pathologist or the laboratory for optimal triage of the specimen and selection of appropriate studies.

Classical cytogenetic studies involve the culture of cells obtained from marrow aspirates and subsequent assessment of the metaphase karyotype. In most instances, routine karyotyping is complemented by the use of fluorescence in situ hybridization (FISH). Fluorescent probes are designed to label certain genes or chromosome regions. Depending on probe design, FISH can be used to detect chromosomal deletions, duplications, rearrangements, and translocations. After hybridizing the FISH probe(s) to interphase cells, up to 200 nuclei are observed by a technologist and the presence of any abnormalities are noted and scored as a percent of all nuclei. For malignancies such as plasma cell myeloma, acute myeloid leukemia, and B-lymphoblastic leukemia, the use of FISH has allowed for improved detection of abnormalities that are not commonly seen in karyotypic analysis, allowing for better risk stratification and optimal therapeutic management.

Increasingly, molecular genetic studies are being routinely used in the clinical setting. Sequencing technologies such as allele-specific oligonucleotide polymerase chain reaction or reverse transcriptase polymerase chain reaction have been used to identify specific recurrent genetic alterations. Common examples include the use of *BCR-ABL* reverse transcriptase polymerase chain reaction to diagnose and/or monitor patients with chronic myeloid leukemia and the use of allele-specific oligonucleotide polymerase chain reaction to detect *KIT* D816V mutations in systemic mastocytosis.

Next-generation sequencing (NGS) is a massively paralleled sequencing platform that allows a multitude of specific genes or even entire exomes to be sequenced and analyzed. Increasingly, laboratories are designing large NGS panels to detect a wide array of gene mutations commonly seen in hematologic malignancies and in solid tumors. Although many NGS panels focus on detecting mutations seen in myeloid and lymphoid malignancies, there is increasing use in the diagnosis of nonneoplastic diseases, such as inherited hemolysis and hemoglobinopathies.

TESTING FOR SPECIFIC CAUSES OF ANEMIA
Renal Disease

The juxtaglomerular apparatus in the afferent arterioles of the kidney produce EPO, the key hormone responsible for inducing the growth and production of erythroid precursors in the bone marrow (**Box 2**). The anemia of renal disease is owing to lack of EPO. The level of renal function at which patients become anemic can vary. Classically, anemia is not seen until the creatinine clearance is less than 30 mL/min. However, in the setting of concurrent inflammation or advanced age, anemia can be seen even with creatinine clearance in the 60 mL/min range. Certain medications can decrease EPO production, with angiotensin-converting enzyme inhibitors and angiotensin II receptor blockers being the most common.[7]

Anemia of Inflammation

The anemia of inflammation, also known as the anemia of chronic disease, is a diagnosis of exclusion. In anemia of chronic disease, iron stores are adequate, but there is impaired iron delivery to the developing red cell. EPO production is suppressed. Therefore, the finding of an insufficiently increased EPO level in the setting of anemia with adequate iron stores is strongly suggestive of anemia of chronic disease. In the

---

Box 2
Testing for specific causes of anemia

Renal disease
- Creatine/blood urea nitrogen
- Erythropoietin level

Anemia of chronic disease
- Erythropoietin
- Ferritin

Nutritional deficiencies
- Iron: ferritin
- Vitamin B_{12}: methylmalonic acid
- Folate: homocysteine
- Copper: serum copper, ceruloplasmin

Thalassemia
- Hemoglobin electrophoresis
- DNA sequencing

Sickle cell disease
- Sickle solubility test
- Hemoglobin electrophoresis

Hemolysis (general screening)
- Haptoglobin
- Lactate dehydrogenase
- Indirect bilirubin
- Reticulocyte count

Myeloma
- Serum protein electrophoresis and immunofixation
- Serum free light chain analysis

future measure of hepcidin levels—the molecular mediator of anemia of chronic disease—will offer direct testing.

Endocrine Disease

Several endocrine diseases can lead to anemia with the etiology related to decreased red cell production. Hypogonadism is an important cause of anemia in men. Testosterone sensitizes erythroid precursors to the effects of EPO. This provides the rationale for why postpubertal males have a 10% to 15% greater hemoglobin concentration, hematocrit, and RBC counts than women.[7] Hypothyroidism can lead to a normocytic or macrocytic anemia.

Iron Deficiency

Over time, a negative iron balance owing to blood loss or increased demand will lead to a reduction in total body iron stores in the reticuloendothelial system and the bone marrow. Three stages in this process have been described. The iron depletion stage shows a decrease in iron stores without a decrease in serum iron levels or hemoglobin concentration outside of the normal range. Serum ferritin is low in this stage. The second stage is characterized by the detection of abnormal iron serologies, such as reduced transferrin saturation, increased total iron-binding capacity, and increased zinc protoporphyrin. The third and final stage demonstrates a hemoglobin concentration of less than the lower limit of the normal range.

Although there are a variety of tests to assess iron stores, studies have shown the most efficient test is the serum ferritin. A serum ferritin level greater than 100 ng/mL essentially rules out iron deficiency.[8] Other "classic" tests such as serum iron levels and transferrin saturation, have low predictive value. Increased total iron binding capacity is specific, but not sensitive for early stages of iron deficiency.

Iron assessment can also be performed on bone marrow aspirate material. Adequate bone marrow spicules must be present to assess for storage iron, which is contained in macrophages. Some investigators suggest a minimum of 7 particles be present to establish the absence of storage iron.[8] In addition to assessment of iron stores, evaluation for increased ring sideroblasts (erythroid precursors containing iron particles that encircle greater than two-thirds of the diameter of the nucleus) can also be performed. An increase in ring sideroblasts can signify a number of different pathologies, such as drugs/toxins (alcohol), heavy metal poisoning (lead), and MDSs.

Other Nutritional Deficiencies

Vitamin B_{12} deficiency

Vitamin B_{12} deficiency produces a megaloblastoid macrocytic anemia, which manifests in the peripheral blood with hypersegmented neutrophils and in the marrow with megaloblastoid maturation of granulocytic and erythroid lineages. There is increasing recognition of the difficulty in using serum vitamin B_{12} levels to determine tissue deficiency. Currently, measurement of methylmalonic acid is recommended. Excess methylmalonic acid is produced in the absence of vitamin B_{12} and is more sensitive and specific for vitamin B_{12} deficiency than direct measurements of serum vitamin B_{12}.[4]

Folate deficiency

Similar to vitamin B_{12} deficiency, folate deficiency manifests as a megaloblastoid macrocytic anemia and shows identical morphologic features. Both serum and red cell folate concentration lack diagnostic specificity and, like vitamin B_{12} deficiency, the use of metabolite assays are more accurate.[4] Lack of folate leads to elevation in serum homocysteine levels. Because vitamin B_{12} deficiency can also lead to elevated homocysteine, methylmalonic acid levels should be incorporated into the workup for folate deficiency.

Copper
Determining copper status is relatively straightforward. Measurement of serum copper and its carrying protein, ceruloplasmin, can aid in determining whether a copper deficiency is present. In most laboratories the ceruloplasmin assay has a faster turn-around time and may be more reflective of copper deficits.[9]

Thalassemia

Thalassemias are inherited genetic disorders that lead to impaired production of hemoglobin. They can range in severity from just a decreased MCV to very severe anemia. Most common types are alpha and beta thalassemia. The hallmark of all thalassemia is a microcytosis owing to decreased production of hemoglobin with a concurrent increase in RBC count. There are many prediction rules based on MCV and red cell count with the most popular being the Mentzer index (MCV/RBC count). A Mentzer index of less than 13 is thought to favor a diagnosis of thalassemia over iron deficiency, but this tends to lack sensitivity and specificity. More complex algorithms have also been derived and improve accuracy.

The diagnosis of beta thalassemia trait is made by hemoglobin electrophoresis. In this assay, hemoglobin is separated by size and charge to assess the presence and quantity of the different hemoglobin species. In beta-thalassemia the levels of a minor hemoglobin component—hemoglobin A2—is increased. In contrast with hemoglobin A, which is composed of 2 alpha chains and 2 beta chains, hemoglobin A2 is composed of 2 alpha chains and 2 delta chains. Increased hemoglobin A2 is a compensatory process owing to decreased production of beta chains.

Alpha thalassemia trait cannot be diagnosis by electrophoresis because there is no increase in hemoglobin A2. Often it is a diagnosis of exclusion in a patient with microcytosis who has normal iron stores and normal hemoglobin electrophoresis. To establish the diagnosis, DNA testing can be performed to determine the presence or absence of the alpha chain gene deletions.

Sickle Cell Disease and Other Hemoglobinopathies

A rapid screening test for sickle cell is the sickle solubility test. In this assay, whole blood is lysed with a reducing agent. If a sickling hemoglobin is present, an insoluble precipitate is produced. Because this is a screening, one cannot differentiate between sickle cell disease, sickle cell trait, or one of the less common sickling hemoglobin species. Definitive diagnosis is made by hemoglobin electrophoresis. Hemoglobin electrophoresis is the standard screening test for hemoglobinopathies. Clues to the presence of hemoglobinopathies are hemolysis, cyanosis, or erythrocytosis. Increasingly, DNA sequencing to find specific mutations is being used to make a precise diagnosis.[10]

Hemolysis

The diagnosis of hemolysis is a 2-step process. The first is to assess for the presence of a hemolytic anemia and the second it to establish the etiology. Screening for hemolysis uses a variety of tests, which often must be interpreted in unison and with knowledge of the patient's medical history.[11]

Haptoglobin is a protein that acts as a scavenger of free hemoglobin, thereby protecting the body from its toxic effects.[12] Low haptoglobin levels are sensitive for hemolysis, but are not specific, because severe liver disease, transfusions, and regular exercise can lead to low levels. An additional cause of absent haptoglobin levels is ahaptoglobinemia. This is an inherited condition that results in total lack of haptoglobin production. This is a relatively common condition that is found in 1:1000 whites and up 4% of African Americans.[13]

Lactate dehydrogenase is an intracellular enzyme found in abundance in the red cell. Although lactate dehydrogenase is sensitive for hemolysis, an increased level can be found in many other disorders, especially liver disease.

Indirect bilirubin increases as the breakdown of heme overwhelms the liver's ability to form conjugated bilirubin and excrete it into the bile. Liver disease can also increase levels and an increased level of indirect bilirubin can only be interpreted to imply hemolysis in the setting of a normal direct bilirubin level. Outside of fulminate hemolysis it is rare to see an indirect bilirubin greater than 4 mg/dL.

As noted, the reticulocyte count will be increased in hemolysis. Sensitivity may be an issue, because some patients will have normal reticulocyte counts owing to nutritional deficiencies, lack of EPO, or destruction of red cell precursors.[14]

Once the presence of hemolysis is established, the next step is to determine the cause. Acquired causes of hemolysis are most often owing to autoimmune disease, mechanical destruction, toxins, or paroxysmal nocturnal hemoglobinuria. The direct antibody test (Coombs test) helps to determine the presence of an antibody-mediated cause, such as might be seen in the setting of autoimmune causes. Inherited etiologies for hemolysis may involve defects in the RBC membrane/cytoskeletal proteins, hemoglobin, or intracellular enzymes. Often the blood smear provides clues to the presence of membrane or cytoskeletal defects, such as those seen in hereditary spherocytosis or elliptocytosis. Hemoglobin electrophoresis is useful for identifying hemoglobinopathies, whereas specific assays are needed to identify enzymatic defects.

Plasma Cell Myeloma

A rare but important cause of anemia, especially in older patients, is plasma cell myeloma. An high index of suspicion for this possibility should be had when evaluating anemic patients with back pain or renal disease. Serum protein electrophoresis with immunofixation and serum free light chain analysis should be obtained when evaluating for myeloma. Assessing for light chain disease is important because 10% of myelomas only excrete light chains.

Myelodysplastic Syndrome

MDS is a group of clonal bone marrow failure disorders that result in anemia and varying degrees of leukopenia and thrombocytopenia. MDS occurs in predominantly older patients, but may occur in younger individuals exposed to cytotoxic chemotherapy for childhood malignancies. Laboratory clues for MDS include a macrocytic anemia with nonelevated reticulocyte count (hypoproliferative anemia). Other cytopenias may be present. A morphologic review of the peripheral blood smear may reveal an oval macrocytosis without an increase in polychromatophilic cells. Neutrophils may show dysplastic features including nuclear hypolobation (unilobed or pseudo-Pelger Huet nuclei) or hypogranular cytoplasm (**Fig. 14**). Platelets may also show dyspoeitic features, including the presence of large or giant forms or those with absent granules.

Bone marrow examination is a requisite in the workup of a patient with suspected MDS. Adequate and well-prepared aspirate smears are of paramount importance, because this allows the pathologist to assess for diagnostic dyspoietic changes in the granulocytic, erythroid, and megakaryocytic lineages and enumerate blasts (see **Fig. 13**; **Figs. 15** and **16**). Cytogenetic studies, including FISH for MDS-related

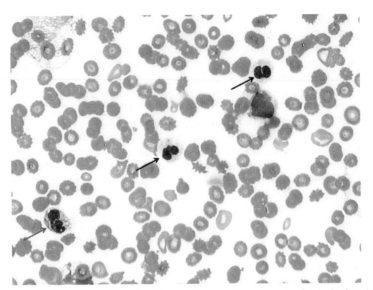

Fig. 14. Dysplastic neutrophils in the setting of acute myeloid leukemia with myelodysplasia-related changes (*black arrows*; original magnification, ×630). These polymorphonuclear leukocytes (PMNs) show bilobed nuclei with "water clear" hypogranular cytoplasm. This is contrast with the pink cytoplasm seen in normal-appearing PMNs (*red arrow*). Identification of such features on peripheral blood film can help to direct the workup and prompt earlier consideration of bone marrow examination.

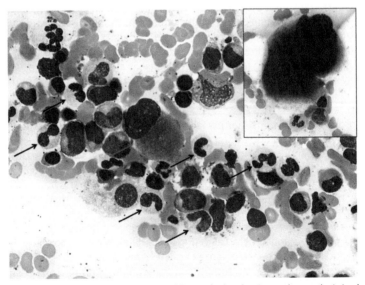

Fig. 15. Multilineage dysplasia in patient with myelodysplastic syndrome (original magnification, ×630). A small megakaryocyte with a hypolobate nucleus (*red arrow*) in a background of granulocytic dysplasia manifest as hypogranular neutrophils (*black arrows*). A normal megakaryocyte is shown for comparison (*inset*; original magnification, ×630).

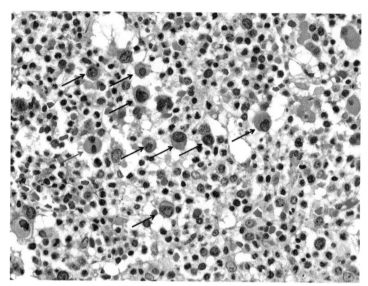

Fig. 16. At greater magnification, megakaryocytes are increased and show prominent dysplastic findings, including small size and hypolobate nuclei (*black arrows*). Rare megakaryocytes also show separated nuclear lobes (*red arrow*), another diagnostic feature of myelodysplasia (stain: hematoxylin and eosin; original magnification, ×630).

abnormalities, are extremely useful for confirming the presence of a clonal disorder, particularly in cases with subtle dyspoietic changes on morphologic examination. NGS panels for genes frequently mutated in myeloid neoplasms are becoming commonly used in routine clinical practice. Similar to cytogenetic studies, pathogenic gene mutations can help to confirm the presence of a clonal disorder and serve as a useful adjunct in cases that show a normal karyotype and lack abnormalities by FISH analysis.

| Box 3 |
| Rational approach to anemia |
| *Basic tests* |
| Complete blood count with indices |
| Reticulocyte count |
| Ferritin |
| Methylmalonic acid |
| Homocysteine |
| Creatinine/blood urea nitrogen |
| *If older or back pain add* |
| Serum protein electrophoresis with immunofixation |
| Serum-free light chain analysis |
| *If neurologic disease present add* |
| Copper |

A Rational Approach to Anemia

By combining clues from the patient history and initial complete blood count one can plot a rational approach to the anemic patient. The reticulocyte counts should be obtained to determine the presence of hemolysis. Given how common iron deficiency is and the lack of specificity of the MCV for this diagnosis, serum ferritin should be tested in every patient. Further specific testing is guided by the results of these initial studies **Box 3.**

REFERENCES

1. Cappellini MD, Motta I. Anemia in clinical practice-definition and classification: does hemoglobin change with aging? Semin Hematol 2015;52(4):261–9.
2. Beutler E, Waalen J. The definition of anemia: what is the lower limit of normal of the blood hemoglobin concentration? Blood 2006;107(5):1747–50.
3. Brugnara C, Mohandas N. Red cell indices in classification and treatment of anemias: from M.M. Wintrobes's original 1934 classification to the third millennium. Curr Opin Hematol 2013;20(3):222–30.
4. Green R, Dwyre DM. Evaluation of Macrocytic Anemias. Semin Hematol 2015;52(4):279–86.
5. Da CL, Galimand J, Fenneteau O, et al. Hereditary spherocytosis, elliptocytosis, and other red cell membrane disorders. Blood Rev 2013;27(4):167–78.
6. Piva E, Brugnara C, Spolaore F, et al. Clinical utility of reticulocyte parameters. Clin Lab Med 2015;35(1):133–63.
7. Pratt MC, Lewis-Barned NJ, Walker RJ, et al. Effect of angiotensin converting enzyme inhibitors on erythropoietin concentrations in healthy volunteers. Br J Clin Pharmacol 1992;34(4):363–5.
8. DeLoughery TG. Microcytic anemia. N Engl J Med 2014;371(14):1324–31.
9. Halfdanarson TR, Kumar N, Li CY, et al. Hematological manifestations of copper deficiency: a retrospective review. Eur J Haematol 2008;80(6):523–31.
10. Harteveld CL. State of the art and new developments in molecular diagnostics for hemoglobinopathies in multiethnic societies. Int J Lab Hematol 2014;36(1):1–12.
11. Ruiz EF, Cervantes MA. Diagnostic approach to hemolytic anemias in the adult. Rev Bras Hematol Hemoter 2015;37(6):423–5.
12. Shih AW, McFarlane A, Verhovsek M. Haptoglobin testing in hemolysis: measurement and interpretation. Am J Hematol 2014;89(4):443–7.
13. Delanghe J, Langlois M, De BM. Congenital anhaptoglobinemia versus acquired hypohaptoglobinemia. Blood 1998;91(9):3524.
14. Liesveld JL, Rowe JM, Lichtman MA. Variability of the erythropoietic response in autoimmune hemolytic anemia: analysis of 109 cases. Blood 1987;69(3):820–6.

Anemia of Inflammation
A Review

Paula G. Fraenkel, MD*

KEYWORDS

- Anemia • Inflammation • Hepcidin • Ferroportin • Interleukin-6 • Erythroferrone
- Iron • Cancer

KEY POINTS

- In anemia of inflammation, proinflammatory cytokines suppress erythropoiesis, cause iron sequestration via effects on the iron regulatory hormone, hepcidin, and promote alteration in the erythrocyte cell membrane leading to shortened red blood cell survival.
- In the setting of critical illness, severe anemia is associated with increased mortality.
- Advanced age, cancer, rheumatologic diseases, chronic infection, and kidney failure are also associated with anemia of inflammation.
- Experimental therapies reverse the effects of anemia of inflammation in animal models, but have not been approved for human use.

EPIDEMIOLOGY

Inflammation is one of the most common causes of anemia in the elderly and chronically ill. In the National Health and Nutrition Examination Study (NHANES III), anemia of inflammation was defined as a low serum iron level (<10.74 μM or <60 μg/dL) without evidence of low iron stores, that is, transferrin saturation greater than 15%, serum ferritin greater than 12 ng/mL, or erythrocyte protoporphyrin concentration greater than 1.24 μM.[1] Other features of anemia of inflammation include inappropriately low levels of erythropoietin, and elevated measures of inflammatory markers, such as C-reactive protein.[2] In the NHANES III, investigators discovered that about 1 million Americans greater than the age of 65 exhibit anemia related to inflammation.

Anemia in Critical Illness

Anemia of inflammation can occur in the setting of acute or chronic inflammation. The CRIT study of anemia and blood transfusion in the critically ill was an observational

Dr P.G. Fraenkel's research is supported by the National Institutes of Health (R01 DK085250 and R01 GM083198). Funding from the Department of Defense Peer-Reviewed Cancer Research Program (CA150529). The funding agencies did not influence the design or interpretation of the studies. Dr P.G. Fraenkel has no relevant financial conflicts of interest.
Department of Medicine, Harvard Medical School, Boston, MA, USA
* Corresponding author. Division of Hematology/Oncology, Cancer Research Institute, Beth Israel Deaconess Medical Center, CLS 434, 330 Brookline Avenue, Boston, MA 02215.
E-mail address: pfraenke@bidmc.harvard.edu

cohort analysis of 4892 patients in intensive care units across the United States.[3] The CRIT study revealed that anemia of inflammation develops in critically ill patients even within 30 days. The mean hemoglobin levels in critically ill individuals decreased over a 30-day period despite the administration of blood transfusions. The CRIT study also demonstrated that severe anemia, hemoglobin less than 9 g/dL, is an independent predictor of increased mortality and length of stay in critically ill patients.

Anemia in the elderly is frequently linked to inflammatory conditions. In a recent study of 191 consecutive hospitalized elderly patients with anemia, 70% of the patients were found to have anemia related to inflammation. Sixteen percent of the patients with anemia of inflammation had concomitant chronic renal failure.[4] Of the patients with inflammatory anemia, 71% were suffering from an acute infection, 12% had cancer, and 16% had a chronic infection, such as a pressure ulcer, or a chronic autoimmune inflammatory disease.[4]

Anemia in Obesity

As the prevalence of obesity is increasing in the United States, more attention is being paid to the potential effect of obesity on erythropoiesis. Obese patients exhibit higher plasma levels of proinflammatory cytokines and acute phase reactants as well as higher rates of iron-restricted erythropoiesis that can result in anemia.[5] Functional iron deficiency is defined as inappropriately low iron stores, despite the presence of inflammation, that is, a normal serum ferritin (12–100 ng/mL for women or 15–100 ng/mL for men) and a serum C-reactive protein greater than 3 mg/L.[6,7] A recent cross-sectional study of 947 obese patients under evaluation for bariatric surgery revealed that 52.5% exhibited functional iron deficiency. Most obese patients with functional iron deficiency appear to have sequestration of iron as manifest by a serum transferrin saturation less than 20%.[6] Weight loss has been associated with an increase in transferrin saturation in overweight individuals,[8] which supports the hypothesis that obesity causes iron sequestration.

Anemia in Cancer

Anemia of inflammation is a common manifestation of advanced cancer. A recent prospective, observational study of 888 patients with a variety of carcinomas revealed that 63.4% of the patients were anemic.[9] The prevalence and severity of anemia correlated with the stage of cancer.[9] The prevalence of increased mean plasma levels of markers of inflammation, including C-reactive protein, fibrinogen, interleukin-6 (IL-6), tumor necrosis factor-α (TNF-α), IL-1β, ferritin, hepcidin, erythropoietin, and reactive oxygen species, was significantly increased in advanced stage compared with patients with early stage cancer. Supporting a role for inflammation in iron sequestration, serum iron levels were significantly reduced in advanced stage patients.[9]

PATHOPHYSIOLOGY

Recent discoveries indicate that both iron sequestration and impaired erythropoiesis cause anemia of inflammation. Erythroid progenitors mature to erythrocytes through a series of stages that require coordination of iron acquisition and cell proliferation. As erythroid progenitors mature to the polychromatophilic stage, transferrin receptor 1 expression on the surface of the red cell membrane increases.[10] Macrophages export iron via ferroportin (fpn). The carrier protein, transferrin, binds free iron with high avidity. Transferrin-bound iron attaches to transferrin receptor 1. In an acidified vacuole, the iron is released from transferrin and exported to the cytoplasm by divalent metal transporter 1, whereas transferrin receptor is recycled to the cell surface (reviewed in Ref. [11]). The iron then enters the mitochondria, where it is attached to protoporphyrin IX in the final step of heme synthesis.

Iron is effectively salvaged in the human body. Macrophages consume senescent erythrocytes, liberate iron from hemoglobin, and store the iron in ferritin for subsequent release of iron to developing erythrocytes via fpn.[10] Studies of the *fpn*-deficient zebrafish, weissherbst,[12,13] and the *fpn*-knockout mouse[14] revealed that fpn is required to export iron from macrophages to developing erythrocytes. In fpn-deficiency, iron remains sequestered in macrophages, resulting in impaired iron delivery to developing erythrocytes and erythroid maturation arrest.[12,13]

Hepcidin is a short, cysteine-rich peptide hormone that regulates the intestinal absorption of iron and its release from macrophage iron stores. Human hepatocytes secrete the iron-regulatory peptide hormone, hepcidin,[15–17] in response to iron overload or inflammation. Hepcidin binds fpn on the surface of macrophages, resulting in the internalization and degradation of both proteins[18] and sequestration of iron in macrophages, away from the developing erythrocytes (**Fig. 1**). Hepcidin appears to be the key regulator of iron homeostasis, because loss of function mutations in genes that regulate *Hepcidin* expression, for example, *Transferrin receptor 2*, *HFE*, *Hemojuvelin*, or *Hepcidin* itself, have each been associated with hereditary iron overload syndromes.[19]

Regulation of Hepcidin

The bone morphogenic protein (BMP) coreceptor, hemojuvelin, and TMPRSS6[20–26] participate in regulating hepcidin transcription in the setting of iron overload. Iron overload enhances BMP signaling and Smad protein phosphorylation, which increases

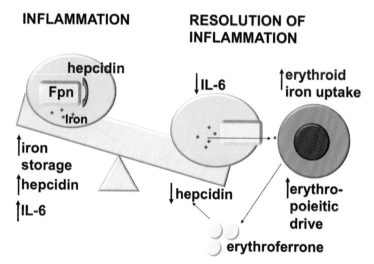

INFLAMMATION

RESOLUTION OF INFLAMMATION

Fig. 1. Inflammation stimulates increased production of the iron-regulatory peptide, hepcidin, by hepatocytes and the proinflammatory cytokine, IL-6, which suppresses erythropoiesis. Hepcidin binds the iron exporter, fpn, causing internalization and degradation of both proteins and decreasing delivery of iron from macrophages to developing erythrocytes. This impairs erythroid development and leads to anemia. Increased erythropoietic drive stimulates erythroid progenitors to release erythroferrone, a hormone that suppresses hepcidin expression. When inflammation resolves, hepcidin and IL-6 levels decline, allowing iron to be exported to from macrophages to erythrocytes and promoting erythropoiesis.

hepcidin transcription. On the other hand, iron deficiency or the acute onset of anemia stimulates release of the hormone, erythroferrone, by erythroid progenitors, and erythropoietin by the kidney.[11,27] Erythroferrone suppresses *hepcidin* expression to promote intestinal iron absorption and macrophage iron release, whereas erythropoietin stimulates proliferation of committed erythroid progenitors.[11,27]

IL-6 and IL-1β[28] are key cytokines that mediate the effects of inflammation on the developing erythrocyte. The transcription factors that mediate the effects of inflammation include Stat3, C/EBPα, and p53[29,30] (**Fig. 2**). IL-6 increases JAK/Stat signaling,[31,32] which promotes phosphorylation of Stat3 and Stat3 binding to the *Hepcidin* promoter.[30,33] IL-1β induces *Hepcidin* expression via the C/EBPα and BMP/SMAD signaling pathways. Hepatocyte damage, via endoplasmic reticulum stress or oxidation, enhances C/EBPα[34,35] or Stat3 activity,[36] respectively, leading to increased *Hepcidin* expression. Lipopolysaccharide (LPS), released by severe

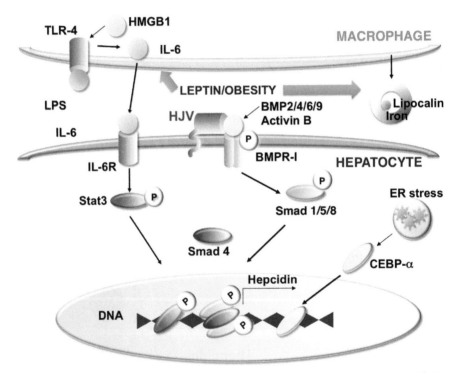

Fig. 2. Inflammation and hepatocyte damage augment *Hepcidin* transcription and iron sequestration via several pathways. LPS, released by bacterial infection, and the proinflammatory cytokine, High mobility growth box 1 (HMGB1), activate TLR4 signaling, which increases IL-6 release by macrophages, whereas leptin and obesity also promote IL-6 release. IL-6 signaling leads to phosphorylation of Stat3 and increased Stat3 binding to the *Hepcidin* promoter, whereas endoplasmic reticulum (ER) stress in hepatocytes promotes CEBP-α binding to the *Hepcidin* promoter. BMP or activin signaling via ligands, including BMP2, 4, 6, and 9 and Activin B, activate receptors, such as BMP receptor-I, causing Smad phosphorylation and Smad binding to the *Hepcidin* promoter, which is required for *Hepcidin* transcription. The BMP coreceptor, hemojuvelin (HJV), interacts with the BMP receptor to enhance BMP signaling. Inflammation or obesity also promotes macrophage release of lipocalin, which can interact with bacterial siderophores to sequester iron. P, Phosphorylation.

bacterial infection, activates toll-like receptor-4 (TLR4) signaling, which, in turn, enhances production of IL-6[37] by macrophages that stimulates hepcidin expression. HMGB1, a proinflammatory cytokine that is produced in patients with critical illness, is associated with increased in-hospital mortality. HMGB1 has been shown to bind the Myeloid differentiation factor2 (MD2)-TLR4 complex[38,39] and to increase expression of TNF and IL-6, cytokines that impair erythropoiesis.[40,41] Inhibition of HMGB1 activity ameliorates anemia of inflammation in mouse models.[38] Recent studies[42] indicate that inflammation in mouse models increases transcript levels of *Activin B*, a member of the transforming growth factor-β superfamily of signaling molecules. Activin B has been shown to increase *hepcidin* transcription in cultured hepatocytes in vitro via Smad signaling.[42]

Iron Sequestration

Hepcidin is not the only protein causing iron sequestration during bacterial infection. Recent studies indicate that stimulation of TLR2 and TLR6 in mouse models decreases expression of fpn in macrophages and causes iron sequestration without increasing macrophage *hepcidin* transcript levels.[43] LPS stimulates macrophages to produce lipocalin 2, which sequesters iron by binding bacterially produced siderophores.[44] Furthermore, infection or inflammation stimulates neutrophil release of the iron binding protein, Lactoferrin. Lactoferrin is internalized by bacteria, sequesters iron, and arrests microbial growth.[45]

Obese individuals exhibit increased plasma levels of proinflammatory cytokines, including leptin, hepcidin, and the iron sequestering protein, lipocalin-2. There are 2 proposed mechanisms by which obesity may contribute to functional iron deficiency and anemia, based on experimental models: (1) leptin and proinflammatory cytokines stimulate hepcidin production in adipocytes and hepatocytes[46]; (2) adipocytes and peripheral blood mononuclear cells in obese patients produce lipocalin 2, which restricts iron availability to developing erythroid cells.[47]

Changes in Erythrocyte Membrane

In addition to effects on iron metabolism, inflammatory cytokines diminish erythropoietin synthesis, impair the differentiation of erythroid progenitors, and shorten the lifespan of mature red blood cells.[48] Incubation of erythrocytes from healthy donors with plasma from patients with septic shock induced hydrolysis of red blood cell membrane phosphatidyl choline to lysophosphatidyl choline and increased erythrocyte phosphatidyl serine exposure,[49] changes that may shorten erythrocyte survival. The presence of renal failure can exacerbate the effects of inflammation. Uremia is associated with reduced levels of albumin, increased levels of nitric oxide, and changes in the levels of erythrocyte membrane proteins that promote the accumulation of reactive oxygen species and oxidation of erythrocyte membrane proteins (reviewed in Ref. [50]). These alterations are thought to accelerate erythrocyte destruction and tissue injury.

NEW EXPERIMENTAL MODELS

In order to develop new therapies for anemia of inflammation, animal models are needed that resemble the findings in human patients. In one recent model, killed *Brucella abortus* (KBA) bacteria are injected once by intraperitoneal injection.[40,51] Fourteen days later, mean murine hemoglobin levels decline by 50%. Erythropoiesis gradually recovers following the injection, just as human patients may recover from the insult of a critical illness, such as sepsis. Hepcidin deficiency blunted the severity of anemia following injection of KBA, whereas IL-6 deficiency protected against

Table 1
Agents with potential activity against anemia of inflammation

Class of Agent	Name	Stage of Development	Route of Administration	Citation
Anti-IL-6	Elsilimomab or BE-8	Decreased thrombocytosis and anemia in patients with metastatic renal cell carcinoma	Intravenous	53,54
Anti-IL-6	Siltuximab	Approved to treat Castleman disease; decreased anemia in patients with Castleman disease; not effective in patients with early stage myelodysplastic syndrome	Intravenous	56,57
Anti-IL-6 receptor	Tocilizumab	Approved to treat rheumatoid arthritis; decreased anemia in patients with Castleman disease	Intravenous	55
BMP receptor antagonist	LDN-193189	Evaluated in mouse models	Oral	58
Anti-hepcidin oligoribonucleotide	Spiegelmer NOX-H94	Evaluated in cynomolgus monkeys and phase I trial in humans published	Intravenous	59,60
Anti-hepcidin antibody	12B9M	Evaluated in cynomolgus monkeys	Intravenous	61

Anti-ferroportin antibody	LY2928057	Phase I trial in humans completed; results unpublished	Intravenous	Clinicaltrials.gov
Anti-hemojuvelin antibody	ABT-207 and h5F9-AM8	Preclinical study in rats	Intravenous	65
Soluble hemojuvelin extracellular domain fused with immunoglobulin Fc	HJV.fc	Preclinical study in rats	Intravenous	66
small interfering RNA (siRNA) against hepatic Egl-9 family hypoxia inducible factor (EglN) prolyl hydroxylases	EglN1+2+3 siRNA lipid nanoparticles	Preclinical study in mice	Intravenous	67
Suppressor of erythroid iron restriction response, bypasses effect of aconitase inactivation	Isocitrate	Preclinical study in rats	Intravenous	68
Inhibitor of activin signaling, decreases LPS or KBA-induced hepcidin expression in mice	Follistatin-315	Preclinical study in mice	Intraperitoneal	42

From Fraenkel PG. Understanding anemia of chronic disease. Hematology Am Soc Hematol Educ Program 2015;2015:16; with permission.

hypoferremia and anemia in murine models. *Hepcidin*-knockout mice exhibited significantly impaired survival compared with wild-type controls following injection of KBA,[51] which supports the long-held theory that anemia of inflammation is protective in critical illness.

EXPERIMENTAL TREATMENTS

The best treatment for anemia of inflammation is to eradicate the underlying disease. When that is not possible, transfusions, intravenous iron supplementation, and erythropoiesis stimulating agents[52] may ameliorate the condition. Newer, experimental approaches target IL-6 activity and the hepcidin-ferroportin axis. In 1993, researchers observed that treating patients with metastatic renal cell carcinoma with a murine anti-IL-6 antibody improved paraneoplastic thrombocytosis and anemia.[53,54] These observations led to the evaluation of antibodies against IL-6 in human patients with inflammatory anemia secondary to multicentric Castleman disease (MCD).

Patients with MCD exhibit generalized lymphadenopathy, systemic chronic inflammation, increased IL-6 activity, and anemia of inflammation.[55] Siltuximab, a human-mouse chimeric anti-IL-6 antibody has been shown to improve anemia in patients with this condition.[56] Siltuximab was subsequently evaluated in a phase II trial in patients with transfusion-dependent, low- or intermediate-risk myelodysplastic syndrome, whose levels of proinflammatory cytokines are often elevated; however, siltuximab failed to reduce transfusion dependence in these patients.[57] Tocilizumab, a humanized monoclonal antibody against the IL-6 receptor that has been approved to treat rheumatoid arthritis, has been found to reduce serum hepcidin levels and improve anemia in patients with Castleman disease and rheumatoid arthritis.[52,55]

Inhibitors of hepcidin production, blockers of hepcidin peptide activity, and antibodies to fpn have also been used to modulate anemia of inflammation. A potent, orally available BMP receptor antagonist, LDN-193189, has been shown to decrease BMP signaling and reduce *hepcidin* mRNA levels in mice in a dose-dependent manner. Furthermore, LDN-193189 ameliorated anemia of inflammation in mice that had been injected with turpentine to generate sterile abscesses.[58] Other efforts have focused on agents that are administered parenterally. NOX-H94, a structured L-oligoribonucleotide that binds human hepcidin with a high affinity, blocked IL-6-induced hypoferremia and moderated the development of anemia in cynomolgus monkey models.[59] In human trials, NOX-H94 prevented LPS-induced hypoferremia.[60] The human antihepcidin antibody, 12B9M, increased serum iron levels in cynomolgus monkeys, but has not been evaluated in a primate model of anemia of inflammation.[61] A phase I trial to evaluate the effect of an antibody against fpn, LY2928057, has been completed, but the results are not yet available (clinicaltrials.gov). **Table 1** summarizes other experimental therapies in development. Conversely, small molecules that increase hepcidin expression may be developed into treatments for iron overload.[62–64]

Knowledge of the interaction between inflammation, iron metabolism, and erythropoiesis has improved the ability to understand anemia of inflammation. Although drugs have not yet been approved to treat this condition, several agents are under investigation, and some agents improve anemia of inflammation in patients with Castleman disease or rheumatoid arthritis. In some cases, anemia of inflammation may be protective; for instance, in animal models of the anemia of critical illness, *hepcidin*-deficient mice exhibited significantly lower rates of survival than wild-type animals.[51] Thus, the best course of action continues to be to identify and treat the underlying causes of the anemia of chronic disease.

REFERENCES

1. Guralnik JM, Eisenstaedt RS, Ferrucci L, et al. Prevalence of anemia in persons 65 years and older in the United States: evidence for a high rate of unexplained anemia. Blood 2004;104(8):2263–8.
2. van Iperen CE, Gaillard CA, Kraaijenhagen RJ, et al. Response of erythropoiesis and iron metabolism to recombinant human erythropoietin in intensive care unit patients. Crit Care Med 2000;28(8):2773–8.
3. Corwin HL, Gettinger A, Pearl RG, et al. The CRIT study: anemia and blood transfusion in the critically ill–current clinical practice in the United States. Crit Care Med 2004;32(1):39–52.
4. Joosten E, Lioen P. Iron deficiency anemia and anemia of chronic disease in geriatric hospitalized patients: how frequent are comorbidities as an additional explanation for the anemia? Geriatr Gerontol Int 2014;15(8):931–5.
5. Coimbra S, Catarino C, Santos-Silva A. The role of adipocytes in the modulation of iron metabolism in obesity. Obes Rev 2013;14(10):771–9.
6. Careaga M, Moizé V, Flores L, et al. Inflammation and iron status in bariatric surgery candidates. Surg Obes Relat Dis 2015;11(4):906–11.
7. Thomas DW, Hinchliffe RF, Briggs C, et al. Guideline for the laboratory diagnosis of functional iron deficiency. Br J Haematol 2013;161(5):639–48.
8. Anty R, Dahman M, Iannelli A, et al. Bariatric surgery can correct iron depletion in morbidly obese women: a link with chronic inflammation. Obes Surg 2008;18(6): 709–14.
9. Maccio A, Madeddu C, Gramignano G, et al. The role of inflammation, iron, and nutritional status in cancer-related anemia: results of a large, prospective, observational study. Haematologica 2015;100(1):124–32.
10. Andrews NC. Forging a field: the golden age of iron biology. Blood 2008;112(2): 219–30.
11. Ganz T, Nemeth E. Iron balance and the role of hepcidin in chronic kidney disease. Semin Nephrol 2016;36(2):87–93.
12. Donovan A, Brownlie A, Zhou Y, et al. Positional cloning of zebrafish ferroportin1 identifies a conserved vertebrate iron exporter. Nature 2000;403(6771):776–81.
13. Fraenkel PG, Traver D, Donovan A, et al. Ferroportin1 is required for normal iron cycling in zebrafish. J Clin Invest 2005;115(6):1532–41.
14. Donovan A, Lima CA, Pinkus JL, et al. The iron exporter ferroportin/Slc40a1 is essential for iron homeostasis. Cell Metab 2005;1(3):191–200.
15. Hentze MW, Muckenthaler MU, Andrews NC. Balancing acts: molecular control of mammalian iron metabolism. Cell 2004;117(3):285–97.
16. Pigeon C, Ilyin G, Courselaud B, et al. A new mouse liver-specific gene, encoding a protein homologous to human antimicrobial peptide hepcidin, is overexpressed during iron overload. J Biol Chem 2001;276(11):7811–9.
17. Bolondi G, Garuti C, Corradini E, et al. Altered hepatic BMP signaling pathway in human HFE hemochromatosis. Blood Cells Mol Dis 2010;45(4):308–12.
18. Nemeth E, Tuttle MS, Powelson J, et al. Hepcidin regulates cellular iron efflux by binding to ferroportin and inducing its internalization. Science 2004;306(5704): 2090–3.
19. Ganz T, Nemeth E. Iron metabolism: interactions with normal and disordered erythropoiesis. Cold Spring Harb Perspect Med 2012;2(5):a011668.
20. Arndt S, Maegdefrau U, Dorn C, et al. Iron-induced expression of bone morphogenic protein 6 in intestinal cells is the main regulator of hepatic hepcidin expression in vivo. Gastroenterology 2010;138(1):372–82.

21. Babitt JL, Huang FW, Wrighting DM, et al. Bone morphogenetic protein signaling by hemojuvelin regulates hepcidin expression. Nat Genet 2006;38(5):531–9.
22. Gibert Y, Lattanzi VJ, Zhen AW, et al. BMP signaling modulates hepcidin expression in zebrafish embryos independent of hemojuvelin. PLoS One 2011;6(1): e14553.
23. Niederkofler V, Salie R, Arber S. Hemojuvelin is essential for dietary iron sensing, and its mutation leads to severe iron overload. J Clin Invest 2005;115(8):2180–6.
24. Zhang AS, Anderson SA, Meyers KR, et al. Evidence that inhibition of hemojuvelin shedding in response to iron is mediated through neogenin. J Biol Chem 2007; 282(17):12547–56.
25. Finberg KE, Heeney MM, Campagna DR, et al. Mutations in TMPRSS6 cause iron-refractory iron deficiency anemia (IRIDA). Nat Genet 2008;40(5):569–71.
26. Melis MA, Cau M, Congiu R, et al. A mutation in the TMPRSS6 gene, encoding a transmembrane serine protease that suppresses hepcidin production, in familial iron deficiency anemia refractory to oral iron. Haematologica 2008;93(10): 1473–9.
27. Kautz L, Jung G, Valore EV, et al. Identification of erythroferrone as an erythroid regulator of iron metabolism. Nat Genet 2014;46(7):678–84.
28. Lee P, Peng H, Gelbart T, et al. Regulation of hepcidin transcription by interleukin-1 and interleukin-6. Proc Natl Acad Sci U S A 2005;102(6):1906–10.
29. Weizer-Stern O, Adamsky K, Margalit O, et al. Hepcidin, a key regulator of iron metabolism, is transcriptionally activated by p53. Br J Haematol 2007;138(2): 253–62.
30. Gkouvatsos K, Papanikolaou G, Pantopoulos K. Regulation of iron transport and the role of transferrin. Biochim Biophys Acta 2012;1820(3):188–202.
31. Kemna E, Pickkers P, Nemeth E, et al. Time-course analysis of hepcidin, serum iron, and plasma cytokine levels in humans injected with LPS. Blood 2005; 106(5):1864–6.
32. Nemeth E, Rivera S, Gabayan V, et al. IL-6 mediates hypoferremia of inflammation by inducing the synthesis of the iron regulatory hormone hepcidin. J Clin Invest 2004;113(9):1271–6.
33. Ganz T, Nemeth E. Hepcidin and iron homeostasis. Biochim Biophys Acta 2012; 1823(9):1434–43.
34. Oliveira SJ, Pinto JP, Picarote G, et al. ER stress-inducible factor CHOP affects the expression of hepcidin by modulating C/EBPalpha activity. PLoS One 2009; 4(8):e6618.
35. Vecchi C, Montosi G, Zhang K, et al. ER stress controls iron metabolism through induction of hepcidin. Science 2009;325(5942):877–80.
36. Millonig G, Ganzleben I, Peccerella T, et al. Sustained submicromolar H_2O_2 levels induce hepcidin via signal transducer and activator of transcription 3 (STAT3). J Biol Chem 2012;287(44):37472–82.
37. Constante M, Jiang W, Wang D, et al. Distinct requirements for HFE in basal and induced hepcidin levels in iron overload and inflammation. Am J Physiol Gastrointest Liver Physiol 2006;291(2):G229–37.
38. Valdes-Ferrer SI, Papoin J, Dancho ME, et al. HMGB1 mediates anemia of inflammation in murine sepsis survivors. Mol Med 2015;21:951–8.
39. Yang H, Wang H, Ju Z, et al. MD-2 is required for disulfide HMGB1-dependent TLR4 signaling. J Exp Med 2015;212(1):5–14.
40. Gardenghi S, Renaud TM, Meloni A, et al. Distinct roles for hepcidin and interleukin-6 in the recovery from anemia in mice injected with Heat-Killed Brucella abortus. Blood 2014;123(8):1137–45.

41. Tracey KJ, Wei H, Manogue KR, et al. Cachectin/tumor necrosis factor induces cachexia, anemia, and inflammation. J Exp Med 1988;167(3):1211–27.
42. Canali S, Core AB, Zumbrennen-Bullough KB, et al. Activin B induces noncanonical SMAD1/5/8 signaling via BMP type I receptors in hepatocytes: evidence for a role in hepcidin induction by inflammation in male mice. Endocrinology 2016; 157(3):1146–62.
43. Guida C, Altamura S, Klein FA, et al. A novel inflammatory pathway mediating rapid hepcidin-independent hypoferremia. Blood 2015;125(14):2265–75.
44. Flo TH, Smith KD, Sato S, et al. Lipocalin 2 mediates an innate immune response to bacterial infection by sequestrating iron. Nature 2004;432(7019):917–21.
45. Kanwar JR, Roy K, Patel Y, et al. Multifunctional iron bound lactoferrin and nano-medicinal approaches to enhance its bioactive functions. Molecules 2015;20(6): 9703–31.
46. Chung B, Matak P, McKie AT, et al. Leptin increases the expression of the iron regulatory hormone hepcidin in HuH7 human hepatoma cells. J Nutr 2007; 137(11):2366–70.
47. Catalan V, Gómez-Ambrosi J, Rodríguez A, et al. Peripheral mononuclear blood cells contribute to the obesity-associated inflammatory state independently of glycemic status: involvement of the novel proinflammatory adipokines chemerin, chitinase-3-like protein 1, lipocalin-2 and osteopontin. Genes Nutr 2015;10(3): 460.
48. Weiss G, Goodnough LT. Anemia of chronic disease. N Engl J Med 2005;352(10): 1011–23.
49. Dinkla S, van Eijk LT, Fuchs B, et al. Inflammation-associated changes in lipid composition and the organization of the erythrocyte membrane. BBA Clin 2016; 5:186–92.
50. Georgatzakou HT, Antonelou MH, Papassideri IS, et al. Red blood cell abnormalities and the pathogenesis of anemia in end stage renal disease. Proteomics Clin Appl 2016;10(8):778–90.
51. Kim A, Fung E, Parikh SG, et al. A mouse model of anemia of inflammation: complex pathogenesis with partial dependence on hepcidin. Blood 2014;123(8): 1129–36.
52. Nemeth E, Ganz T. Anemia of inflammation. Hematol Oncol Clin North Am 2014; 28(4):671–81, vi.
53. Blay JY, Favrot M, Rossi JF, et al. Role of interleukin-6 in paraneoplastic thrombocytosis. Blood 1993;82(7):2261–2.
54. Rossi JF, Lu ZY, Jourdan M, et al. Interleukin-6 as a therapeutic target. Clin Cancer Res 2015;21(6):1248–57.
55. Song SN, Tomosugi N, Kawabata H, et al. Down-regulation of hepcidin resulting from long-term treatment with an anti-IL-6 receptor antibody (tocilizumab) improves anemia of inflammation in multicentric Castleman disease. Blood 2010; 116(18):3627–34.
56. van Rhee F, Wong RS, Munshi N, et al. Siltuximab for multicentric Castleman's disease: a randomised, double-blind, placebo-controlled trial. Lancet Oncol 2014;15(9):966–74.
57. Garcia-Manero G, Gartenberg G, Steensma DP, et al. A phase 2, randomized, double-blind, multicenter study comparing siltuximab plus best supportive care (BSC) with placebo plus BSC in anemic patients with International Prognostic Scoring System low- or intermediate-1-risk myelodysplastic syndrome. Am J Hematol 2014;89(9):E156–62.

58. Mayeur C, Kolodziej SA, Wang A, et al. Oral administration of a bone morphogenetic protein type I receptor inhibitor prevents the development of anemia of inflammation. Haematologica 2015;100(2):e68–71.

59. Schwoebel F, van Eijk LT, Zboralski D, et al. The effects of the anti-hepcidin Spiegelmer NOX-H94 on inflammation-induced anemia in cynomolgus monkeys. Blood 2013;121(12):2311–5.

60. van Eijk LT, John AS, Schwoebel F, et al. Effect of the antihepcidin Spiegelmer lexaptepid on inflammation-induced decrease in serum iron in humans. Blood 2014; 124(17):2643–6.

61. Cooke KS, Hinkle B, Salimi-Moosavi H, et al. A fully human anti-hepcidin antibody modulates iron metabolism in both mice and nonhuman primates. Blood 2013; 122(17):3054–61.

62. Gaun V, Patchen B, Volovetz J, et al. A chemical screen identifies small molecules that regulate hepcidin expression. Blood Cells Mol Dis 2014;53(4):231–40.

63. Zhen AW, Nguyen NH, Gibert Y, et al. The small molecule, genistein, increases hepcidin expression in human hepatocytes. Hepatology 2013;58(4):1315–25.

64. Alkhateeb AA, Buckett PD, Gardeck AM, et al. The small molecule ferristatin II induces hepatic hepcidin expression in vivo and in vitro. Am J Physiol Gastrointest Liver Physiol 2015;308(12):G1019–26.

65. Boser P, Seemann D, Liguori MJ, et al. Anti-repulsive guidance molecule C (RGMc) antibodies increases serum iron in rats and cynomolgus monkeys by hepcidin downregulation. AAPS J 2015;17(4):930–8.

66. Theurl I, Schroll A, Sonnweber T, et al. Pharmacologic inhibition of hepcidin expression reverses anemia of chronic inflammation in rats. Blood 2011; 118(18):4977–84.

67. Querbes W, Bogorad RL, Moslehi J, et al. Treatment of erythropoietin deficiency in mice with systemically administered siRNA. Blood 2012;120(9):1916–22.

68. Richardson CL, Delehanty LL, Bullock GC, et al. Isocitrate ameliorates anemia by suppressing the erythroid iron restriction response. J Clin Invest 2013;123(8): 3614–23.

Megaloblastic Anemias
Nutritional and Other Causes

 CrossMark

Ralph Green, MD, PhD*, Ananya Datta Mitra, MD

KEYWORDS

- Anemia • Megaloblastic • Vitamin B_{12} • Folate • Pernicious anemia
- Methylmalonic acid • Homocysteine • Transcobalamin

KEY POINTS

- Vitamin B_{12} and folate deficiencies are the most important causes of megaloblastic anemia.
- The main cause of vitamin B_{12} deficiency that results in megaloblastic anemia is pernicious anemia caused by autoimmune destruction of gastric parietal cells.
- The prevalence of folate deficiency has decreased because of widespread food folate fortification, but it still occurs among the poor, elderly, and alcoholics, particularly in countries that do not fortify the diet. It can also result from malabsorption or increased cell turnover and increased demand.
- Nuclear-cytoplasmic asynchrony from the ineffective DNA synthesis causes megaloblastic changes in the bone marrow with resulting anemia and cytopenias.

MEGALOBLASTIC ANEMIAS: NUTRITIONAL AND OTHER CAUSES

Introduction

Ineffective DNA synthesis in hematopoietic precursor cells is the primary mechanism that leads to megaloblastic anemia. The most frequent causes of megaloblastic anemia are deficiencies of either vitamin B_{12} or folate within a long list that includes deficiency of other micronutrients, congenital disorders, myelodysplastic syndromes, and acquired DNA synthesis defects as seen in the settings of chemotherapy (**Box 1**).[1] The ineffective hematopoiesis resulting from the asynchrony between nuclear and cytoplasmic development is most evident on Wright-Giemsa–stained bone marrow aspirate smears. Megaloblastic erythroid precursors are larger than normal and their nuclei are larger and appear immature with granular chromatin. During the initial stages of cellular differentiation, the slow condensation of chromatin results in an open sievelike vesicular nucleus. In subsequent stages there is more cytoplasm in

Disclosures: The authors have nothing to disclose.
Department of Pathology and Laboratory Medicine, UC Davis Medical Center, University of California Davis Health System, 4400 V. Street, Sacramento, CA 95817, USA
* Corresponding author.
E-mail address: rgreen@UCDAVIS.EDU

Med Clin N Am 101 (2017) 297–317
http://dx.doi.org/10.1016/j.mcna.2016.09.013
0025-7125/17/© 2016 Elsevier Inc. All rights reserved.

medical.theclinics.com

Box 1
Causes of megaloblastic anemia

Vitamin deficiencies

Deficiency of folate
1. Decreased intake
   a. Nutritional deficiency (elderly, alcoholics, poverty)
   b. Diet induced: goat's milk, synthetic diets
   c. Infants with prematurity
   d. Hyperalimentation
2. Decreased absorption
   a. Celiac disease and tropical sprue
3. Increased demand
   a. Pregnancy
   b. Puberty
   c. Chronic hemolytic anemia
   d. Exfoliative dermatitis
   e. Hemodialysis

Deficiency of vitamin B_{12}
1. Impaired absorption
   a. Pernicious anemia
   b. After gastrectomy or ileal resection
   c. Zollinger-Ellison syndrome
   d. Blind loop syndrome
   e. Fish tapeworm infestation
   f. Pancreatic insufficiency
2. Decreased intake
   a. Vegans
   b. Vegetarians

Other causes

1. Drugs (eg, antibiotics, anticancer agent, anticonvulsants and oral contraceptives)

2. Inborn errors of metabolism

3. Acute megaloblastic anemia
   a. Nitrous oxide exposure
   b. Acute illness

4. Idiopathic (congenital dyserythropoietic anemia, erythroleukemia, and refractory megaloblastic anemia)

5. Thiamine-responsive megaloblastic anemia

---

the megaloblastic erythroid precursors relative to the size of the nucleus. The granulocytic precursors also show nuclear-cytoplasmic dyssynchrony with the development of so-called giant metamyelocytes and bands, which have a characteristic horseshoe-shaped nucleus and open chromatin. The development of megakaryocytes is also affected, as reflected by abnormal large polylobated megaloblastic megakaryocytes with a lack of cytoplasmic granules. Corresponding changes in the blood smear include anemia with oval macrocytes, anisocytosis, poikilocytosis, leukopenia with hypersegmented polymorphonuclear cells, and thrombocytopenia.

Pathogenesis of Megaloblastic Anemia

Deficiencies of folate and vitamin B_{12} are the leading causes of megaloblastic anemia worldwide. In the era of food folic acid fortification, there is a decreasing trend of folate deficiency prevalence in most developed countries. Classically, in megaloblastosis, there is defective DNA synthesis in rapidly dividing hematopoietic precursors.[2,3] To a lesser extent, RNA and protein synthesis are impaired and these cells generally have much more cytoplasm and RNA than do their normal counterparts, suggesting that cytoplasmic constituents are synthesized faster than DNA. There is prolongation of the S-phase of DNA synthesis because of the delay in migration of the DNA replication fork and the connection of DNA fragments synthesized from the lagging strand (Okazaki fragments).[4,5] Evidence suggests that, because of this nuclear maturation arrest, unbalanced cell growth and impaired cell division occur.[6] There is substantial loss of defective hematopoietic precursors through apoptosis.[7] The metabolic interrelationship between folate and B_{12} has been implicated in the development of the megaloblastic anemia observed in either of the 2 vitamin deficiencies because B_{12} is necessary to regenerate tetrahydrofolate (THF) through the methionine synthase reaction and this is required for the production of methylene-THF, which is essential for thymidine and hence DNA synthesis.[3] Vitamin B_{12} is the cofactor for both the cytoplasmic methionine synthase and the mitochondrial l-methylmalonyl–coenzyme A mutase reactions.[8,9]

Clinical Picture

Anemia develops gradually with sufficient time for cardiopulmonary and intraerythrocytic compensation to occur before symptoms develop.[10] Symptoms generally develop in severely anemic patients. The main symptoms include weakness, palpitation, fatigue, light-headedness, and shortness of breath caused by low hematocrit. Jaundice can occur from intramedullary and extravascular hemolysis. Leukopenia or thrombocytopenia are generally present, but do not typically cause any clinical concern. With B_{12} deficiency, there are often neurologic symptoms as well as autonomic gastrointestinal disturbances. The neurologic symptoms result from symmetric paresthesias, numbness, and impaired vibration and position sense leading to gait disturbances.[11,12] About 10% of B_{12}-deficient patients show hyperpigmentation and some patients with pernicious anemia have associated autoimmune vitiligo. There may be cerebral manifestations in B_{12} deficiency, including mental confusion, paranoia, dementia, and even frank psychosis.[13] Other associated symptoms encountered rarely with vitamin B_{12} deficiency include generalized malabsorption caused by intestinal megaloblastosis, infertility, glossitis, and cerebral venous thrombosis.[14,15] A greater risk of thrombosis may occur as a result of hyperhomocysteinemia in severe B12 deficiency.

Laboratory Features

Megaloblastic anemia is suspected based on consideration of the clinical features described earlier in conjunction with the results of a blood count and examination of the blood smear showing anemia, and increased red cell indices (mean corpuscular volume [MCV], mean corpuscular hemoglobin) together with anisocytosis, poikilocytosis, and hypersegmented neutrophils.[16] However, the presence of hypersegmented neutrophils is not diagnostic of megaloblastic anemia because they can also be encountered in iron deficiency anemia. Thus studies for iron deficiency should also be considered in cases of megaloblastic anemia.[17] The initial tests that should be performed to evaluate megaloblastic anemia are the measurement of plasma or serum levels of vitamin B_{12} and folate as well as red cell folate.[18] Because of folic acid fortification programs in the United States and many other parts of the world, vitamin B_{12} deficiency is more commonly encountered than folate deficiency. For this reason, B_{12} deficiency is considered first.

B_{12} deficiency is suggested by a B_{12} level of less than 200 pg/mL. However, B_{12} levels may be low without underlying deficiency because of low or absent levels of the major plasma B_{12} binding protein, haptocorrin,[19] or can be spuriously normal in patients with pernicious anemia if they have excessive levels of circulating intrinsic factor antibodies. Intrinsic factor antibodies can interact with the intrinsic factor binder that is used in most B_{12} assays.[20] Borderline B_{12} levels (200–400 ng/L) should be followed up with measuring metabolite levels that increase in B_{12} deficiency.[21,22] Increased methylmalonic acid (MMA) levels are widely considered to be a highly sensitive and specific test for identifying B_{12} deficiency and, when MMA levels are not increased, this is strongly suggestive of normal B_{12} status.[21,22] The levels of MMA always decrease with vitamin B_{12} therapy when there is underlying B_{12} deficiency.[23,24] MMA can increase (300–700 nmol/L) in renal failure and is refractory to B_{12} administration.[24,25] B_{12} deficiency also leads to high plasma homocysteine levels. However, this is not a specific indicator of B_{12} deficiency, because high homocysteine levels are also caused by folate deficiency.[18,21] The fraction of the B_{12} in circulation that is bound to the B_{12} transport protein transcobalamin as opposed to the other plasma B_{12}-binding protein, haptocorrin, has been proposed as a more reliable indicator of functional B_{12} status because it is responsible for cellular delivery and uptake of the vitamin.[26] However, because of problems with other indices of B_{12} status assessment used alone, there has been a trend to combine the use of 2 or more analytes, such as total B_{12} with either transcobalamin or MMA.[27] More recently, use of a combined indicator of B_{12} status, cB_{12} (where $cB_{12} = \log_{10} [(\text{holotranscobalamin} \cdot B_{12})/(\text{MMA} \cdot \text{total homocysteine})]$), has been successfully applied in population studies to identify B_{12} deficiency. However, this approach awaits validation in patients with megaloblastic anemia suspected of being caused by B_{12} deficiency.[28] In B_{12} deficiency, serum folate levels are frequently increased because of the trapping of folate in the form of methylfolate.[29] Because megaloblastic anemia is usually associated with considerable extravascular hemolysis, including intramedullary destruction of erythroid precursors, serum bilirubin and lactate dehydrogenase (LDH) levels are typically increased.[17]

There are many causes of B_{12} deficiency and a good understanding of the physiology of B_{12} absorption is necessary to evaluate the several possible underlying disorders that can lead to B_{12}-deficient megaloblastic anemia. Complete and detailed considerations of the causes of B_{12} deficiency are well described elsewhere.[3,22] In general, causes of B_{12} deficiency may be divided into gastric and ileal causes, because the key components of the normal pathway for B_{12} absorption require a functioning stomach for production of the protein intrinsic factor and an intact cubilin receptor for the intrinsic factor–B_{12} complex in the terminal ileum.[3,22] Preeminent among the several causes of B_{12} deficiency is the disease pernicious anemia, caused by autoimmune destruction of the gastric parietal cells that produce intrinsic factor. The presence of circulating anti–intrinsic factor I antibodies is highly specific for the diagnosis of pernicious anemia. However, the test has a poor sensitivity, being positive in only 60% of patients with pernicious anemia.[30,31] Chronic atrophic gastritis, which is associated with pernicious anemia, can be diagnosed by endoscopic biopsy, an increased fasting serum gastrin level, and decreased serum pepsinogen I levels.[32,33] Causes of B_{12} deficiency are discussed in further detail later.

The initial tests for possible folate deficiency include a plasma or serum level of less than 4 μg/L, which indicates folate deficiency. However, occasionally, a borderline folate level (4–8 μg/L) might be associated with high plasma levels of homocysteine consistent with underlying folate deficiency being responsible for megaloblastic change in the marrow. In contrast, borderline serum folate levels with normal homocysteine level are not considered deficient.[21,34] An increased level of serum total homocysteine is less specific for folate deficiency because homocysteine level is also increased in vitamin B_{12} deficiency,[21,35,36] classic homocystinuria, hypothyroidism, and renal failure. Although low red blood cell folate level is seen in folate deficiency, it is not specific, because B_{12} deficiency can also be associated with a low red cell folate level. Thus, red blood cell folate testing should be combined with serum or plasma B_{12} and folate testing. The major advantage of measuring red blood cell folate level is that it reflects average folate status of the individual during the 3-month to 4-month period that corresponds with normal red cell lifespan and is not influenced by recent dietary intake of folate.[3,18]

In the evaluation of megaloblastic anemias, clinical signs and symptoms should be considered apart from the laboratory parameters. Although patients with folate deficiency mainly present with hematologic symptoms, those with B_{12} deficiency often have predominantly neurologic signs and symptoms. Also, long-term consequences of folate deficiency can lead to cardiovascular, developmental, cerebral, and immunologic defects.[37]

CONDITIONS THAT MAY CONFUSE OR OBSCURE THE PICTURE OF MEGALOBLASTIC ANEMIA
Coexistent Microcytic Anemia

Coexisting microcytic anemias resulting from iron deficiency anemia, the anemia of chronic disease, or thalassemia minor can obscure the megaloblastic features in the bone marrow or peripheral blood.[38,39] Peripheral blood may show a dimorphic picture with marked anisocytosis and the blood count showing a normal MCV but a markedly increased red cell distribution width (RDW). Intermediate megaloblasts,[40] which look smaller than the usual megaloblastic cells, predominate in the marrow. However, in these situations, there are still hypersegmented neutrophils in the blood and giant metamyelocytes and bands in the marrow. Coexistence of a megaloblastic and microcytic process can also be encountered in celiac disease,[41] gastric bypass surgery for morbid obesity,[42] and chronic *Helicobacter pylori* infection.[43,44]

Acute Leukemia and Myelodysplasia

A hypercellular and dysplastic bone marrow with bizarre bone marrow morphology seen in severe nutritional megaloblastic anemia can be mistaken for signs of acute leukemia or myelodysplasia.[17,45,46] Rarely, the erythroid series show little or no maturation, and megaloblastic pronormoblasts predominate in the marrow with dysmorphic forms and prominent mitotic figures. There are often associated severe cytopenias. This picture resembles erythroid leukemia and, because the treatment and prognosis differ greatly between the conditions, a high level of awareness and suspicion as well as suitable testing to exclude a possible megaloblastic anemia should be undertaken if megaloblastic features are prominent before treatment of acute leukemia is instituted.

Attenuated Megaloblastic Anemia

Megaloblastic changes may be attenuated if patients with advanced megaloblastic anemia receive B_{12} or folate therapy or blood transfusion before marrow aspiration; the anemia continues until the marrow has responded to the hematinic therapy but the megaloblastic changes may be masked within 36 to 48 hours.

Acute Megaloblastic Anemia

A serious megaloblastic state can develop acutely within a few days because of tissue folate or B_{12} deficiency. These patients present with thrombocytopenia and/or leukopenia with minimal effects in red cell counts because of the higher longevity of red blood cells. The commonest cause of acute megaloblastic anemia is nitrous oxide (N_2O) anesthesia, which destroys the methylcobalamin form of B_{12}, leading to a megaloblastic state in the bone marrow within 12 to 24 hours.[47,48] Hypersegmented neutrophils generally appear after 5 days of exposure but then persist for several days.[49] If the source is removed, the effects of N_2O generally disappear over a few days and the removal can be expedited by the use of folinic acid or cobalamin.[50] Sometimes acute megaloblastic anemia can develop in seriously ill patients in intensive care units,[51] patients receiving massive transfusion at surgery,[52] those on dialysis or total parenteral nutrition, and those who are receiving folate antagonists such as trimethoprim or low-dose methotrexate. Levels of red cell folate and serum vitamin B_{12} might be normal but the marrow shows megaloblastosis. There is always a prompt response to therapeutic doses of parenteral folate and B_{12} in these patients.

CAUSES OF VITAMIN B_{12} DEFICIENCY

There are several causes and varying degrees of severity of B_{12} deficiency[17,22] (see **Box 1**).

Impaired Absorption

Pernicious anemia is an autoimmune gastritis, occurring in middle-aged to elderly adults, leading to the destruction of gastric parietal cells and failure of intrinsic factor production,[53] resulting in achlorhydria.[32,54] Susceptibility to pernicious anemia is associated with human leukocyte antigen types A2, A3, B7, and B_{12},[55] and with blood group A.[56]

Helicobacter pylori Infection

Very commonly, H pylori infects the gastric mucosa and causes gastritis and peptic ulcers. However, the role of H pylori in the pathogenesis of pernicious anemia is still a mystery. Previous studies have shown a very low incidence of H pylori infection in patients with pernicious anemia.[57] An interesting proposition has been put forward, that chronic infection with H pylori may trigger an autoimmune process directed against the host H+/K+-ATPase protein.[44,58]

Gastrectomy Syndromes

Gastric resections for any cause as well Roux-en-Y gastric bypass surgery for morbid obesity lead to multiple nutritional deficiencies.[3] Iron deficiency anemia is the most common anemia to occur after gastric surgery; however, B_{12} deficiency with megaloblastic anemia occurs occasionally. B_{12} deficiency usually develops 5 to 6 years postsurgery because of the lack of intrinsic factor and the gradual depletion of the body's B_{12} stores.[59] In classic B_{12} deficiency serum iron levels are usually high. In contrast, postgastrectomy patients with low serum B_{12} levels typically have low serum iron levels.[60] After partial gastrectomy, B_{12} deficiency might develop because of mucosal atrophy[61] or bacterial overgrowth, classically known as blind loop syndrome.[62] B_{12} malabsorption in blind loop syndrome occurs because of intestinal colonization with bacteria, which thrive on cobalamin. This cause of B_{12} deficiency is therefore amenable to antibiotic therapy.[63]

Hyperchlorhydria

Zollinger-Ellison syndrome, results from a gastrin-secreting tumor in the pancreas, which stimulates the gastric mucosa to secrete immense amounts of hydrochloric acid. The large quantities of acid acidify the duodenal contents, thus preventing the binding of B_{12} to the intrinsic factor.[64]

Diseases of the Small Intestine

Because the terminal ileum is the eventual site for B_{12} absorption; intestinal disorders such as ileal resection,[65] ileitis of any cause (inflammatory bowel disease, radiation),[66] lymphoma arising in the terminal ileum, drug-related or toxin-related disorders,[67] or tropical sprue[68] can lead to B_{12} deficiency.

Inherited Disorders of Vitamin B_{12} Absorption

Imerslund-Graesbeck syndrome (IGS) is a rare genetic pediatric disorder resulting in vitamin B_{12} malabsorption in the terminal ileum.[69] Usually clinically evident during the first 6 years of life, IGS usually results in megaloblastic anemia and may be accompanied by neurologic defects of variable severity with/without proteinuria. The disorder results from defects in one of 2 genes (cub or amn) that together code for the cubilin protein, which comprises the receptor for the intrinsic factor–B_{12} complex.[70]

Hereditary intrinsic factor deficiency (HIFD) occurs because of recessive mutations as well as a partial gene deletion in the intrinsic factor gene,[71] and results in decreased intrinsic factor leading to B_{12} malabsorption.

Definitive diagnosis of IGS and HIFD can only be confirmed by genetic testing. Treatment consists of parenteral vitamin B_{12} supplementation, which should be administered without confirmation of diagnosis.

Miscellaneous Causes

Infestation by the fish tapeworm Diphyllobothrium latum, arising from the ingestion of uncooked or partially cooked fish, can lead to B_{12} deficiency caused by competition between the worm and the host for ingested B_{12}.[72]

Patients with acquired immunodeficiency syndrome sometimes present with low serum B_{12} levels caused by B_{12} malabsorption.[73] This malabsorption can have a combination of intestinal and gastric causes.[74,75]

Patients with pancreatic diseases can have B_{12} deficiency caused by malabsorption from pancreatic insufficiency.[76] Pancreatic proteases, which are lacking in pancreatic insufficiency, are required for digestion of the salivary B_{12}-binding protein haptocorrin and transfer of B_{12} to intrinsic factor for absorption.[77]

Dietary insufficiency of B_{12} is common among vegans and vegetarians and this can lead to reduced B_{12} status, but true deficiency of B_{12}, sufficient to cause megaloblastic anemia, is very rare among even strict vegetarians who do not consume milk or eggs.[78] Low serum B_{12} levels can be found in 50% to 60% of patients among this group. Depletion of the body's B_{12} store occurs slowly, caused by efficient reabsorption of biliary B_{12} by the enterohepatic pathway.[79,80] It may take 10 to 20 years for a vegan to manifest features of megaloblastic anemia caused by B_{12} deficiency.[81,82]

In addition, B_{12} deficiency may occur in severe general malnutrition. A megaloblastic anemia can develop without B_{12} deficiency in protein calorie malnutrition, such as kwashiorkor or marasmus.[83]

Inherited Disorders of B_{12} Metabolism

Several inherited disorders of cobalamin metabolism involving various steps in the cellular processing of B_{12} and its conversion to active forms have been identified and designated as the cobalamin mutants. These mutants have been extensively described in several reviews.[84,85]

Methylmalonic aciduria is an autosomal condition caused by complete or partial deficiency of the enzyme methylmalonyl-coenzyme A mutase.[85] Patients present early in life with lethargy, vomiting, hypotonia, hypothermia, respiratory distress, ketoacidosis, hyperammonemia, neutropenia, and thrombocytopenia without megaloblastic anemia and are fatal within the first 4 weeks of life.

Homocystinuria

The defect lies in the enzyme N5-methyltetrahydrofolate-homocysteine methyltransferase (MTR; methionine synthase), resulting in decreased production of methylcobalamin.[86] Patients present early in life, or rarely in adult life, with vomiting, mental retardation, megaloblastic anemia, severe homocystinuria, and hyperhomocysteinemia without methylmalonic aciduria or methylmalonic acidemia. Prenatal diagnosis in infants followed by B_{12} treatment usually results in normal development.

Methylmalonic Aciduria and Homocystinuria

When there is a defect in the reduction of the cobalt atom in the cobalamin molecule from Co2+ to Co1+ this leads to combined hyperhomocysteinemia and methylmalonic acidemia. Onset of the manifestations ranges from the neonatal period to adolescence with lethargy; failure to thrive; neurologic abnormalities in infants; and psychological abnormalities, progressive dementia, and motor defect in older patients.[85] Megaloblastic anemia occurs in about half the cases and patients are partially responsive to B_{12}.

CLINICAL FEATURES OF B_{12} DEFICIENCY

The main features include megaloblastic anemia, cytopenias, glossitis, cardiomyopathy, yellow discoloration of skin, weight loss, neurologic abnormalities, and immunologic defects.[87,88] Other effects of B_{12} deficiency include combined degeneration of the spinal cord, increased risk of vascular disease caused by hyperhomocysteinemia, potential increase in breast cancer risk in premenopausal women,[89] and osteoporosis.[90,91]

Neurologic Abnormalities

The neurologic manifestations include gradual onset of paresthesias, involving the tips of fingers and toes, along with lancinating pains caused by peripheral neuropathy. This stage is followed by loss of vibratory sense and proprioception resulting in abnormalities of gait. Progressive demyelination of the dorsal and lateral columns of the spinal cord leads to spastic ataxia in untreated patients.[92] There may also be development of somnolence, dysgeusia, and visual disturbances caused by optic atrophy and dementia of the Alzheimer type.[93] There are also psychological disturbances resulting from B_{12} deficiency that include psychotic depression, paranoid schizophrenia, and frank psychosis.[94]

Concealed B_{12} Deficiency

Some patients have a B_{12}-responsive neuropsychiatric disease with normal, borderline, or low serum B_{12} levels.[12] These patients present with peripheral neuropathy, gait disturbance, memory loss, and psychiatric symptoms. Although their B_{12} levels are within the normal range, they have increased levels of serum MMA and/or homocysteine, suggesting a tissue B_{12} deficiency. These patients typically are responsive to B_{12} therapy.

MANAGEMENT AND PROGNOSIS

The required daily allowance of vitamin B_{12} is 2.4 µg.[95,96] Patients with clinical vitamin B_{12} deficiency have a resolution of megaloblastic anemia and resolution of or improvement in neurologic symptoms with adequate supplementation of B_{12}; however, most of these patients have malabsorption and require parenteral or high-dose oral replacement therapy.[95]

Injected Vitamin B_{12}

Injections of vitamin B_{12}, known as cyanocobalamin in the United States and hydroxocobalamin in Europe,[95,97] are recommended in different dosage schedules. Depending on the dose, only approximately 10% of the injected dose of the drug is retained in the body. Patients with severe abnormalities require frequent doses of 1000 µg of B_{12} numerous times per week for 1 to 2 weeks followed by once a week and then once a month, after clinical improvement. Hematologic response is brisk, with an increase in the reticulocyte count in 1 week and rapid improvement of megaloblastic erythroid changes in the bone marrow, which returns to normal within 36 to 48 hours of treatment. However, the abnormal giant granulocytic forms may persist for 1 to 2 weeks. Neutropenia and thrombocytopenia, if present, generally resolve within a week. Total recovery from the anemia occurs within 6 to 8 weeks. The effect of therapy on neurologic disease depends on the severity and duration of the neurologic abnormalities before initiation of treatment.[11,12] Treatment of PA, or any B_{12} deficiency that is caused by malabsorption, needs to be maintained lifelong. In patients in whom vitamin B_{12} therapy is discontinued after clinical recovery, neurologic symptoms generally relapse within 6 months, and megaloblastic anemia reappears within 1 to several years.[95,97]

High-dose Oral Treatment

Studies have shown that high-dose oral (2000 µg of B_{12} daily) and parenteral therapy are equally effective in producing excellent hematologic and neurologic remissions.[12,98] More information is required from long-term studies to assess whether oral treatment is effective when doses are administered less frequently than daily. Patients must be informed of the advantages and disadvantages of oral versus parenteral therapy, and, irrespective of the form of treatment, those with pernicious anemia or malabsorption should be made aware of the need for lifelong replacement.

Special Circumstances

B_{12} is always recommended after a total gastrectomy, although it is not required after a partial gastrectomy, but patients should be followed diligently for any evidence of B_{12} deficiency or anemia, because megaloblastic changes can be masked by postgastrectomy iron deficiency.[99,100] Blind loop syndrome anemia can be treated with parenteral B_{12} therapy following a week's therapy with oral broad-spectrum antibiotics.[101] Surgical correction of the anatomic lesion also cures the syndrome. Fish tapeworm treatment consists of a single oral dose of a 50 mg/kg of niclosamide or a dose of 5 to 10 mg/kg of praaziquantel, followed by B_{12} replacement.[3]

CAUSES OF FOLATE DEFICIENCY
Cause and Pathogenesis

The most common causes of folate deficiency are nutritional deficiency, impaired absorption, and loss or increased requirements. However, the prevalence of folate deficiency has decreased dramatically as a result of mandated fortification of the food supply with folic acid in many countries.

Dietary Deficiency

Before the mid-1990s, inadequate intake was one of the most common causes of deficiency of folate. The feasibility of folic acid fortification of a staple grain or cereal,[102] together with the discovery that correction of folate deficiency during pregnancy could reduce the risk of neural tube defect pregnancies,[103] led to the mandated fortification of the diet with folic acid in many countries. Excessive cooking can destroy dietary folate and aggravate folate deficiency. Because of limitation of folate stores, folate deficiency develops rapidly in malnourished individuals and chronic alcoholics. Other causes of folate deficiency include hyperalimentation[104] and subtotal gastrectomy.[105] Premature infants are at increased risk of folate deficiency during infection, diarrhea, or hemolytic anemia.[106] Children on synthetic diets[107] and infants exclusively fed on goat's milk[108] also develop folate deficiency. Megaloblastic anemia in alcoholic cirrhosis is usually the result of folate deficiency,[109] although megaloblastic changes occur even when large doses of folate supplementation are given and alcohol consumption is maintained, suggesting that there is a metabolic effect of alcohol beyond its nutritional effects.[110]

Impaired Absorption

Folate deficiency can occur in nontropical sprue or celiac disease caused by chronic inflammation of the proximal small intestinal mucosa caused by dietary intake of gluten.[111] The patients typically have weight loss, glossitis, diarrhea, steatorrhea, iron deficiency, hypocalcemia, and other fat-soluble vitamin deficiencies. The serum folate levels are low, resulting in megaloblastic anemia.[112] Another entity that might lead to folate deficiency is tropical sprue, an idiopathic malabsorptive disease endemic to the Caribbean, south India, parts of southern Africa, and southeast Asia.[113] This condition can be promptly corrected by folate therapy together with systemic antibiotics, suggesting an infectious source of the disease.[114]

Other Intestinal Defects

Regional enteritis,[115] surgical resection of the small intestine,[116] lymphoma or leukemic infiltration of the small intestine,[117] Whipple disease,[117] scleroderma and amyloidosis,[118] and diabetes mellitus[119] can all lead to impairment of folate absorption.

Increased Requirements

Folate deficiency is one of the major cause of megaloblastic anemia of pregnancy,[120] mostly in developing countries.[121] In pregnancy, there is a 5-fold to 10-fold increased requirement of folate caused by transmission of folate to the growing fetus.[122,123] This requirement intensifies with multiple pregnancies, poor nutrition, infection, concomitant hemolytic anemia, or anticonvulsant medication. Folate deficiency is challenging to diagnose in pregnancy because of the development of physiologic anemia associated with physiologic macrocytosis; MCV may increase to 120 fL.[124] Serum and red cell folate levels decrease gradually during pregnancy, even in healthy women not on folic acid supplementation.[125] Hypersegmented neutrophils, usually a consistent indicator of early megaloblastic anemia, are less prominent in early megaloblastic anemia of pregnancy.[126] Folate deficiency also occurs during lactation and is aggravated by protracted lactation.[127] Folic acid fortification of the diet has been shown to be effective in ameliorating the folic acid deficiency and hence the risk of megaloblastic anemia during pregnancy.[128]

Increase in Cell Turnover

Folate requirement increases abruptly in chronic hemolytic anemia because of increased bone marrow turnover.[129] The bone marrow becomes megaloblastic within days during episodes of acute hemolysis. Folate deficiency can also occur in chronic exfoliative dermatitis, in which there is folate loss of 5 to 20 μg/d.[130] Folate supplementation in patients with psoriasis before initiation of methotrexate therapy can prevent the development of folate deficiency from methotrexate without diminishing its therapeutic effect.[130] There can be significant folate loss in dialysis fluid during hemodialysis.[131]

CLINICAL FEATURES OF FOLATE DEFICIENCY

Clinical manifestations of folate-deficient megaloblastic anemia typically include a history of nutritional deficiency with no neurologic signs and response to folate therapy.

LABORATORY FEATURES OF FOLATE DEFICIENCY

The initial test for folate deficiency is the presence of low serum or plasma folate levels (<3 ng/mL). Although an increase in homocysteine level often precedes low plasma folate levels, it is a less specific indicator.[21] Another indicator that is useful for identifying folate deficiency is the red cell folate.[132] Red cell folate remains comparatively unaffected by sudden changes in folate intake, because it reflects folate status over the lifespan of red cells. However, red cell folate cannot reliably distinguish between folate and B_{12} deficiency and also cannot detect acutely developing megaloblastic anemia.[133]

OTHER EFFECTS OF FOLATE DEFICIENCY
Neural Tube Closure

Folate deficiency results in congenital anomalies of the fetus, most notably defects in neural tube closure.[134] This outcome may also be related to antibodies against folate receptors, which have been detected in some women and may be overcome by higher folate intake.[134,135] Mutations in the enzymes of folate metabolism[136] result in an increase in the risk of congenital anomalies caused by the diminished conversion of methylene-tetrahydrofolate to methyl-tetrahydrofolate, which is essential for embryonic development. Fortification of folate has been successful in reducing the incidence of neural tube defects by between 20% and 50% in North America.[137,138] In addition to the hematological complications, there are other detrimental effects of folate deficiency affecting the brain and vascular system, as well as cancer risk. These effects have been reviewed elsewhere.[37]

INBORN ERRORS OF FOLATE METABOLISM
Hereditary Folate Malabsorption

Hereditary folate malabsorption is an uncommon congenital disorder in which there is impairment in the intestinal absorption of folate, often associated with impaired folate transportation through the choroid plexus into the cerebrospinal fluid (CSF).[139,140] This defect involves the proton-coupled folate transporter. Patients typically present with severe megaloblastic anemia and central nervous system (CNS) symptoms (seizures and mental retardation) with low serum folate and undetectable CSF folate levels.[141] Although parenteral folate corrects the anemia it has no effect on CSF folate concentration and neurologic symptoms. Daily folinic acid therapy restores CSF folate level and reduces CNS manifestations.[142]

Dihydrofolate Reductase Deficiency

Deficiency of the enzyme dihydrofolate reductase results in folate-refractory megaloblastic anemia responsive to folinic acid within days or weeks of birth.[143]

Methionine Synthase (MTR) Deficiency

Diminished MTR activity results in megaloblastic anemia and mental retardation. The anemia is refractory to folate, cobalamin, or pyridoxal phosphate.[144]

Methylene Tetrahydrofolate Reductase Deficiency

This is a rare autosomal recessive disorder characterized by severe hyperhomocysteinemia and homocystinuria without megaloblastic anemia or methylmalonic aciduria. Patients generally present with neurologic and vascular complications.[142]

MANAGEMENT AND PROGNOSIS

Folic acid supplementation, 1 to 5 mg/d, given orally, is usually adequate to correct anemia. Parenteral preparation (5 mg/mL) of folate should be used in patients with malabsorption. Tropical sprue is usually treated with folate, together with antibiotics and with additional doses of B_{12} if indicated. Treatment should be continued for a minimum of 2 years to prevent relapse. During pregnancy the required allowance of folate is 400 μg/d because higher doses can obscure B_{12} deficiency.[145] Mothers with nutritional deficiency or with malabsorption may be given 1 mg of vitamin B_{12} parenterally every 3 months to prevent any associated B_{12} deficiency during gestation. Evaluation of serum folate and B_{12} levels is mandatory in the treatment of megaloblastic anemia because monotherapy with folate may partly correct the hematologic abnormalities caused by B_{12} deficiency, but may lead to progressive and catastrophic neurologic consequences.[146] In cases of emergency when identification of the cause of the deficiency is ambiguous, both folate and B_{12} supplementation must be given, ideally after obtaining serum samples.

DRUG-INDUCED MEGALOBLASTIC ANEMIA

The structural similarity of aminopterin and methotrexate to folic acid leads to the entry of these drugs into the cells via the folate carrier.[147] As suitable substrates for the polyglutamyl synthase enzyme, these folate analogues then acquire a polyglutamate chain,[148] which makes them strong inhibitors of dihydrofolate reductase, resulting in the blocking of the conversion of dihydrofolate to tetrahydrofolate. This inhibition of one-carbon metabolism causes a decrease in nucleotide (particularly thymidine) biosynthesis that leads to a major derangement in DNA replication.[149] Drug toxicity often presents with mouth and esophageal ulcerations, abdominal pain, vomiting and diarrhea, ulcerations throughout the large and small intestines, alopecia, hyperpigmentation, and megaloblastic anemia. Toxicity from the use of folate antagonists is treated with folinic acid (N5-formyl tetrahydrofolate) 3 to 6 mg/d intramuscularly. This treatment is known as folinic acid rescue and is often used in chemotherapy to rescue patients receiving high doses of methotrexate.[150] Another antifolate compound, pemetrexed, used in the treatment of lung cancer and mesothelioma, can cause megaloblastic anemia that is treatable with cobalamin and folate. Zidovudine (azidothymidine [AZT]), used in acquired immunodeficiency syndrome therapy, is another agent that has the side effect of severe megaloblastic anemia.[151] Hydroxyurea is sometimes still used in the treatment of myeloproliferative disorders, including chronic myelogenous leukemia, polycythemia vera, and essential thrombocythemia, as well as psoriasis, rheumatoid arthritis, and sickle cell disease, and inhibits conversion of ribonucleotides to deoxy-ribonucleotides,[152] resulting in megaloblastosis in the marrow. This condition de-velops within a few days of initiating hydroxyurea therapy and is promptly reversible after the withdrawal of the drug. Chronic use of proton pump inhibitors causes inhibition of parietal cell function leading to low serum levels of B_{12}.[153] Trimethoprim is a microbial dihydrofolate reductase inhibitor that is reported to have only a minimal effect on the human enzyme. However, trimethoprim does induce a biochemical state of megaloblastosis[154] and can aggravate a state of folate deficiency in patients with borderline folate status.[155]

OTHER RARE CAUSES OF MEGALOBLASTIC ANEMIA
Congenital Dyserythropoietic Anemia

These are inherited dysplastic anemias affecting the erythroid lineage only, leading to the development of multinucleated normoblasts. The underlying molecular defect in these anemias is in the glycosylation of polylactosaminoglycans associated with membrane proteins and ceramides.[156]

Refractory Megaloblastic Anemia

Sideroblastic anemia and myelodysplastic disorders can manifest as refractory mega-loblastic anemia.[157] Atypical megaloblastic changes are confined to the erythroid line-age. Very rarely, some patients with sideroblastic anemia are responsive to pyridoxine (200 mg/d).[158]

Acute Erythroid Leukemia

In this form of acute myelogenous leukemia[159] nucleated red cells with marked macro-cytosis appear in the peripheral blood. There is prominent erythroid hyperplasia in the bone marrow with unusual vacuolated and multinucleated red cell precursors with increased numbers of blasts.

Thiamine-responsive Megaloblastic Anemia

Thiamine-responsive megaloblastic anemia is an autosomal recessive disease and it is typically associated with diabetes and deafness. It is thought to be caused by a defect in the thiamine (vitamin B_1) transport mechanism that results in reduced nucleic acid production through impaired transketolase catalysis,[160] which induces cell cycle arrest or apoptosis in bone marrow. The condition generally responds to therapeutic doses of thiamine, resulting in improvement of diabetes and correction of anemia. However, the advanced sensorineural deafness is irreversible.

These unusual causes of megaloblastic anemia should be considered in the differ-ential diagnosis in cases of megaloblastic anemia refractory to folate and B_{12} therapy and when all the common and correctable causes are excluded.

REFERENCES

1. Oberley MJ, Yang DT. Laboratory testing for cobalamin deficiency in megalo-blastic anemia. Am J Hematol 2013;88(6):522–6.
2. Bertaux O, Mederic C, Valencia R. Amplification of ribosomal DNA in the nucle-olus of vitamin B12-deficient Euglena cells. Exp Cell Res 1991;195(1):119–28.
3. Green R. Folate, Cobalamin, and Megaloblastic Anemias. In: Kaushansky K, Lichtman MA, Prchal JT, et al, editors. Williams Hematology. 9th edition. New York: McGraw-Hill; 2015.

4. Steinberg SE, Fonda S, Campbell CL, et al. Cellular abnormalities of folate deficiency. Br J Haematol 1983;54(4):605–12.

5. Wickremasinghe RG, Hoffbrand AV. Reduced rate of DNA replication fork movement in megaloblastic anemia. J Clin Invest 1980;65(1):26–36.

6. Rondanelli EG, Gorini P, Magliulo E, et al. Differences in proliferative activity between normoblasts and pernicious anemia megaloblasts. Blood 1964;24: 542–52.

7. Koury MJ, Horne DW, Brown ZA, et al. Apoptosis of late-stage erythroblasts in megaloblastic anemia: association with DNA damage and macrocyte production. Blood 1997;89(12):4617–23.

8. Stabler SP. Megaloblastic anemias: pernicious anemia and folate deficiency. In: Young NS, Gerson SL, High KA, editors. Clinical hematology. Philadelphia: Mosby; 2006. p. 242–51.

9. Stabler SP. Vitamin B_{12}. In: Erdman JW Jr, MacDonald IA, Zeisel SH, editors. Present knowledge in nutrition. 10th edition. New York: Wiley-Blackwell; 2012. p. 343–58.

10. Fernandes-Costa FJ, Green R, Torrance JD. Increased erythrocytic diphosphoglycerate in megaloblastic anaemia. A compensatory mechanism? S Afr Med J 1978;53(18):709–12.

11. Healton EB, Savage DG, Brust JC, et al. Neurologic aspects of cobalamin deficiency. Medicine 1991;70(4):229–45.

12. Lindenbaum J, Healton EB, Savage DG, et al. Neuropsychiatric disorders caused by cobalamin deficiency in the absence of anemia or macrocytosis. N Engl J Med 1988;318(26):1720–8.

13. Smith AD. Megaloblastic madness. Br Med J 1960;2(5216):1840–5.

14. Remacha AF, Souto JC, Pinana JL, et al. Vitamin B12 deficiency, hyperhomocysteinemia and thrombosis: a case and control study. Int J Hematol 2011;93(4): 458–64.

15. Limal N, Scheuermaier K, Tazi Z, et al. Hyperhomocysteinaemia, thrombosis and pernicious anaemia. Thromb Haemost 2006;96(2):233–5.

16. Lindenbaum J, Nath BJ. Megaloblastic anaemia and neutrophil hypersegmentation. Br J Haematol 1980;44(3):511–3.

17. Green R, Dwyre DM. Evaluation of macrocytic anemias. Semin Hematol 2015; 52(4):279–86.

18. Green R. Indicators for assessing folate and vitamin B12 status and for monitoring the efficacy of intervention strategies. Food Nutr Bull 2008;29(2 Suppl): S52–63 [discussion: S64–6].

19. Carmel R. Mild transcobalamin I (haptocorrin) deficiency and low serum cobalamin concentrations. Clin Chem 2003;49(8):1367–74.

20. Carmel R, Agrawal YP. Failures of cobalamin assays in pernicious anemia. N Engl J Med 2012;367(4):385–6.

21. Green R. Metabolite assays in cobalamin and folate deficiency. Baillieres Clin Haematol 1995;8(3):533–66.

22. Stabler SP. Clinical practice. Vitamin B12 deficiency. N Engl J Med 2013;368(2): 149–60.

23. Pennypacker LC, Allen RH, Kelly JP, et al. High prevalence of cobalamin deficiency in elderly outpatients. J Am Geriatr Soc 1992;40(12):1197–204.

24. Stabler SP, Marcell PD, Podell ER, et al. Assay of methylmalonic acid in the serum of patients with cobalamin deficiency using capillary gas chromatography-mass spectrometry. J Clin Invest 1986;77(5):1606–12.

25. Rasmussen K, Vyberg B, Pedersen KO, et al. Methylmalonic acid in renal insufficiency: evidence of accumulation and implications for diagnosis of cobalamin deficiency. Clin Chem 1990;36(8 Pt 1):1523–4.
26. Herzlich B, Herbert V. Depletion of serum holotranscobalamin II. An early sign of negative vitamin B12 balance. Lab Invest 1988;58(3):332–7.
27. Miller JW, Garrod MG, Rockwood AL, et al. Measurement of total vitamin B12 and holotranscobalamin, singly and in combination, in screening for metabolic vitamin B12 deficiency. Clin Chem 2006;52(2):278–85.
28. Fedosov SN, Brito A, Miller JW, et al. Combined indicator of vitamin B12 status: modification for missing biomarkers and folate status and recommendations for revised cut-points. Clin Chem Lab Med 2015;53(8):1215–25.
29. Herbert V, Zalusky R. Interrelations of vitamin B12 and folic acid metabolism: folic acid clearance studies. J Clin Invest 1962;41:1263–76.
30. Samloff IM, Kleinman MS, Turner MD, et al. Blocking and binding antibodies to intrinsic factor and parietal call antibody in pernicious anemia. Gastroenterology 1968;55(5):575–83.
31. Ardeman S, Chanarin I. A method for the assay of human gastric intrinsic factor and for the detection and titration of antibodies against intrinsic factor. Lancet 1963;2(7322):1350–4.
32. Toh BH, Chan J, Kyaw T, et al. Cutting edge issues in autoimmune gastritis. Clin Rev Allergy Immunol 2012;42(3):269–78.
33. Lewerin C, Jacobsson S, Lindstedt G, et al. Serum biomarkers for atrophic gastritis and antibodies against *Helicobacter pylori* in the elderly: implications for vitamin B12, folic acid and iron status and response to oral vitamin therapy. Scand J Gastroenterol 2008;43(9):1050–6.
34. De Bruyn E, Gulbis B, Cotton F. Serum and red blood cell folate testing for folate deficiency: new features? Eur J Haematol 2014;92(4):354–9.
35. Savage DG, Lindenbaum J, Stabler SP, et al. Sensitivity of serum methylmalonic acid and total homocysteine determinations for diagnosing cobalamin and folate deficiencies. Am J Med 1994;96(3):239–46.
36. Stabler SP, Marcell PD, Podell ER, et al. Elevation of total homocysteine in the serum of patients with cobalamin or folate deficiency detected by capillary gas chromatography-mass spectrometry. J Clin Invest 1988;81(2):466–74.
37. Green R, Miller JW. Folate deficiency beyond megaloblastic anemia: hyperhomocysteinemia and other manifestations of dysfunctional folate status. Semin Hematol 1999;36(1):47–64.
38. Spivak JL. Masked megaloblastic anemia. Arch Intern Med 1982;142(12): 2111–4.
39. Green R, Kuhl W, Jacobson R, et al. Masking of macrocytosis by alphathalassemia in blacks with pernicious anemia. N Engl J Med 1982;307(21): 1322–5.
40. Fudenberg H, Estren S. Non-Addisonian megaloblastic anemia; the intermediate megaloblast in the differential diagnosis of pernicious and related anemias. Am J Med 1958;25(2):198–209.
41. Harper JW, Holleran SF, Ramakrishnan R, et al. Anemia in celiac disease is multifactorial in etiology. Am J Hematol 2007;82(11):996–1000.
42. Green R. Anemias beyond B12 and iron deficiency: the buzz about other B's, elementary, and nonelementary problems. Hematology Am Soc Hematol Educ Program 2012;2012:492–8.
43. Bunn HF. Vitamin B12 and pernicious anemia–the dawn of molecular medicine. N Engl J Med 2014;370(8):773–6.

44. Hershko C, Ronson A, Souroujon M, et al. Variable hematologic presentation of autoimmune gastritis: age-related progression from iron deficiency to cobalamin depletion. Blood 2006;107(4):1673–9.

45. Dalsania CJ, Khemka V, Shum M, et al. A sheep in wolf's clothing. Am J Med 2008;121(2):107–9.

46. Parmentier S, Meinel J, Oelschlaegel U, et al. Severe pernicious anemia with distinct cytogenetic and flow cytometric aberrations mimicking myelodysplastic syndrome. Ann Hematol 2012;91(12):1979–81.

47. Amess JA, Burman JF, Rees GM, et al. Megaloblastic haemopoiesis in patients receiving nitrous oxide. Lancet 1978;2(8085):339–42.

48. Kondo H, Osborne ML, Kolhouse JF, et al. Nitrous oxide has multiple deleterious effects on cobalamin metabolism and causes decreases in activities of both mammalian cobalamin-dependent enzymes in rats. J Clin Invest 1981;67(5):1270–83.

49. Skacel PO, Hewlett AM, Lewis JD, et al. Studies on the haemopoietic toxicity of nitrous oxide in man. Br J Haematol 1983;53(2):189–200.

50. Kano Y, Sakamoto S, Sakuraya K, et al. Effects of leucovorin and methylcobalamin with N2O anesthesia. J Lab Clin Med 1984;104(5):711–7.

51. Easton DJ. Severe thrombocytopenia associated with acute folic acid deficiency and severe hemorrhage in two patients. Can Med Assoc J 1984;130(4):418–20, 422.

52. Beard ME, Hatipov CS, Hamer JW. Acute onset of folate deficiency in patients under intensive care. Crit Care Med 1980;8(9):500–3.

53. Toh BH, van Driel IR, Gleeson PA. Pernicious anemia. N Engl J Med 1997; 337(20):1441–8.

54. Nielsen MJ, Rasmussen MR, Andersen CB, et al. Vitamin B12 transport from food to the body's cells–a sophisticated, multistep pathway. Nature reviews. Gastroenterol Hepatol 2012;9(6):345–54.

55. Ungar B, Mathews JD, Tait BD, et al. HLA-DR patterns in pernicious anaemia. Br Med J 1981;282(6266):768–70.

56. Hoskins LC, Loux HA, Britten A, et al. Distribution of ABO blood groups in patients with pernicious anemia, gastric carcinoma and gastric carcinoma associated with pernicious anemia. N Engl J Med 1965;273(12):633–7.

57. Karnes WE Jr, Samloff IM, Siurala M, et al. Positive serum antibody and negative tissue staining for *Helicobacter pylori* in subjects with atrophic body gastritis. Gastroenterology 1991;101(1):167–74.

58. Green R. Protean *H. pylori*: perhaps "pernicious" too? Blood 2006;107(4):1247.

59. Maclean LD, Sundberg RD. Incidence of megaloblastic anemia after total gastrectomy. N Engl J Med 1956;254(19):885–93.

60. Van der Weyden M, Rother M, Firkin B. Megaloblastic maturation masked by iron deficiency: a biochemical basis. Br J Haematol 1972;22(3):299–307.

61. Lees F, Grandjean LC. The gastric and jejunal mucosae in healthy patients with partial gastrectomy. AMA Arch Intern Med 1958;101(5):943–51.

62. Chen M, Krishnamurthy A, Mohamed AR, et al. Hematological disorders following gastric bypass surgery: emerging concepts of the interplay between nutritional deficiency and inflammation. Biomed Res Int 2013;2013:205467.

63. Murphy MF, Sourial NA, Burman JF, et al. Megaloblastic anaemia due to vitamin B12 deficiency caused by small intestinal bacterial overgrowth: possible role of vitamin B12 analogues. Br J Haematol 1986;62(1):7–12.

64. Shimoda SS, Rubin CE. The Zollinger-Ellison syndrome with steatorrhea. I. Anticholinergic treatment followed by total gastrectomy and colonic interposition. Gastroenterology 1968;55(6):695–704.
65. Kennedy HJ, Callender ST, Truelove SC, et al. Haematological aspects of life with an ileostomy. Br J Haematol 1982;52(3):445–54.
66. Anderson CG, Walton KR, Chanarin I. Megaloblastic anaemia after pelvic radiotherapy for carcinoma of the cervix. J Clin Pathol 1981;34(2):151–2.
67. Waxman S, Corcino JJ, Herbert V. Drugs, toxins and dietary amino acids affecting vitamin B12 or folic acid absorption or utilization. Am J Med 1970; 48(5):599–608.
68. Sheehy TW, Perez-Santiago E, Rubini ME. Tropical sprue and vitamin B12. N Engl J Med 1961;265:1232–6.
69. Grasbeck R, Tanner SM. Juvenile selective vitamin B_{12} malabsorption: 50 years after its description-10 years of genetic testing. Pediatr Res 2011;70(3):222–8.
70. Kozyraki R, Kristiansen M, Silahtaroglu A, et al. The human intrinsic factor-vitamin B12 receptor, cubilin: molecular characterization and chromosomal mapping of the gene to 10p within the autosomal recessive megaloblastic anemia (MGA1) region. Blood 1998;91(10):3593–600.
71. Tanner SM, Li Z, Perko JD, et al. Hereditary juvenile cobalamin deficiency caused by mutations in the intrinsic factor gene. Proc Natl Acad Sci U S A 2005;102(11):4130–3.
72. Nyberg W. The influence of *Diphyllobothrium latum* on the vitamin B12-intrinsic factor complex. I. In vivo studies with Schilling test technique. Acta Med Scand 1960;167:185–7.
73. Harriman GR, Smith PD, Horne MK, et al. Vitamin B12 malabsorption in patients with acquired immunodeficiency syndrome. Arch Intern Med 1989;149(9): 2039–41.
74. Herzlich BC, Schiano TD, Moussa Z, et al. Decreased intrinsic factor secretion in AIDS: relation to parietal cell acid secretory capacity and vitamin B12 malabsorption. Am J Gastroenterol 1992;87(12):1781–8.
75. Remacha AF, Cadafalch J. Cobalamin deficiency in patients infected with the human immunodeficiency virus. Semin Hematol 1999;36(1):75–87.
76. Gueant JL, Champigneulle B, Gaucher P, et al. Malabsorption of vitamin B12 in pancreatic insufficiency of the adult and of the child. Pancreas 1990;5(5): 559–67.
77. Toskes PP, Deren JJ, Conrad ME. Trypsin-like nature of the pancreatic factor that corrects vitamin B12 malabsorption associated with pancreatic dysfunction. J Clin Invest 1973;52(7):1660–4.
78. Gilois C, Wierzbicki AS, Hirani N, et al. The hematological and electrophysiological effects of cobalamin. Deficiency secondary to vegetarian diets. Ann N Y Acad Sci 1992;669:345–8.
79. Green R, Jacobsen DW, van Tonder SV, et al. Enterohepatic circulation of cobalamin in the nonhuman primate. Gastroenterology 1981;81(4):773–6.
80. Green R, Jacobsen DW, Van Tonder SV, et al. Absorption of biliary cobalamin in baboons following total gastrectomy. J Lab Clin Med 1982;100(5):771–7.
81. Ford MJ. Megaloblastic anaemia in a vegetarian. Br J Clin Pract 1980;34(7):222.
82. Michaud JL, Lemieux B, Ogier H, et al. Nutritional vitamin B12 deficiency: two cases detected by routine newborn urinary screening. Eur J Pediatr 1992; 151(3):218–20.

83. Wickramasinghe SN, Akinyanju OO, Grange A, et al. Folate levels and deoxyuridine suppression tests in protein-energy malnutrition. Br J Haematol 1983; 53(1):135–43.

84. Carmel R, Green R, Rosenblatt DS, et al. Update on cobalamin, folate, and homocysteine. Hematol Education Program Am Soc Hematol 2003;62–81.

85. Fowler B. Genetic defects of folate and cobalamin metabolism. Eur J Pediatr 1998;157(Suppl 2):S60–6.

86. Rosenblatt DS, Cooper BA, Pottier A, et al. Altered vitamin B12 metabolism in fibroblasts from a patient with megaloblastic anemia and homocystinuria due to a new defect in methionine biosynthesis. J Clin Invest 1984;74(6):2149–56.

87. Katka K. Immune functions in pernicious anaemia before and during treatment with vitamin B12. Scand J Haematol 1984;32(1):76–82.

88. Katka K, Eskola J, Granfors K, et al. Serum IgA deficiency and anti-IgA antibodies in pernicious anemia. Clin Immunol Immunopathol 1988;46(1):55–60.

89. Zhang SM, Willett WC, Selhub J, et al. Plasma folate, vitamin B6, vitamin B12, homocysteine, and risk of breast cancer. J Natl Cancer Inst 2003;95(5):373–80.

90. Dhonukshe-Rutten RA, Lips M, de Jong N, et al. Vitamin B-12 status is associated with bone mineral content and bone mineral density in frail elderly women but not in men. J Nutr 2003;133(3):801–7.

91. Stone KL, Bauer DC, Sellmeyer D, et al. Low serum vitamin B-12 levels are associated with increased hip bone loss in older women: a prospective study. J Clin Endocrinol Metab 2004;89(3):1217–21.

92. Di Lazzaro V, Restuccia D, Fogli D, et al. Central sensory and motor conduction in vitamin B12 deficiency. Electroencephalogr Clin Neurophysiol 1992;84(5): 433–9.

93. Fraser TN. Cerebral manifestations of Addisonian pernicious anaemia. Lancet 1960;2(7148):458–9.

94. Shulman R. Psychiatric aspects of pernicious anaemia: a prospective controlled investigation. Br Med J 1967;3(5560):266–70.

95. Stabler SP. Vitamin B12 deficiency. N Engl J Med 2013;368(21):2041–2.

96. Dietary reference intakes for thiamin, riboflavin, niacin, vitamin B6, folate, vitamin B12, pantothenic acid, biotin, and choline, vol. 446. Washington, DC: The National Academies Press; 2000.

97. Carmel R. How I treat cobalamin (vitamin B12) deficiency. Blood 2008;112(6): 2214–21.

98. Kuzminski AM, Del Giacco EJ, Allen RH, et al. Effective treatment of cobalamin deficiency with oral cobalamin. Blood 1998;92(4):1191–8.

99. Green R. Screening for vitamin B12 deficiency: caveat emptor. Ann Intern Med 1996;124(5):509–11.

100. Sumner AE, Chin MM, Abrahm JL, et al. Elevated methylmalonic acid and total homocysteine levels show high prevalence of vitamin B12 deficiency after gastric surgery. Ann Intern Med 1996;124(5):469–76.

101. Paulk EA Jr, Farrar WE Jr. Diverticulosis of the small intestine and megaloblastic anemia: intestinal microflora and absorption before and after tetracycline administration. Am J Med 1964;37:473–80.

102. Colman N, Green R, Metz J. Prevention of folate deficiency by food fortification. II. Absorption of folic acid from fortified staple foods. Am J Clin Nutr 1975;28(5): 459–64.

103. Smithells RW, Sheppard S, Schorah CJ, et al. Possible prevention of neural-tube defects by periconceptional vitamin supplementation. Lancet 1980;1(8164): 339–40.

104. Ballard HS, Lindenbaum J. Megaloblastic anemia complicating hyperalimentation therapy. Am J Med 1974;56(5):740–2.

105. Mollin DL, Hines JD. Late post-gastrectomy syndromes. Observations on the nature and pathogenesis of anaemia following partial gastrectomy. Proc R Soc Med 1964;57:575–80.

106. Hoffbrand AV. Folate deficiency in premature infants. Arch Dis Child 1970; 45(242):441–4.

107. Royston NJ, Parry TE. Megaloblastic anaemia complicating dietary treatment of phenylketonuria in infancy. Arch Dis Child 1962;37(194):430–5.

108. Becroft DM, Holland JT. Goat's milk and megaloblastic anaemia of infancy: a report of three cases and a survey of the folic acid activity of some New Zealand milks. N Z Med J 1966;65(405):303–7.

109. Savage D, Lindenbaum J. Anemia in alcoholics. Medicine 1986;65(5):322–38.

110. Lindenbaum J, Lieber CS. Hematologic effects of alcohol in man in the absence of nutritional deficiency. N Engl J Med 1969;281(7):333–8.

111. Trier JS. Celiac sprue. N Engl J Med 1991;325(24):1709–19.

112. Hjelt K, Krasilnikoff PA. The impact of gluten on haematological status, dietary intakes of haemopoietic nutrients and vitamin B12 and folic acid absorption in children with coeliac disease. Acta Paediatr Scand 1990;79(10):911–9.

113. Klipstein FA. Tropical sprue in New York City. Gastroenterology 1964;47:457–70.

114. Klipstein FA, Schenk EA, Samloff IM. Folate repletion associated with oral tetracycline therapy in tropical sprue. Gastroenterology 1966;51(3):317–32.

115. Chanarin I, Bennett MC. Absorption of folic acid and D-xylose as tests of small-intestinal function. Br Med J 1962;1(5283):985–9.

116. Booth CC. The metabolic effects of intestinal resection in man. Postgrad Med J 1961;37:725–39.

117. Pitney WR, Joske RA, Mackinnon NL. Folic acid and other absorption tests in lymphosarcoma, chronic lymphocytic leukaemia, and some related conditions. J Clin Pathol 1960;13:440–7.

118. Hoskins LC, Norris HT, Gottlieb LS, et al. Functional and morphologic alterations of the gastrointestinal tract in progressive systemic sclerosis (scleroderma). Am J Med 1962;33:459–70.

119. Vinnik IE, Kern F Jr, Struthers JE Jr. Malabsorption and the diarrhea of diabetes mellitus. Gastroenterology 1962;43:507–20.

120. Streiff RR, Little AB. Folic acid deficiency in pregnancy. N Engl J Med 1967; 276(14):776–9.

121. de Benoist B. Conclusions of a WHO technical consultation on folate and vitamin B12 deficiencies. Food Nutr Bull 2008;29(2 Suppl):S238–44.

122. Shojania AM. Folic acid and vitamin B12 deficiency in pregnancy and in the neonatal period. Clin perinatology 1984;11(2):433–59.

123. Landon MJ, Eyre DH, Hytten FE. Transfer of folate to the fetus. Br J Obstet Gynaecol 1975;82(1):12–9.

124. Chanarin I, McFadyen IR, Kyle R. The physiological macrocytosis of pregnancy. Br J Obstet Gynaecol 1977;84(7):504–8.

125. Avery B, Ledger WJ. Folic acid metabolism in well-nourished pregnant women. Obstet Gynecol 1970;35(4):616–24.

126. Giles C. An account of 335 cases of megaloblastic anaemia of pregnancy and the puerperium. J Clin Pathol 1966;19(1):1–11.

127. Shapiro J, Alberts HW, Welch P, et al. Folate and vitamin B-12 deficiency associated with lactation. Br J Haematol 1965;11:498–504.

128. Colman N, Larsen JV, Barker M, et al. Prevention of folate deficiency by food fortification. III. Effect in pregnant subjects of varying amounts of added folic acid. Am J Clin Nutr 1975;28(5):465–70.

129. Lindenbaum J, Klipstein FA. Folic acid deficiency in sickle-cell anemia. N Engl J Med 1963;269:875–82.

130. Hild DH. Folate losses from the skin in exfoliative dermatitis. Arch Intern Med 1969;123(1):51–7.

131. Whitehead VM, Comty CH, Posen GA, et al. Homeostasis of folic acid in patients undergoing maintenance hemodialysis. N Engl J Med 1968;279(18):970–4.

132. Hoffbrand AV, Newcombe FA, Mollin DL. Method of assay of red cell folate activity and the value of the assay as a test for folate deficiency. J Clin Pathol 1966; 19(1):17–28.

133. Lindenbaum J. Status of laboratory testing in the diagnosis of megaloblastic anemia. Blood 1983;61(4):624–7.

134. Prevention of neural tube defects: results of the Medical Research Council Vitamin Study. MRC Vitamin Study Research Group. Lancet 1991;338(8760): 131–7.

135. Rothenberg SP, da Costa MP, Sequeira JM, et al. Autoantibodies against folate receptors in women with a pregnancy complicated by a neural-tube defect. N Engl J Med 2004;350(2):134–42.

136. van der Put NM, Gabreels F, Stevens EM, et al. A second common mutation in the methylenetetrahydrofolate reductase gene: an additional risk factor for neural-tube defects? Am J Hum Genet 1998;62(5):1044–51.

137. Honein MA, Paulozzi LJ, Mathews TJ, et al. Impact of folic acid fortification of the US food supply on the occurrence of neural tube defects. JAMA 2001;285(23):2981–6.

138. De Wals P, Tairou F, Van Allen MI, et al. Reduction in neural-tube defects after folic acid fortification in Canada. N Engl J Med 2007;357(2):135–42.

139. Qiu A, Jansen M, Sakaris A, et al. Identification of an intestinal folate transporter and the molecular basis for hereditary folate malabsorption. Cell 2006;127(5): 917–28.

140. Zhao R, Matherly LH, Goldman ID. Membrane transporters and folate homeostasis: intestinal absorption and transport into systemic compartments and tissues. Expert Rev Mol Med 2009;11:e4.

141. Min SH, Oh SY, Karp GI, et al. The clinical course and genetic defect in the PCFT gene in a 27-year-old woman with hereditary folate malabsorption. J Pediatr 2008;153(3):435–7.

142. Whitehead VM. Acquired and inherited disorders of cobalamin and folate in children. Br J Haematol 2006;134(2):125–36.

143. Zittoun J. Congenital errors of folate metabolism. Bailliere's Clin Haematol 1995; 8(3):603–16.

144. Arakawa T, Narisawa K, Tanno K, et al. Megaloblastic anemia and mental retardation associated with hyperfolic-acidemia: probably due to N5 methyltetrahydrofolate transferase deficiency. Tohoku J Exp Med 1967;93(1):1–22.

145. Rosenberg IH. Folic acid and neural-tube defects–time for action? N Engl J Med 1992;327(26):1875–7.

146. Vilter CF, Vilter RW, Spies TD. The treatment of pernicious and related anemias with synthetic folic acid; observations on the maintenance of a normal hematologic status and on the occurrence of combined system disease at the end of one year. J Lab Clin Med 1947;32(3):262–73.

147. Henderson GB, Suresh MR, Vitols KS, et al. Transport of folate compounds in L1210 cells: kinetic evidence that folate influx proceeds via the high-affinity

transport system for 5-methyltetrahydrofolate and methotrexate. Cancer Res 1986;46(4 Pt 1):1639–43.

148. Schoo MM, Pristupa ZB, Vickers PJ, et al. Folate analogues as substrates of mammalian folylpolyglutamate synthetase. Cancer Res 1985;45(7):3034–41.

149. Kesavan V, Sur P, Doig MT, et al. Effects of methotrexate on folates in Krebs ascites and L1210 murine leukemia cells. Cancer Lett 1986;30(1):55–9.

150. Spiegel RJ, Cooper PR, Blum RH, et al. Treatment of massive intrathecal methotrexate overdose by ventriculolumbar perfusion. N Engl J Med 1984;311(6): 386–8.

151. Yarchoan R, Broder S. Development of antiretroviral therapy for the acquired immunodeficiency syndrome and related disorders. A progress report. N Engl J Med 1987;316(9):557–64.

152. Krakoff IH, Brown NC, Reichard P. Inhibition of ribonucleoside diphosphate reductase by hydroxyurea. Cancer Res 1968;28(8):1559–65.

153. Termanini B, Gibril F, Sutliff VE, et al. Effect of long-term gastric acid suppressive therapy on serum vitamin B12 levels in patients with Zollinger-Ellison syndrome. Am J Med 1998;104(5):422–30.

154. Sive J, Green R, Metz J. Effect of trimethoprim on folate-dependent DNA synthesis in human bone marrow. J Clin Pathol 1972;25(3):194–7.

155. Spector I, Green R, Bowes D, et al. Trimethoprim-sulphamethoxazole therapy and folate nutrition. S Afr Med J 1973;47(28):1230–2.

156. Zdebska E, Mendek-Czajkowska E, Ploski R, et al. Heterozygosity of CDAN II (HEMPAS) gene may be detected by the analysis of erythrocyte membrane glycoconjugates from healthy carriers. Haematologica 2002;87(2):126–30.

157. Najfeld V, McArthur J, Shashaty GG. Monosomy 7 in a patient with pancytopenia and abnormal erythropoiesis. Acta haematologica 1981;66(1):12–8.

158. Camaschella C. Recent advances in the understanding of inherited sideroblastic anaemia. Br J Haematol 2008;143(1):27–38.

159. Roggli VL, Saleem A. Erythroleukemia: a study of 15 cases and literature review. Cancer 1982;49(1):101–8.

160. Fleming JC, Tartaglini E, Steinkamp MP, et al. The gene mutated in thiamine-responsive anaemia with diabetes and deafness (TRMA) encodes a functional thiamine transporter. Nat Genet 1999;22(3):305–8.

Iron Deficiency Anemia

Thomas G. DeLoughery, MD, MACP, FAWM

KEYWORDS

- Iron • Ferritin • Inflammatory bowel disease • Ulcers • TMPRSS6

KEY POINTS

- Iron deficiency can lead to symptoms independent of anemia.
- The serum ferritin is the most efficient test for iron deficiency.
- Oral iron is best given once a day with vitamin C.

INTRODUCTION

Iron deficiency anemia is the most common and most treatable of all anemias. There is an evolving understanding that iron deficiency can lead to symptoms independent of anemia and can be associated with a variety of diseases. This review covers iron metabolism as well as the epidemiology, diagnosis, and treatment of this common anemia.

IRON METABOLISM

Iron is found in a variety of foods, with meat being the richest source. Iron in food is largely in the ferric form (Fe^{3+}), which is reduced by stomach acid to the ferrous from (Fe^{2+}). In the jejunum, 2 receptors on the mucosal cells absorb iron. One receptor is specific for heme-bound iron and absorbs 30% to 40% of ingested heme iron. The other receptor, divalent metal transporter (DMT1), takes up inorganic iron but is 1% to 10% less efficient at absorption. Iron is exported from the enterocyte via ferroportin and is then delivered to plasma transferrin, the main transport molecule for iron. Transferrin can deliver iron to the marrow for use in red cell production or to the liver for storage, which is done by binding to the transferrin receptor on the red cell membrane. Ferritin is the storage protein for iron. The ferritin protein consists of 24 ferritin subunits that create a shell that can store up to 4500 iron molecules.[1] Iron that is contained in hemoglobin in senescent red cells is recycled by binding to ferritin in the macrophage.

Author reports no conflicts of interest.
Division of Hematology/Medical Oncology, Department of Medicine, Knight Cancer Institute, Oregon Health and Science University, MC L586, 3181 Southwest Sam Jackson Park Road, Portland, OR 97239, USA
E-mail address: delought@ohsu.edu

It is then transferred to transferrin for recycling into developing red cells or is sent to storage. This system is extremely efficient and loses less than 5% of the iron contained in total red cell mass.

The protein hepcidin controls iron absorption and iron's release from stores.[1] Hepcidin binds to ferroportin, leading to its degradation. When hepcidin degrades ferroportin, iron cannot be released from the enterocyte or hepatocytes, leading to both a lack of iron absorption and a halt in iron release to developing red cells. Hepcidin synthesis is upregulated not only by iron but also by inflammation. Levels are reduced by hypoxia, increased erythropoiesis, and iron deficiency.

Recommended dietary iron intake is 8 mg daily for adult men and 18 mg for premenopausal women, increasing to 27 mg daily during pregnancy.[2] Meats are rich in heme iron, and iron in meat is much more effectively absorbed. Nonmeat sources of iron are poorer in iron stores, the iron is less effectively absorbed, and it is difficult to ingest large enough amounts to meet iron requirements.

EPIDEMIOLOGY AND ETIOLOGIES

Given that there is no natural mechanism for the body to excrete iron, the predominant mechanism for iron deficiency is blood loss, most commonly from menstrual periods or from gastrointestinal bleeding (**Box 1**). The next major causes are issues with the absorption of iron. Both of these can be compounded by the influence of iron-poor diets. In the United States, the incidence of iron deficiency in men is approximately 1%, but is at least 11% and often higher in women.[3]

Women are at greater risk for developing iron deficiency due to obligate iron losses through menstruation, with an average loss of 35 mL of blood equivalent to 16 mg of iron per period.[2,4,5] The average iron requirements per day in women average 1 to 3 mg, with higher needs for those with heavier periods. Compounding this iron loss is that dietary iron intake is often inadequate to maintain a positive iron balance.[6,7] Several studies demonstrate high levels of iron deficiency in women, with the most

---

Box 1
Etiologies of iron deficiency

Menstrual losses

Pregnancy and delivery

Gastrointestinal losses
  Cancer
  Gastritis
  Helicobacter pylori
    Atrophic gastritis
    Ulcers
  Hookworm and other parasites
  Inflammatory bowel disease
  Meckel diverticulum
  Vascular malformations

Obesity

Celiac disease

Hematuria

Bariatric surgery

striking being a 1967 study that showed 25% of healthy college-age women had no marrow iron stores and 33% had reduced stores.[8] Pregnancy adds to demands on iron, with requirements rising to 6 mg per day at the end of pregnancy.[9]

Gastrointestinal loss is the next major source of iron deficiency. Gastrointestinal lesions lead to iron deficiency by gradual blood loss over long periods of time. Neoplasm is the most feared source of blood loss, with incidence found in up to 10% of older patients with iron deficiency anemia. Colon cancer is the most common tumor, followed by upper tract lesions, such as gastric cancer. Small bowel tumors are rare and are usually not screened for unless there is refractory iron deficiency or bleeding. Ulcer and gastritis are also common causes of blood loss. Patients who use aspirin or nonsteroidal anti-inflammatory agents have an increased incidence of iron deficiency. A subtle cause are Cameron ulcers, lineal ulcerations in hiatal hernias, that can be missed on routine endoscopy.

Helicobacter pylori infections lead to iron deficiency by several mechanisms.[10] The first is that infection is a risk factor for ulcers, especially gastric. Second, infection results in achlorhydria, which results in impaired iron absorption, leading to inability to convert ferric to ferrous iron. *H pylori* infections also may lead to autoimmune gastritis, which in early stages leads to iron deficiency and later on to B_{12} deficiency.[11]

The increase in surgical interventions to attempt to correct the obesity epidemic is becoming a major cause of iron deficiency. Obese patients are often iron deficient, one study showing a 7.9% incidence, with elevated hepcidin levels implicated in reducing iron absorption.[12,13] After bariatric surgery, the incidence of iron deficiency can be as high as 50%, with a meta-analysis showing 23%.[14] Because the main site of iron absorption is the duodenum, surgeries that involve bypassing this part of the bowel are associated with a higher incidence of deficiency, but iron deficiency is seen as a sequela of most types of bariatric surgeries.[15]

Athletes are another group at risk for iron deficiency.[16] Studies have shown that the gastrointestinal tract is the main source of iron loss.[17] Augmenting this is exercise-induced hemolysis leading to urinary iron losses.[18] This hemolysis is not only caused by foot strike but perhaps also by intense muscle contractions, as signs of hemolysis are also seen in competitive swimmers. Recently, decreased iron absorption also has been implicated as a cause of deficiency, as levels of hepcidin are often elevated in athletes due to training-induced inflammation.[16] Although it is clear that frank anemia can affect performance, there is increasing evidence that nonanemic iron deficiency also may be detrimental.[16,19–21]

Patients who have inflammatory bowel disease have a high incidence of iron deficiency.[22] Iron insufficiencies are due to the presence of inflamed bowel losing blood, as well as the marked inflammatory state leading to a rise in hepcidin levels blocking iron absorption. In those patients who require bowel surgery, this also adds to the stress on iron stores.

Celiac disease is triggered by gluten ingestion and results in an immune response classically thought to affect the gastrointestinal tract but also causing systemic effects.[23] Severe iron deficiency can be a presentation of celiac disease. Classically the pathophysiology was thought to be lack of absorption due to villous blunting, but there is also gastrointestinal blood loss and increased hepcidin levels.[24]

Vascular malformations commonly occur in the bowel, and bleeding from these lesions can lead to iron deficiency. Patients suffering from hereditary hemorrhagic telangiectasia, a genetic disease with arteriovenous malformations (AVMs) spread through the bowel, often have ongoing severe iron loss. Aortic stenosis may lead to AVM formation (Heyde syndrome). AVMs can lead to blood loss in patients with ventricular assist devices (VADs) and are reported in 17.5% to 30.0% of bleeding patients.[25]

The lack of pulse pressure in both patients with VAD and those with severe aortic stenosis appears to be the key risk factor for AVM formation. AVMs can be due to increased sympathetic tone leading to smooth muscle relaxants or hypoperfusion leading to vascular dilatation.[26]

Both aspirin and nonsteroidal anti-inflammatory agents can lead to iron deficiency through overt bleeding from ulcers and/or increased gastrointestinal blood loss.[27,28] One study showed the use of daily aspirin increased blood loss from 0.8 mL per day to 5.0 mL per day.[28] With the use of these drugs, there is also a higher incidence of small bowel lesions, which can add to blood loss.[19]

New research demonstrates that there are differences in how patients absorb iron. Rare patients present in childhood suffering from iron-refractory iron deficiency due to defects with an iron metabolism protein, TMRPSS6, leading to very high levels of hepcidin, which blocks iron absorption.[29] This protein exists in the population with many polymorphisms that can affect iron absorption, suggesting that an individual's ability to absorb iron can vary greatly.[30] For example, a TMRPSS6 polymorphism has been shown to be protective against iron deficiency in menstruating women, whereas others increase the risk.[30,31]

SYMPTOMS

Iron deficiency can lead to symptoms both due to the lack of iron itself and due to the resultant anemia. Symptoms of anemia can include fatigue, tachycardia, and lack of endurance. Pica, unusual cravings for eating ice or clay, can occur.

Increasingly recognized are symptoms in iron-depleted but nonanemic patients. Given the key role of iron in many cellular proteins and enzymes, especially cytochromes and myoglobin, it is not surprising that symptoms can be seen before anemia occurs.

The most profound symptom is fatigue, which can occur with even modest reductions in iron stores. Two studies show that oral iron supplementation in iron-deficient, but not anemic, women whose ferritins were less than 50 ng/mL improves fatigue,[32,33] whereas a third study shows improvement of fatigue with parenteral iron in women with ferritins less than 15 or iron saturation less than 20%.[34] Another recent study also showed improvement in fatigue with iron supplementation to iron-deficient but nonanemic fatigued adolescents.[35] These studies, along with improvements in athletic performance cited previously, clearly demonstrate the role of iron in well-being beyond hemoglobin level.

Another common symptom of lack of iron is cold intolerance.[36] Some of these symptoms are due to the anemia, as they often correct when the anemia is corrected. However, some patients notice cold intolerance with nonanemic iron deficiency. This may be due to decreased efficacy of thyroid hormone. The effectiveness of intracellular thyroid is dependent on iron stores, so lack of iron reduces the effectiveness of the hormone.

Patients with heart failure are found to have an increased incidence of both overt and functional iron deficiency. Incidence of iron deficiency can be as high as 13% to 42%, with a higher percentage having functional iron deficiency.[37,38] Repletion of the deficient iron stores has been shown to improve cardiac function and quality of life, and also to reduce hospitalization.[38,39]

Another group in which iron deficiency may play a detrimental role is patients with pulmonary hypertension.[40,41] Cellular response to hypoxia is dependent on iron, as iron chelation mimics hypoxia via upregulation of genes that control the hypoxic response.[42] Iron has been shown to play a crucial role in regulating pulmonary vascular resistance. A study of iron-deficient patients showed an exaggerated hypoxic rise in pulmonary artery pressures compared with healthy controls.[43] Low iron stores have been seen in patients with pulmonary hypertension, with the finding that repletion lowers pulmonary artery pressure.[44]

Restless leg syndrome is a condition in which patients have leg cramps, unpleasant leg sensations, and the need to move the legs at night.[45] Low iron stores are seen in many of these sufferers, with studies of brain iron also showing low iron stores.[46] In many patients, iron repletion controls symptoms, suggesting these low iron stores are pathogenic in at least some patients with restless leg syndrome.[31,47]

A common complaint in iron-deficient women is hair loss, with increased loss reported in women with ferritins less than 100 ng/dL.[48] The pattern most associated with iron deficiency is diffuse nonscarring scalp alopecia.

DIAGNOSIS

Many tests are proposed for the diagnosis of iron deficiency, but the serum ferritin is currently the most efficient and cost-effective[12,49] (**Box 2**). The anemia of iron deficiency is classically a microcytic anemia, but this finding is not sensitive or specific. The red cell mean corpuscular volume (MCV) is low with severe iron deficiency, but concurrent medical issues, such as liver disease, may blunt the decrease in red cell size. A fall in MCV is also a late finding in iron deficiency. Thalassemia and the anemia of inflammation can lead to microcytosis as well.

Free zinc protoporphyria is generated when there is inadequate iron delivered to the developing red cells.[50] Lack of iron for the heme molecule will result in free protoporphyrin to be released, making this a marker of lack of red cell iron. Given that the anemia of inflammation is also marked by decreased red cell iron delivery, this will be elevated in both iron deficiency and the anemia of inflammation. Although much less common, lead poisoning also leads to a raised free protoporphyrin.

Serum iron as a diagnostic test is suboptimal, as it is low in the anemia of inflammation and can be falsely elevated with oral iron intake in iron-deficient patients. Also there is tremendous variation in day-to-day levels. A raised total iron binding capacity (TIBC) is specific for iron deficiency, but because it is reduced by inflammation, aging, and poor nutrition, its sensitivity is low. Iron saturation also suffers due to its dependence on both the TIBC and serum iron, with saturation being low in both iron deficiency and anemia of chronic disease. Serum levels of soluble transferrin receptor will be increased in iron deficiency and this test is not affected by inflammation.[51] However, levels can be increased in any condition associated with increased red cell mass, such as hemolytic anemias or in patients with chronic lymphocytic leukemia, and one can miss some overt cases of iron deficiency.[52] Although the "gold standard" for iron deficiency is the bone marrow iron stain, this is an invasive and expensive procedure and rarely needs to be used.

Box 2
Diagnosis of iron deficiency

Ferritin: most efficient diagnostic test

Mean corpuscular volume: may be normal or elevated, not that useful

Free erythrocyte protoporphyria: increased in iron deficiency, anemia of chronic disease, and lead poisoning

Serum iron: (too) variable

Total iron binding capacity: sensitive but not specific

Ferritin plasma levels correlate with body iron stores in healthy patients. There has been concern raised that, since ferritin is an acute phase reactant, this will affect its usefulness in diagnosing iron deficiency anemia. Although the transcription of ferritin mRNA is upregulated by inflammation, the synthesis of the ferritin protein is regulated by cellular iron content, with ferritin mRNA being translated to protein only when the cell is iron replete.[7] Therefore, an iron-replete patient may have a very high ferritin with inflammation, but it is rare for an iron-deficient patient to have a ferritin more than 100 ng/mL. The lower limits of "normal" depend on the clinical situation. Although a level of 15 ng/mL is very specific for iron deficiency, in older patients or in those with inflammatory states, one cannot rule out iron deficiency until the ferritin is greater than 100 ng/dL. The thorough 1992 review by Guyatt and colleagues[53] showed that the likelihood ratio of iron deficiency is positive up to a ferritin of 40 ng/mL and up to 70 ng/mL in the setting of inflammation. Consequently, the serum ferritin is the one test most likely to provide information about the patient's iron status. Of course, one must consider the patient's age and clinical condition when interpreting results.

TREATMENT

Eating a diet higher in bioavailable iron can help treat iron deficiency, but is unlikely in and of itself to replete iron stores, although it can help maintain them. The food richest in iron is meat. Cooking with iron skillets can also increase dietary iron but the amount of iron enrichment can be variable.[54,55]

The long-established treatment of iron deficiency has been ferrous sulfate given 3 times a day. This has been challenged recently by studies suggesting that lower doses of iron, such as 15 to 20 mg elemental iron daily can be as effective as higher doses and is better tolerated with fewer gastrointestinal side effects.[56,57] For example, a trial comparing 15, 50, and 150 mg oral elemental iron showed that there was no difference in ferritin rise with any dose and showed less gastrointestinal toxicity with the smallest dose. The reason that low-dose iron is effective may be that enterocyte iron absorption appears to be saturable, and that 1 dose of iron can "block" absorption of further iron doses for the rest of the day.[58] This mechanism was highlighted by a recent study that showed an abrupt rise in hepcidin levels with iron consumption.[59] Taking the iron supplement with meat protein (cow, pork, and fish) can also increase iron absorption.[60] Vitamin C aids absorption in several ways.[61] First, as a reducing agent, vitamin C helps keeps iron in the more soluble ferrous form. Second, iron and vitamin C can form a soluble complex. Concomitant calcium and fiber can decrease iron absorption, but this can be overcome by taking vitamin C.[62] Importantly, a potent inhibitor of iron absorption is tea; ingestion can reduce absorption by 90%.[63] Coffee also decreases iron absorption to about two-thirds the degree that tea does.[61,63]

Multiple oral iron preparations exist, and no one compound appears to be superior to another.[64] A sensible approach to oral iron replacement is to start with a single ferrous sulfate taken with a meal that (if not vegetarian) contains meat (**Table 1**). Avoiding tea and coffee plus taking 500 units of vitamin C with that meal will also aid iron absorption. If ferrous sulfate is not tolerated, then ferrous gluconate, which has less elemental iron per tablet, can be tried. The reticulocyte count should rise in 1 week and hemoglobin should start rising by the second week of therapy. If the hemoglobin has not responded by this time, it is unlikely the patient will respond to oral iron.[65] Iron should be continued until iron stores are replete with a goal ferritin of 50 to 100 ng/dL.

Gastrointestinal side effects of oral iron are common, with 30% to 50% of patients reporting symptoms.[66] Endoscopy in patients taking oral iron often shows esophageal erosions and gastritis.[67,68]

Table 1
Treatment of iron deficiency

1. One iron pill per day: can be cheapest brand (should have more than 18 mg of elemental iron)
   a. Example: Ferrous sulfate (65 mg elemental iron), Ferrous gluconate (37.5 mg elemental iron)
2. Take iron with 500 mg vitamin C: helps absorption
3. Take with meals: if a meat eater, take iron with meat because this will improve absorption of iron
4. Avoid drinking tea or coffee with iron pills.

Nonmeat Sources of Iron		
Food	Amount	Iron, mg
Blackstrap molasses	2 tablespoons	7.2
Lentils, cooked	1 cup	6.6
Tofu	4 ounces	6.4
Spinach, cooked	1 cup	6.4
Bagel, enriched	1 medium	6.4
Chickpeas, cooked	1 cup	4.7
Tempeh	1 cup	4.5
Lima beans, cooked	1 cup	4.5
Black-eyed peas, cooked	1 cup	4.3
Swiss chard, cooked	1 cup	4.0
Kidney beans, cooked	1 cup	3.9
Black beans, cooked	1 cup	3.6
Pinto beans, cooked	1 cup	3.6
Turnip greens, cooked	1 cup	3.2
Prune juice	8 ounces	3.0
Quinoa, cooked	1 cup	2.8
Beet greens, cooked	1 cup	2.7
Tahini	2 tablespoons	2.7
Veggie hot dog, iron-fortified	1 hot dog	2.7
Peas, cooked	1 cup	2.5
Cashews	1/4 cup	2.1
Bok choy, cooked	1 cup	1.8
Bulgur, cooked	1 cup	1.7
Raisins	1/2 cup	1.6
Apricots, dried	15 halves	1.4
Veggie burger,	1 patty	1.4
Watermelon	1/8 medium	1.4
Almonds	1/4 cup	1.3
Kale, cooked	1 cup	1.2
Sunflower seeds	1/4 cup	1.2

When patients do not respond to oral iron, several factors should be considered. The side effects of stomach pain and constipation can hinder compliance. Taking a smaller dose of iron and even decreasing to every other day may reduce these symptoms. The patient's history also should be reviewed regarding use of tea, coffee, or vitamin C. In patients who have ongoing bleeding, such as from AVMs, the iron loss may be too great for oral iron to overcome. Bowel issues, such as surgical resection or inflammatory bowel disease, also can lead to oral iron resistance. *H pylori* infection and celiac disease lead to impaired absorption of iron.

INTRAVENOUS IRON

Over the past few years, the indications for intravenous iron have rapidly expanded (**Table 2**).[69] Parenteral iron should be used in any iron-deficient patient who is not responding to or cannot tolerate oral iron. Patients with known absorption problems, such as history of bowel surgery or bariatric procedures, should preferentially receive intravenous iron. Ongoing blood loss, such as from hereditary hemorrhagic telangiectasia, will require ongoing iron infusions, as these patients cannot keep up with their gastrointestinal iron losses. For several reasons, patients suffering from inflammatory bowel disease should be preferentially treated with intravenous iron. First is that many patients have ongoing gastrointestinal blood loss that can outstrip oral iron intake. Second is that these patients already have many gastrointestinal issues and there is low tolerance of oral iron. Studies have shown both better tolerance and effectiveness of intravenous iron over iron.[70] Third, oral iron can lead to gastritis and this can have adverse effects of worsening the bowel disease and changing the microbiome.[71]

The major disadvantage with intravenous iron is infusion reactions, but both the incidence and severity of these is often overstated.[72] These reactions are not true allergic reactions but are related to complement activation by the labile free iron.[73] Recently detailed advice about treating these reactions has been published[74]; in general, for mild reactions, the infusion is stopped and then resumed at a slower rate once symptoms resolve. For more severe reactions, fluids and steroids are used. Diphenhydramine should be avoided, as this can worsen symptoms. Studies show rates of mild reactions are approximately 1:200 and major ones are approximately 1:200,000.[75]

Because free iron is toxic, all intravenous iron contains carbohydrates that bind the elemental iron to prevent reactions. There are 2 forms of intravenous iron. One is iron that can be given as single-dose repletion. The other form is iron salts that must be given over multiple doses for full replacement. The iron salts are ferrous gluconate and iron sucrose. Ferrous gluconate is approved as a 125-mg dose, but in practice 250 mg is given as a single dose. Iron sucrose is approved as a single 100-mg dose, but often 200 to 300 mg is given in clinic practice.

There are 4 single replacement dose irons available: low molecular weight iron dextran, ferumoxytol, ferric carboxymaltose, and iron isomaltoside (currently only available in Europe). The advantages of these agents is that single replacement doses can be given in 1 to 2 sessions. For example, low molecular weight iron dextran has abundant data for a 1-hour 1000-mg single replacement dose.[76,77] Iron

Table 2	
Intravenous iron	
Agent	**Typical single dose**
Low molecular weight iron dextran	1000 mg
Ferric gluconate	125 mg
Iron sucrose	300 mg
Ferumoxytol	510 mg
Ferric carboxymalate	1000 mg

carboxymaltose can be given as a 1000-mg single dose, but this vial size is not available in the United States, so 750 mg given a week apart is the standard dosing. Ferumoxytol is a superparamagnetic iron oxide coated with carbohydrate that is marketed as both iron replacement and as an MRI contrast agent. The approved use is 510 mg over 15 minutes, repeated once in 3 to 8 days, although there is increasing experience with a single 1020-mg dose.[78] Patients needing MRI scans in the ensuing 3 months need to let radiologists know they received ferumoxytol, as it can function as a contrast agent and alter MRIs. Finally, iron isomaltoside allows infusions of up to 1000 mg in 15 minutes.

Formulas calculating total iron deficit tend to be unreliable, so the most pragmatic approach is to use a 1000-mg replacement dose. Patients with severe iron deficiency anemia may have deficits that exceed 1 g, so a ferritin should be checked 2 to 4 weeks after an infusion. If the ferritin is not higher than 50 ng/dL at that time, another iron dose should be given. After a patient receives intravenous iron, long-term follow-up is essential. The ferritin should be checked every 3 to 4 months, and if it falls below 50, iron infusions should be repeated. Patients with ongoing gastrointestinal bleeding should have ferritin checked more often and may require frequent infusions.

DETERMINING THE ETIOLOGY OF IRON DEFICIENCY

A priority in iron deficiency is determining the cause. Given that there are no natural mechanisms for ridding the body of iron, blood loss must always be assumed. As little as 5 mL of blood loss per day can lead to iron deficiency. The finding of melena or bloody stools is not sensitive, as studies have shown that those with up to 100 mL of blood loss per day may have normal-colored stool.[79] As noted previously, the incidence of gastrointestinal lesions are high and this must always be considered as a source of the iron loss. Risk factors for presence of tumor are age older than 50, male sex, and hemoglobin less than 9 g/dL.[80] In general, any man with unexplained iron deficiency or any woman older than 40 should undergo upper endoscopy and colonoscopy.[21] Routine gastric biopsy may diagnose atrophic gastritis or *H pylori* infections.[81] For premenopausal women, the recommendations are that women older than 40 should undergo testing, as well as those with gastrointestinal symptoms, weight loss, or blood in the stool.[82] Testing the stool for blood can identify patients with blood loss, but the sensitivity of testing varies, with tests that detect heme-porphyrin (example HemoQuant) being more sensitive to upper tract bleeding.[79] Also, most stool tests require 10 mL or more of daily blood loss to be positive, and losses less than this can still lead to iron deficiency.[83] A urinalysis also should be checked, as hematuria may rarely be persistent enough to lead to iron deficiency.

In patients with iron deficiency not responsive to oral iron, adherence to and tolerability of oral iron should be assessed. The clinical issues to consider are celiac disease, autoimmune gastritis, *H pylori* infections along with menorrhagia, and ongoing gastrointestinal losses.[11] Testing for celiac disease is by serology (antitissue glutaminase antibodies) and for *H pylori*. Autoimmune gastritis is screened for by obtaining a serum gastrin, which will be markedly elevated, and antiparietal cell antibodies.

There are several options for further gastrointestinal workup in patients with ongoing iron needs.[79] Pill endoscopy, the use of a small television camera taken orally, can find lesions in 30% of patients. Vascular ectasia is the most common source of bleeding found by pill endoscopy in older patients, whereas inflammatory bowel disease, small bowel tumors, and celiac disease are more common in younger patients.[81] Patients with known gastrointestinal blood loss have higher yields of 50% to 90%.[79] Push endoscopy is also widely available and allows for therapy, but is more invasive and may have a lower yield than capsule endoscopy. This should be considered for patients who have evidence of gastrointestinal bleeding despite negative capsule endoscopy.[84]

SUMMARY

Iron deficiency is one of the most common causes of anemia. Increasingly it is being recognized that iron lack can lead to a wide variety of clinical problems, such as fatigue and restless legs. Diagnosis is made by the use of the serum ferritin, and treatment can be oral or intravenous iron. Key to management is to try to identify and treat any source of blood loss in these patients.

REFERENCES

1. Evstatiev R, Gasche C. Iron sensing and signalling. Gut 2012;61(6):933–52.
2. Miller EM. The reproductive ecology of iron in women. Am J Phys Anthropol 2016; 159(Suppl 61):S172–95.
3. Looker AC, Dallman PR, Carroll MD, et al. Prevalence of iron deficiency in the United States. JAMA 1997;277:973–6.
4. Hallberg L, Hogdahl AM, Nilsson L, et al. Menstrual blood loss and iron deficiency. Acta Med Scand 1966;180(5):639–50.
5. Levi M, Rosselli M, Simonetti M, et al. Epidemiology of iron deficiency anaemia in four European countries: a population-based study in primary care. Eur J Haematol 2016. [Epub ahead of print].
6. Hunt JR, Zito CA, Johnson LK. Body iron excretion by healthy men and women. Am J Clin Nutr 2009;89(6):1792–8.
7. Pantopoulos K, Porwal SK, Tartakoff A, et al. Mechanisms of mammalian iron homeostasis. Biochemistry 2012;51(29):5705–24.
8. Scott DE, Pritchard JA. Iron deficiency in healthy young college women. JAMA 1967;199(12):897–900.
9. Pavord S, Myers B, Robinson S, et al. UK guidelines on the management of iron deficiency in pregnancy. Br J Haematol 2012;156(5):588–600.
10. Hudak L, Jaraisy A, Haj S, et al. An updated systematic review and meta-analysis on the association between Helicobacter pylori infection and iron deficiency anemia. Helicobacter 2016. [Epub ahead of print].
11. Hershko C, Camaschella C. How I treat unexplained refractory iron deficiency anemia. Blood 2014;123(3):326–33.
12. Mei Z, Cogswell ME, Parvanta I, et al. Hemoglobin and ferritin are currently the most efficient indicators of population response to iron interventions: an analysis of nine randomized controlled trials. J Nutr 2005;135(8):1974–80.
13. Weng TC, Chang CH, Dong YH, et al. Anaemia and related nutrient deficiencies after Roux-en-Y gastric bypass surgery: a systematic review and meta-analysis. BMJ Open 2015;5(7):e006964.
14. Love AL, Billett HH. Obesity, bariatric surgery, and iron deficiency: true, true, true and related. Am J Hematol 2008;83(5):403–9.
15. Ruz M, Carrasco F, Rojas P, et al. Heme- and nonheme-iron absorption and iron status 12 mo after sleeve gastrectomy and Roux-en-Y gastric bypass in morbidly obese women. Am J Clin Nutr 2012;96(4):810–7.
16. Peeling P, Dawson B, Goodman C, et al. Athletic induced iron deficiency: new insights into the role of inflammation, cytokines and hormones. Eur J Appl Physiol 2008;103(4):381–91.

17. Nickerson HJ, Holubets MC, Weiler BR, et al. Causes of iron deficiency in adolescent athletes. J Pediatr 1989;114(4 Pt 1):657–63.
18. Amitrano L, Guardascione MA, Brancaccio V, et al. Coagulation disorders in liver disease. Semin Liver Dis 2002;22(1):83–96.
19. Allison MC, Howatson AG, Torrance CJ, et al. Gastrointestinal damage associated with the use of nonsteroidal antiinflammatory drugs. N Engl J Med 1992; 327(11):749–54.
20. Lisman T, Bijsterveld NR, Adelmeijer J, et al. Recombinant factor VIIa reverses the in vitro and ex vivo anticoagulant and profibrinolytic effects of fondaparinux. J Thromb Haemost 2003;1(11):2368–73.
21. Low MS, Speedy J, Styles CE, et al. Daily iron supplementation for improving anaemia, iron status and health in menstruating women. Cochrane Database Syst Rev 2016;(4):CD009747.
22. Murawska N, Fabisiak A, Fichna J. Anemia of chronic disease and iron deficiency anemia in inflammatory bowel diseases: pathophysiology, diagnosis, and treatment. Inflamm Bowel Dis 2016;22(5):1198–208.
23. Fasano A, Catassi C. Clinical practice. Celiac disease. N Engl J Med 2012; 367(25):2419–26.
24. Hershko C, Patz J. Ironing out the mechanism of anemia in celiac disease. Haematologica 2008;93(12):1761–5.
25. French JB, Pamboukian SV, George JF, et al. Gastrointestinal bleeding in patients with ventricular assist devices is highest immediately after implantation. ASAIO J 2013;59(5):480–5.
26. Stulak JM, Lee D, Haft JW, et al. Gastrointestinal bleeding and subsequent risk of thromboembolic events during support with a left ventricular assist device. J Heart Lung Transplant 2014;33(1):60–4.
27. Hreinsson JP, Bjarnason I, Bjornsson ES. The outcome and role of drugs in patients with unexplained gastrointestinal bleeding. Scand J Gastroenterol 2015; 50(12):1482–9.
28. Ridolfo AS, Rubin A, Crabtree RE, et al. Effects of fenoprofen and aspirin on gastrointestinal microbleeding in man. Clin Pharmacol Ther 1973;14(2):226–30.
29. Donker AE, Raymakers RA, Vlasveld LT, et al. Practice guidelines for the diagnosis and management of microcytic anemias due to genetic disorders of iron metabolism or heme synthesis. Blood 2014;123(25):3873–86.
30. Pei SN, Ma MC, You HL, et al. TMPRSS6 rs855791 polymorphism influences the susceptibility to iron deficiency anemia in women at reproductive age. Int J Med Sci 2014;11(6):614–9.
31. Cho YW, Allen RP, Earley CJ. Lower molecular weight intravenous iron dextran for restless legs syndrome. Sleep Med 2013;14(3):274–7.
32. Vaucher P, Druais PL, Waldvogel S, et al. Effect of iron supplementation on fatigue in nonanemic menstruating women with low ferritin: a randomized controlled trial. CMAJ 2012;184(11):1247–54.
33. Verdon F, Burnand B, Stubi CL, et al. Iron supplementation for unexplained fatigue in non-anaemic women: double blind randomised placebo controlled trial. BMJ 2003;326(7399):1124.
34. Krayenbuehl PA, Battegay E, Breymann C, et al. Intravenous iron for the treatment of fatigue in nonanemic, premenopausal women with low serum ferritin concentration. Blood 2011;118(12):3222–7.
35. Sharma R, Stanek JR, Koch TL, et al. Intravenous iron therapy in non-anemic iron-deficient menstruating adolescent females with fatigue. Am J Hematol 2016; 91(10):973–7.

36. Brigham D, Beard J. Iron and thermoregulation: a review. Crit Rev Food Sci Nutr 1996;36(8):747–63.
37. Cohen-Solal A, Leclercq C, Deray G, et al. Iron deficiency: an emerging therapeutic target in heart failure. Heart 2014;100(18):1414–20.
38. von HS, Jankowska EA, van Veldhuisen DJ, et al. Iron deficiency and cardiovascular disease. Nat Rev Cardiol 2015;12(11):659–69.
39. Qian C, Wei B, Ding J, et al. The efficacy and safety of iron supplementation in patients with heart failure and iron deficiency: a systematic review and meta-analysis. Can J Cardiol 2016;32(2):151–9.
40. Robinson JC, Graham BB, Rouault TC, et al. The crossroads of iron with hypoxia and cellular metabolism. Implications in the pathobiology of pulmonary hypertension. Am J Respir Cell Mol Biol 2014;51(6):721–9.
41. Sutendra G, Michelakis ED. The metabolic basis of pulmonary arterial hypertension. Cell Metab 2014;19(4):558–73.
42. Gassmann M, Muckenthaler MU. Adaptation of iron requirement to hypoxic conditions at high altitude. J Appl Physiol (1985) 2015;119(12):1432–40.
43. Frise MC, Cheng HY, Nickol AH, et al. Clinical iron deficiency disturbs normal human responses to hypoxia. J Clin Invest 2016;126(6):2139–50.
44. Smith TG, Talbot NP, Privat C, et al. Effects of iron supplementation and depletion on hypoxic pulmonary hypertension: two randomized controlled trials. JAMA 2009;302(13):1444–50.
45. Trenkwalder C, Allen R, Hogl B, et al. Restless legs syndrome associated with major diseases: a systematic review and new concept. Neurology 2016;86(14):1336–43.
46. Earley CJ, Barker B, Horska A, et al. MRI-determined regional brain iron concentrations in early- and late-onset restless legs syndrome. Sleep Med 2006;7(5):458–61.
47. Rinaldi F, Galbiati A, Marelli S, et al. Treatment options in Intractable Restless Legs Syndrome/Willis-Ekbom Disease (RLS/WED). Curr Treat Options Neurol 2016;18(2):7.
48. St Pierre SA, Vercellotti GM, Donovan JC, et al. Iron deficiency and diffuse non-scarring scalp alopecia in women: more pieces to the puzzle. J Am Acad Dermatol 2010;63(6):1070–6.
49. Zimmermann MB, Hurrell RF. Nutritional iron deficiency. Lancet 2007;370(9586):511–20.
50. Bruno M, De FL, Iolascon A. How I diagnose non-thalassemic microcytic anemias. Semin Hematol 2015;52(4):270–8.
51. Harms K, Kaiser T. Beyond soluble transferrin receptor: old challenges and new horizons. Best Pract Res Clin Endocrinol Metab 2015;29(5):799–810.
52. Mast AE, Blinder MA, Gronowski AM, et al. Clinical utility of the soluble transferrin receptor and comparison with serum ferritin in several populations. Clin Chem 1998;44(1):45–51.
53. Guyatt GH, Oxman AD, Ali M, et al. Laboratory diagnosis of iron-deficiency anemia: an overview. J Gen Intern Med 1992;7:145–53.
54. Brittin HC, Nossaman CE. Iron content of food cooked in iron utensils. J Am Diet Assoc 1986;86(7):897–901.
55. Kroger-Ohlsen MV, Trugvason T, Skibsted LH, et al. Release of iron into food cooked in an iron pot: effects of pH, salt, and organic acids. J Food Sci 2002;67(9):3301–3.
56. Rimon E, Kagansky N, Kagansky M, et al. Are we giving too much iron? Low-dose iron therapy is effective in octogenarians. Am J Med 2005;118(10):1142–7.

57. Zhou SJ, Gibson RA, Crowther CA, et al. Should we lower the dose of iron when treating anaemia in pregnancy? A randomized dose-response trial. Eur J Clin Nutr 2009;63(2):183–90.

58. O'Neil-Cutting MA, Crosby WH. Blocking of iron absorption by a preliminary oral dose of iron. Arch Intern Med 1987;147(3):489–91.

59. Moretti D, Goede JS, Zeder C, et al. Oral iron supplements increase hepcidin and decrease iron absorption from daily or twice-daily doses in iron-depleted young women. Blood 2015;126(17):1981–9.

60. Cook JD, Monsen ER. Food iron absorption in human subjects. III. Comparison of the effect of animal proteins on nonheme iron absorption. Am J Clin Nutr 1976; 29(8):859–67.

61. Morck TA, Cook JD. Factors affecting the bioavailability of dietary iron. Cereal Food World 1981;26(12):667–72.

62. Hurrell R, Egli I. Iron bioavailability and dietary reference values. Am J Clin Nutr 2010;91(5):1461S–7S.

63. Hurrell RF, Reddy M, Cook JD. Inhibition of non-haem iron absorption in man by polyphenolic-containing beverages. Br J Nutr 1999;81(4):289–95.

64. Comparison of oral iron supplements. Pharm Lett 2008;24(8):240811.

65. Okam MM, Koch TA, Tran MH. Iron deficiency anemia treatment response to oral iron therapy: a pooled analysis of five randomized controlled trials. Haematologica 2016;101(1):e6–7.

66. Tolkien Z, Stecher L, Mander AP, et al. Ferrous sulfate supplementation causes significant gastrointestinal side-effects in adults: a systematic review and meta-analysis. PLoS One 2015;10(2):e0117383.

67. Kaye P, Abdulla K, Wood J, et al. Iron-induced mucosal pathology of the upper gastrointestinal tract: a common finding in patients on oral iron therapy. Histopathology 2008;53(3):311–7.

68. Laine LA, Bentley E, Chandrasoma P. Effect of oral iron therapy on the upper gastrointestinal tract. A prospective evaluation. Dig Dis Sci 1988;33(2):172–7.

69. Auerbach M, DeLoughery TG. Single-dose intravenous iron for iron deficiency: a new paradigm. Hematol Am Soc Hematol Educ Program 2016.

70. Bonovas S, Fiorino G, Allocca M, et al. Intravenous versus oral iron for the treatment of anemia in inflammatory bowel disease: a systematic review and meta-analysis of randomized controlled trials. Medicine (Baltimore) 2016;95(2):e2308.

71. Lee T, Clavel T, Smirnov K, et al. Oral versus intravenous iron replacement therapy distinctly alters the gut microbiota and metabolome in patients with IBD. Gut 2016. [Epub ahead of print].

72. DeLoughery TG, Auerbach M. Is low-molecular weight iron dextran really the most risky iron? Unconvincing data from an unconvincing study. Am J Hematol 2016;91(5):451–2.

73. Szebeni J, Fishbane S, Hedenus M, et al. Hypersensitivity to intravenous iron: classification, terminology, mechanisms and management. Br J Pharmacol 2015;172(21):5025–36.

74. Rampton D, Folkersen J, Fishbane S, et al. Hypersensitivity reactions to intravenous iron: guidance for risk minimization and management. Haematologica 2014; 99(11):1671–6.

75. Avni T, Bieber A, Grossman A, et al. The safety of intravenous iron preparations: systematic review and meta-analysis. Mayo Clin Proc 2015;90(1):12–23.

76. Auerbach M, Pappadakis JA, Bahrain H, et al. Safety and efficacy of rapidly administered (one hour) one gram of low molecular weight iron dextran (INFeD) for the treatment of iron deficient anemia. Am J Hematol 2011;86(10):860–2.

77. Okam MM, Mandell E, Hevelone N, et al. Comparative rates of adverse events with different formulations of intravenous iron. Am J Hematol 2012;87(11):E123–4.
78. Auerbach M, Strauss W, Auerbach S, et al. Safety and efficacy of total dose infusion of 1,020 mg of ferumoxytol administered over 15 min. Am J Hematol 2013; 88(11):944–7.
79. Rockey DC. Occult and obscure gastrointestinal bleeding: causes and clinical management. Nat Rev Gastroenterol Hepatol 2010;7(5):265–79.
80. Kim BS, Li BT, Engel A, et al. Diagnosis of gastrointestinal bleeding: a practical guide for clinicians. World J Gastrointest Pathophysiol 2014;5(4):467–78.
81. Koulaouzidis A, Yung DE, Lam JH, et al. The use of small-bowel capsule endoscopy in iron-deficiency anemia alone; be aware of the young anemic patient. Scand J Gastroenterol 2012;47(8–9):1094–100.
82. Green BT, Rockey DC. Gastrointestinal endoscopic evaluation of premenopausal women with iron deficiency anemia. J Clin Gastroenterol 2004;38(2):104–9.
83. Zhu A, Kaneshiro M, Kaunitz JD. Evaluation and treatment of iron deficiency anemia: a gastroenterological perspective. Dig Dis Sci 2010;55(3):548–59.
84. Crabol Y, Terrier B, Rozenberg F, et al. Intravenous immunoglobulin therapy for pure red cell aplasia related to human parvovirus b19 infection: a retrospective study of 10 patients and review of the literature. Clin Infect Dis 2013;56(7): 968–77.

Myelodysplastic Syndromes: Updates and Nuances

Kim-Hien T. Dao, DO, PhD

KEYWORDS

- Myelodysplastic syndrome • Anemia • Azacitidine
- Therapy-related myelodysplastic syndrome • Blood and marrow transplant

KEY POINTS

- Myelodysplastic syndrome (MDS) is characterized by low blood cell counts, abnormal blood cell development, clonal genetic markers, and increased propensity toward AML.
- The recent genetic characterization of MDS has advanced various aspects of clinical management.
- Novel therapies are emerging to address common drivers of MDS development and disease progression.
- Patients with MDS should always be considered for clinical trial participation whenever possible to support scientific discoveries toward improving outcomes.

INTRODUCTION

In this review article, I discuss anemia caused by underlying MDS, a hematologic malignancy associated with widely varying clinical presentations, mutation patterns, and patient outcomes. *Myelo* means marrow and *dysplasia* means abnormal development. MDS is characterized by low blood cell counts, abnormal blood cell development, clonal genetic markers, and increased propensity toward acute myeloid leukemia (AML). The general incidence in the US population is approximately 4.8 per 100,000 per year but is as high as 30 to 60 per 100,000 per year in people over 70 years old (Surveillance, Epidemiology, and End Results Cancer Statistics Review, 1975–2010. National Cancer Institute; 2013). There is a slight male-to-female predominance (1.26–1). Risk-adapted monitoring and therapy are essential cornerstones of MDS clinical management. Over the past 5 years, advances in massive parallel sequencing technology have enabled genetic characterization of MDS to a point where the focus has now shifted toward translating these findings to improve patient outcomes. This will require, for example, integration of genetic data and disease behavior to help

Disclosure Statement: The author has no conflict of interest to disclose.
Hematology and Medical Oncology, Knight Cancer Institute, Oregon Health & Science University, Mail Code: UHN73C, 3181 South West Sam Jackson Park Road, Portland, OR 97239, USA
E-mail address: daok@ohsu.edu

choose/design better therapies, exploitation of synthetic lethality based on mutational exclusivity, and defining the genetic and biologic determinants of the good responders versus poor responders to various existing therapies. The use of genetic markers to predict and monitor risk for disease relapse may improve the selection of conditioning regimens and maintenance therapies in the setting of allogeneic blood and marrow transplant (BMT). The availability of molecular genetic testing has also helped with the diagnosis of MDS and other prediagnostic conditions, especially when dysplasia is not overtly present or World Health Organization (WHO) criteria are not met based on absolute cutoffs (eg, >10% dysplasia in a cell lineage). I present these discussions points using clinical vignettes that broadly represent common situations. I will not provide in-depth coverage of the genetics of MDS, prognostic systems, treatment options, allogeneic BMT, and drugs in the pipeline. The discussion points focus on integrating genetic data into diagnostic and prognostic considerations, managing patients who fail DNA methyltransferase (DNMT) inhibitors, and evaluating patients for allogeneic BMT. I discuss potential future directions in clinical management and translational research in MDS.

CLINICAL VIGNETTE 1: DIAGNOSTIC CONSIDERATIONS IN MYELODYSPLASTIC SYNDROME

A previously healthy 37-year-old man presented with progressive fatigue and dyspnea on exertion over the course of a few weeks. He was found to have a hypoproliferative anemia with hemoglobin level of 6.3 g/dL and reticulocyte of 0.15%. His platelet count, white blood cell count (WBC), and WBC differential were unremarkable. His blood smear was otherwise unremarkable. There was no laboratory evidence of hemolysis. He also reported intermittent fevers and diffuse body aches. His bone marrow biopsy showed hypercellular marrow (100% cellularity), marked myeloid hyperplasia, mild dysplasia in granulocytes (dyspoeisis in <10%), mild reticulin fibrosis, 3% blasts enumerated by morphology, slightly increased megakaryocytes with occasional clusters and small forms, scant erythropoiesis, and focally increased plasma cells (overall 2%). He had a normal male karyotype, and *BCR-ABL* and *JAK2*-V617F were not detected. He required frequent red blood cell transfusions to maintain hemoglobin above 7.0 g/dL. He was referred for discussion of treatment recommendations for newly diagnosed MDS.

ASSESSMENT OF CLINICAL VIGNETTE 1

The patient is relatively young with rapid onset of symptoms mainly due to symptomatic anemia. The median age of MDS diagnosis is 76 years old[1] and the typical clinical presentation tends to be indolent and progressive over months not weeks. However, approximately 6% of cases of MDS are diagnosed in people under 50 years old.[1] The patient does not have the standard risk factors for MDS, including, for example, advanced age, hereditary marrow failure syndromes, industrial benzene or other solvent exposure, and prior chemotherapy and radiation.[2] In addition to cytopenias, the complete blood cell count and a blood smear in an MDS patient may also reveal bilobed (pseudo–Pelger-Huët), hypersegmented, or hypogranulated neutrophils, unexplained macrocytosis (>100 fL) and oval-shaped red blood cells (macro-ovalocytes), elevated red blood cell distribution width, and giant or hypogranulated platelets. The patient did not have any of these findings. Thus, even before looking closer at his outside bone marrow biopsy slides and ordering molecular testing on his blood, I had already considered other possible diagnoses of anemia.

The patient's marrow is abnormal but the findings are nonspecific. At 37 years old, the patient's marrow cellularity, the hematopoietic cellular component expressed as a percentage relative to fatty tissue, should be approximately 50% based on the general approximation that a typical normal bone marrow cellularity percentage is 100−age.[3] Referring to the 2008 WHO criteria,[4] the following are required for a conclusive diagnosis of MDS: persistent cytopenias(s), greater than or equal to 10% dysplasia in one or more cell lineage, and MDS-associated clonal cytogenetic or molecular marker. In this case, the cytopenia (anemia) has been present for only a few weeks since diagnosis, the dysplasia is not apparently a prominent finding (granulocytic dyspoiesis in <10% of cells), and the lack of a clonal cytogenetic marker was not helpful for a diagnosis of MDS. Approximately 50% of cases of de novo MDS (cases of MDS not associated with prior chemotherapy, radiation, or antecedent hematologic malignancy) are associated with a cytogenetic marker.[5,6] Therefore, not having a cytogenetic marker does not exclude the possibility of a diagnosis of MDS. It is also not uncommon to come across a pathology report that lacks qualitative and/or quantitative description of dysplasia, which is inherently important for evaluating the WHO criteria for diagnosing MDS. Some of the morphologic manifestations of MDS are less specific for MDS (eg, increased megaloblastoid changes or cytoplasmic vacuolization) and some are more specific for MDS, including nuclear hypolobation in granulocytes and multiple separated nuclei in megakaryocytes.[4,7] Thus, so far, the patient does not seem to meet the criteria for a conclusive diagnosis of MDS. Furthermore, sequencing of a 42-gene hematologic malignancy panel from a blood sample returned without any mutations. It has been estimated that more than 90% of MDS harbor mutations in at least 1 of the genes listed in **Fig. 1**.[8,9] In my clinical practice, if a patient has suspected MDS but does not have a conclusive diagnosis of MDS by WHO criteria and has no mutation in this gene panel, I reconsider other differential diagnoses for anemia and proceed with work-up accordingly.

The patient does not fulfill the basic criterion for one of the prediagnostic stages associated with MDS and other hematologic malignancies (**Table 1**) because he does not have a clonal molecular or cytogenetic marker. These prediagnostic stages

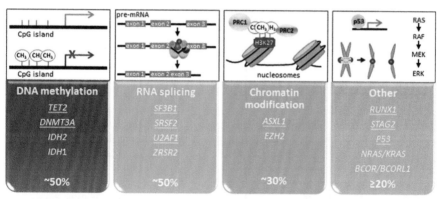

Fig. 1. Categories of commonly mutated genes in MDS. In the figure, the estimated frequency of MDS cases carrying a mutation in each category is indicated. Approximately 90% of patients with MDS have at least one mutation in one of the genes involved in DNA methylation, RNA splicing, chromatin modification, or in the other category. The other category include genes involved in DNA damage and stress response pathway, transcriptional regulation, RAS/RAF/MEK/ERK pathway, and sister chromatid separation (cohesion complex). Each of the genes underlined is typically reported as present in 10% or more cases of MDS.

Table 1
Prediagnostic stages toward myelodysplastic syndrome

	Idiopathic Cytopenia of Undetermined Significance	Nonrandom X-inactivation[a] Without Mutation	Nonrandom X-inactivation[a] with Mutation	Clonal Hematopoiesis of Indeterminate Potential[b]	Clonal Cytopenia of Undetermined Significance	Low-risk Myelodysplastic Syndrome	High-risk Myelodysplastic Syndrome
Cytopenia(s)	+	–	–	–	+	+	+
Dysplasia	–	–	–	–	–	+/–	+
Molecular drivers	–	–	+	+	+	+	+
Nonrandom X-inactivation	+/–	+	+	+/–	+	+	+
Neoplastic transformation							

[a] Determined by differentiating polymorphic alleles of HUMARA or G6PD genes on X chromosome.
[b] The vast majority of mutations associated with CHIP involve ASXL1, DNTM3A, or TET2.

were only recently defined with the aid of high throughput, more cost-effective massive parallel sequencing of samples from existing cohort studies.[10–13] Given the patient's clinical presentation was highly unusual for MDS and he had symptoms suggestive of systemic inflammation, I checked an erythrocyte sedimentation rate, which was profoundly elevated at 120 mm/h (normal range 0–15 mm/h). I considered a diagnosis of immune-mediated pure red cell aplasia given the scant erythropoiesis observed in the marrow. This is a condition associated with the destruction of precursors of red blood cells but without the typical laboratory findings of hemolytic anemia. I had ruled out aplastic anemia because he had preserved WBC and platelets and a hypercellular marrow. A paroxysmal nocturnal hemoglobinuria screen by flow cytometry was negative. HIV antibody screen, Epstein-Barr virus detection by polymerase chain reaction, and parvovirus B19 detection by polymerase chain reaction were negative. Thus, I treated the patient with prednisone (60 mg daily for 2 weeks, then rapidly tapered him off) and cyclosporine (trough level 200–250 ng/mL). Within 3 weeks, he had a brisk erythropoiesis with a hemoglobin rise to 10.3 g/dL without transfusion support and then achieved a normal hemoglobin level after 5 weeks of treatment. He was treated with cyclosporine alone for 1 year, then tapered off, and has maintained normal blood counts for more than 2 years.

In summary, this case highlights the importance of carefully considering the clinical presentation, degree and type of dysplasia present, lack of a clonal genetic marker, and other causes of anemia in those patients without a conclusive diagnosis of MDS by WHO criteria.

CLINICAL VIGNETTE 2: EVALUATING PATIENTS WHO FAIL HYPOMETHYLATING AGENTS

A 78-year-old woman was diagnosed with low-risk myelodysplasia (International Prognostic Scoring System [IPSS] score of 0; estimated median overall survival [OS] of 5.7 years).[14] She initially presented with a hemoglobin of 5.8 g/dL. Her WBC and platelets were in the normal range. Review of her bone marrow biopsy findings confirmed the WHO criteria diagnosis of MDS. Her marrow was markedly hypercellular at 90%. She had mild megaloblastoid changes in the erythroid lineage and prominent bilobed and unilobed megakaryocytic forms. Blasts were 3% to 4% by morphology and she had a normal female karyotype. JAK2-V617F and BCR-ABL were negative. No other molecular studies were done. The patient was highly dependent on red blood cell transfusions. Because of the degree of anemia, she was treated with azacitidine, 75 mg/m^2/d, subcutaneously on days 1 to 7 of every 28-day cycle. After the second cycle, her hemoglobin rose to 11.3 g/dL and she achieved transfusion independence. She proceeded with the third and fourth cycles as scheduled and was referred at the end of her fourth cycle due to persistent pancytopenia, with a clinical determination of azacitidine failure and disease progression. At her first consult visit, she had a fever in the setting of severe neutropenia and was promptly admitted to the hospital for further evaluation.

ASSESSMENT OF CLINICAL VIGNETTE 2

This patient had low-risk MDS using the original IPSS scoring system. If her risk group is compared using a revised IPSS (IPSS-R) scoring system incorporating the degree of anemia as a variable, her score is 3.5 (intermediate risk, median OS of 3 years).[15] Other risk scoring systems and common cytogenetic findings observed in MDS are listed in **Table 2**. Several low-risk scoring systems have emerged and may better delineate patients within the low-risk group.[19–21] Generally, the standard approach is to consider azacitidine for treatment of high-risk patients (intermediate-2 or high-risk IPSS categories) given the survival benefit of median 9.5 months observed in a multicenter, randomized

Table 2
Prognostic scoring systems in myelodysplastic syndrome

System	Risk Factors Evaluated	Validated Application
International prognostic scoring system (IPSS), International Working Group for Prognosis in MDS[16]	• 4 Risk groups • Factors: blasts, cytogenetics, and number of cytopenias	• At diagnosis • Patients not on therapy • De novo MDS (not to be used for therapy-related or secondary MDS or CMML) • Lower-risk group is highly variable
World Health Organisation Classification-based prognosis scoring system (WPSS)[17]	• 5 Risk groups • Factors: WHO category, cytogenetics, and red blood cell transfusion dependence ≥q8wk for ≥4 mo	• Applied at any time • Patients not on therapy • De novo MDS (not to be used for therapy-related or secondary MDS or CMML)
MD Anderson scoring system (MDACC)[18]	• 4 Risk groups • Factors: cytogenetics, performance status, age, hemoglobin, platelet count, WBC, marrow blasts, prior transfusion	• At diagnosis only • Patients not on therapy • De novo MDS, therapy-related and secondary MDS, and CMML • Delineation of the low to intermediate-1 IPSS groups better
International prognostic scoring system, revised (IPSS-R), International Working Group for Prognosis in MDS[15]	• 5 Risk groups • In addition to IPSS risk factors, increased delineation of the cytogenetic subgroups[a]	• At diagnosis • Patients not on therapy • De novo MDS (not to be used for therapy-related or secondary MDS or CMML) • Lower-risk group is highly variable

[a] Cytogenetic subgroups: very good: Y, del(11q); good: normal, del(5q), del(12p), del(20q), double, including del(5q). Intermediate: del(7q), +8, +19, i(17q), any other single or double independent clones; poor: −7, inv(3)/t(3q)/del(3q), double, including −7/del(7q), complex: 3 abnormalities; and very poor: complex: greater than 3 abnormalities.

phase 3 trial comparing azacitidine with best supportive care.[22] Azacitidine and decitabine are cytosine nucleoside analogs that inhibit DNMT at lower dose ranges. DNMT catalyzes methylation of cytosines in CpG islands involved in transcriptional regulation of genes. Azacitidine is also considered in low-risk patients (low or intermediate-1 risk IPSS categories) who display significant cytopenias and/or have failed other treatment options. Treating low-risk patients with azacitidine has been studied in a large phase II study using various dosing strategies.[23] MDS treatment options for various clinical aspects of MDS are listed in **Table 3**. For example, for anemia, treatment might include danazol, erythropoiesis-stimulating agents, immunosuppression, and/or lenalidomide. Given the patient's high erythropoietin level of greater than 500 ng/mL and degree of anemia and transfusion dependence, however, it was unlikely that she would have an adequate, if any, response to erythropoiesis-stimulating agents.[24,25] Thus, she was treated with azacitidine (Food and Drug Administration [FDA]-approved in 2004 for MDS) with the hope that this would significantly improve her anemia.

Although azacitidine was studied with the dose/schedule used in this patient, there are no consensus guidelines on how to manage patients on azacitidine specifically.

Table 3
Treatment options for various issues encountered in myelodysplastic syndrome

Condition	Treatment
Anemia	• Erythropoiesis-stimulating agents ± granulocyte colony-stimulating factor • Anabolic steroids or Danazol • Lenalidomide (most effective in 5q minus syndrome) or similar agents • Immunosuppressive agents • DNMT inhibitors • Transfusions (generally, for hematocrit <21%; for select patients, hematocrit <24%); generally, iron chelation is considered in select patients but the survival benefit has not been proven in a prospective, randomized controlled study
Thrombocytopenia	• Immunosuppressive agents • Thrombopoietin receptor agonists • Anabolic steroids or Danazol • DNMT inhibitors • Transfusions (generally, for platelet counts of <10,000/μL)
Neutropenia	• Granulocyte colony-stimulating factor • Antimicrobial prophylaxis refer to "infection prevention" • DNMT inhibitors

Infection prevention	• Prolonged severe neutropenia, for example, absolute neutrophil count of <500 cells/μL expected for ≥7 d
	  ○ Levaquin or similar
	  ○ Posaconazole or similar
	• Acyclovir (prophylaxis dose) indefinitely for periodic or prolonged neutropenia

Bleeding prevention	• Antifibrinolytic agents (topical or systemic)
Disease-modifying therapies	• DNMT inhibitors • Lenalidomide or similar
Disease burden reduction	• DNMT inhibitors • Cytotoxic chemotherapy (usually in setting of high-risk disease with excessive blasts)

Therefore, I highlight some important considerations and provide a "how I evaluate and treat" guideline that I routinely apply in my patients (**Fig. 2**).

In this schematic, I summarize my general approach to patients with MDS. I provide additional details on how I choose the dose/schedule of azacitidine and monitor for response on a practical level. Many patients at the beginning of therapy (eg, first and second cycles) will need close monitoring of their blood counts (eg, two or three times a week) but this is usually adjusted during later cycles based on a patient's typical length and depth of nadir. Whenever possible, all patients, regardless of their IPSS-R risk group should be considered for clinical trial participation.

Treatment with azacitidine:
1. Dose/schedule:
   - Consider azacitidine 75 mg/m^2 daily for 5 days, every 28-day cycle (LOW RISK, elderly, frail or vulnerable patients)
   - Consider azacitidine 75 mg/m^2 daily for 7 days, every 28-day cycle (HIGH RISK patients)
2. Assess response:

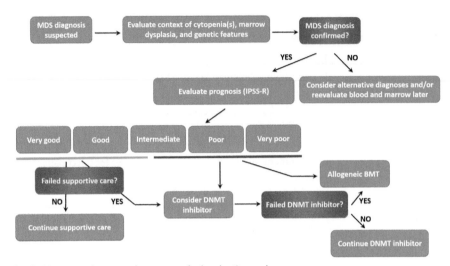

Fig. 2. How I evaluate and treat myelodysplastic syndrome.

- Evaluate platelet doubling as a simple marker of response after first cycle
- Evaluate typical length and depth of nadir
- Evaluate marrow after 3–4 cycles or after any cycle thereafter that result in more pronounced nadir than usual
- If hypocellular marrow, allow additional time for recovery (lengthen cycle) and/or adjust total dose given per cycle
- If hypercellular marrow with dysplasia, consider standard dosing of azacitidine if not already at 75 mg/m^2 daily for 7 days, every 28-day cycle for at least 3 more cycles; or consider possibility of DNMT inhibitor failure

3. Consider stopping if no response after 6 cycles; continue indefinitely, if possible, in patients with any hematologic response
4. Consider antimicrobial prophylaxis (**Table 3**) if nadir is expected to be ≥7 days

Allogeneic BMT:

Allogeneic BMT may be an option for some patients with certain disease characteristics, good organ function and performance status, and suitable donor options. Disease characteristics warranting consideration of allogeneic BMT: patients in the poor and very poor IPSS-R risk groups, select patients in the intermediate IPSS-R risk group, select patients with therapy-related MDS, patients with secondary MDS, select patients who fail DNMT inhibitors, select patients with persistent/progressive severe cytopenias, and patients displaying clonal evolution with increasing blasts and/or new genetic markers.

The guideline covers some key principles and is not meant to replace clinical assessment and judgment. There are specific disease/patient characteristics to consider when managing patients with MDS, including active comorbidities, overall health, goals of care, caregiver support, and access to clinic/infusion services. In this guideline, I consider the existing data on azacitidine in low-risk MDS, the fact that older patients have increased toxicity and altered drug metabolism, the kinetics of clinical responses with azacitidine in clinical trial studies, and the molecular and hematologic markers that predict clinical responses. Hematologic responses are higher in those patients harboring TET2[26,27] or DNMT3A mutations.[28,29] Approximately 90%

of clinical responses occur within 4 cycles of a 28-day cycle.[23] This is a point when I re-evaluate risks/benefits with my patients, especially those who have experienced significant quality-of-life decrement and/or side effects or toxicities. If there has been no appreciable response after 6 cycles, the patient is unlikely to achieve a response with additional cycles but not impossible. Decitabine (FDA-approved in 2006 for MDS) is not my first choice in patients with intermediate-2 and high-risk MDS, mainly due to the lack of a phase 3, randomized controlled trial showing a clear survival benefit.[30–32] The exact reason for this is unknown but some investigators have proposed that the current dosing strategies may favor cytotoxic effects over DNMT inhibitory effects,[33] the ideal dose/schedule has not been determined,[34,35] and the fact that decitabine has a different mechanism of action because it only incorporates into DNA, whereas aza-citidine incorporates into both DNA and RNA.[36] Overall, decitabine is thought to have similar rates of progression-free survival and hematologic responses compared with azacitidine in retrospective studies but may be associated with slightly more neutro-penic/infectious complications especially in an older patient population.[37]

In this clinical vignette, the patient had a deeper and longer nadir (period of lowest blood cell counts) during the third cycle compared with the previous two cycles when she had an excellent hematologic response and marrow recovery between the first and second cycles and the second and third cycles. She had not fully recovered counts on day 1 of the fourth cycle, however, but was given this cycle at full dose, on time. During her fourth cycle, she ended up having her deepest and longest nadir yet and presented with neutropenic fever. Work-up in the hospital revealed she had aspergillus pneumonia, an infection associated with high mortality rates in patients with hematologic malignancies.[38] Her marrow evaluation revealed a hypocellular marrow (approximately 10% cellularity) with trilineage hypoplasia, megaloblastoid erythropoiesis, megakaryocytic dysplasia, no increase in blasts (1%), and no evidence of acute leukemia. Thus, she was experiencing a cumulative azacitidine toxicity effect leading to severe pancytopenia and marrow hypoplasia. She had not been on prophylaxis antibiotics. I indicate the antibiotic prophylaxis regimen I use in my clinical practice (see **Fig. 2**). In this case, I would have evaluated her marrow after the third cycle and considered reducing her azacitidine dose (eg, to a 5-day regimen) or lengthening her cycles to a 35-day or 42-day cycle. The patient survived this critical illness and eventually recovered her counts approximately 8 weeks later. She had one additional year of transfusion independence but had to restart azacitidine when her anemia returned. She maintained some degree of response for another year before her disease progressed to a highly proliferative chronic myelomonocytic leukemia (CMML)-like disease.

In summary, there may be multifactorial reasons for patients who fail DNMT inhibitors. The reasons may not be strictly due to disease characteristics. The reasons for failing DNMT inhibitors should be looked at carefully to avoid a premature conclusion of DNMT inhibitor failure when actually the treatment had worked too well. Appropriate marrow evaluation, dose/schedule adjustment, and supportive care should be instituted. Patients who fail DNMT inhibitors due to disease characteristics have a poor prognosis,[39,40] including those patients initially thought to have low-risk MDS.[41]

CLINICAL VIGNETTE 3: RISK-ADAPTED TREATMENT AND ALLOGENEIC BLOOD AND MARROW TRANSPLANT

A 70-year-old man with history of chronic lymphocytic leukemia (normal karyotype) and diffuse large B-cell lymphoma transformation presented with progressive neutropenia and a new clonal derivative chromosome 7, resulting in del7q and gain in 1q in approximately 10% of marrow cells. He had received 5 different multiagent cytotoxic chemotherapy regimens over the course of 6 years, including the last regimen consisting of carmustine, etoposide, cytarabine, and melphalan as high-dose chemotherapy followed by autologous stem cell rescue. He had a DNMT3A p.R635L mutation. Dysplasia was prominent (>10% level) in the granulocytic series (cytoplasmic to nuclear asynchrony and abnormal granulation) and in the megakaryocytes (separate nuclear lobes and hyperchromatic nuclei). Blasts were less than 5%. These findings are most compatible with therapy-related MDS. He is being referred for evaluation of treatment options.

ASSESSMENT OF CLINICAL VIGNETTE 3

This is a patient with therapy-related MDS. His cytogenetic findings suggest that of the two pathways toward therapy-related MDS (**Table 4**), the disease pathogenesis was

Table 4
Therapy-related myelodysplastic syndrome and their genetic and clinical pathways

Pathway	Clinical Features	Genetic and Biologic Features
Alkylating agents[a] Interstrand and intrastrand DNA crosslinks	• Longer latency, median 5–7 y • Older patients • Preceded by dysplastic phase • Deletion or loss of 5q and/or 7q or complete loss of chromosome 5 and 7 • Poor response to standard induction chemotherapy	• Alkylating agents have reactive groups that interact covalently with nucleophilic sites in DNA • Diadduct/monoadduct ratio proportional to leukemogenicity • Melphalan induces nonrandom chromosome breaks, for example, chromosomes 5, 7, 11, and 17 • Clustering of break points at centromeric or pericentric region of several chromosomes, including chromosomes 5 and 7
Topoisomerase II inhibitors[b] Intercalate double-stranded DNA	• Short latency, median 1–3 y • Younger patients • No dysplastic phase • Balanced chromosome aberrations, for example, MLL 11q23, RUNX1/AML1 21q22, PML-RARA t(15;17) • More favorable response to standard induction chemotherapy	• Antitumor antibiotics and epipodophyllotoxins • Intercalate double-stranded DNA → stabilize DNA-topoisomerase complex, which collides with the replication fork or transcriptional machinery → double-strand breaks • Double-strand breaks occur frequently at loci of hematopoietic transcription factors for example, *MLL, AML1, CBFB, RARA, NUP98* • Double-strand breaks colocalize with DNaseI hypersensitivity sites that have open chromatin structure

[a] Alkylating agents examples include melphalan, cyclophosphamide, busulfan, carmustine, cisplatin, carboplatin, dacarbazine, and chlorambucil.
[b] Antitumor antibiotics and epipodophyllotoxins, examples include etoposide, doxorubicin, daunorubicin, and mitoxantrone.

more consistent with the alkylating agent–driven pathway. He had received both types of chemotherapy in the past (alkylating and topoisomerase II inhibitors). In **Table 4** I compare and contrast the typical features of these 2 pathways.[42–45] Recently, prognostic systems specific for therapy-related MDS were validated.[46,47] High-risk features include age greater than or equal to 65 years, Eastern Cooperative Oncology Group performance status 2 to 4, poor-risk cytogenetics (−7 and/or complex), WHO MDS subtype (refractory anemia with ring sideroblasts or refractory anemia with excess blasts type 1 or 2), presence of cytopenias, and transfusion dependency. Cytogenetic abnormalities are present in approximately 80% to 90% of patients with therapy-related MDS[42–44] versus approximately 50% of patients with de novo MDS (patients without prior chemotherapy or radiation).[5,6] MDS with complex cytogenetics (defined as 3 or more cytogenetic abnormalities) and monosomy karyotype (defined as 2 or more monosomies or a single monosomy with other structural abnormalities) carry a very poor prognosis and are characteristically associated with low responses to cytotoxic chemotherapy and poor survival outcomes after allogeneic BMT.[48–56] Mutations in *TP53* are more common in therapy-related MDS than in de novo MDS.[57,58] Secondary MDS/AML, as referred to herein, is a condition in which MDS/AML develops after having another type of hematologic malignancy, such as primary myelofibrosis. Secondary MDS has similar poor-risk characteristics to therapy-related MDS, both having higher frequency of complex and monosomy karyotypes and higher rates of AML transformation compared with de novo MDS.[59–61]

Due to prior cumulative chemotherapy toxicities, patients who have therapy-related MDS/AML may have increased risks for organ toxicities and infectious complications with intensive chemotherapy. The decision to treat therapy-related or secondary MDS/AML patients with multiagent cytotoxic chemotherapy should be carefully reviewed because those with high-risk cytogenetic disease may not realize any survival benefit from multiagent cytotoxic chemotherapy either as the only therapy or as cytoreductive therapy ahead of allogeneic BMT.[62] Various calculators are available to estimate in-hospital and/or early mortality rates after multiagent cytotoxic chemotherapy to aid with more patient-specific risk/benefit discussions.[63–65] Many of these calculators include prognostic factors, such as age, functional status, kidney function, cytogenetics, blast counts, and de novo versus therapy-related or secondary MDS/AML. Incorporation of genetic mutations into these risk calculators are likely forthcoming.

Thus, this patient should be considered for allogeneic BMT if he has a suitable donor option. In addition to therapy-related and secondary MDS, allogeneic BMT should be considered early in disease course for de novo MDS patients in the IPSS intermediate-2 and high-risk groups.[66] A question that often comes up is whether azacitidine treatment should be used as a bridge to transplant.[67,68] Treatment with azacitidine ahead of allogeneic BMT may serve several purposes, including improving marrow function, reducing blast counts, and delaying disease transformation to AML. Generally, if a patient has disease characteristics that warrant allogeneic BMT, is an allogeneic BMT candidate, and has less than 10% marrow myeloblasts, proceeding with transplant in the short term as upfront therapy is recommended because there may be increased adverse outcomes with a prolonged pretransplant period, such as immunosuppression, infectious complications, transfusion dependence, transfusion-related alloimmunization, and iron overload that may delay or affect transplant success. The strongest predictors of relapse after allogeneic BMT are related to disease cytogenetics and marrow myeloblasts.[69] Although reducing marrow myeloblasts to less than 10% has been cited as an optimal goal before proceeding with transplant conditioning chemotherapy and is often included as an inclusion criterion for BMT clinical trials, there are no prospective, randomized controlled studies based on disease characteristics to support that giving azacitidine or chemotherapy to achieve this goal provides OS benefit if the marrow myeloblasts are just above this value (eg, 10%–20%) or if the disease is associated with high-risk cytogenetics. High-risk cytogenetics and high percentage of marrow myeloblasts reflect disease biology; therefore, those patients with these characteristics have worse outcomes compared with those without these characteristics, perhaps regardless of the preallogeneic BMT treatment.[62]

Curing patients of their high-risk hematologic malignancies requires an adequate and steady graft-versus-leukemia effect. Although the donor and host are typically matched at key HLA loci to minimize acute graft rejection by the host and acute graft-versus-host disease, the unmatched antigens (including tumor antigens) not considered in identifying a matched donor ideally induce donor immunogenic responses against host leukemia cells (graft-versus-leukemia effect) more so than against other host tissues (graft-versus-host disease). In this case, the patient had an HLA-identical sibling donor. A majority of transplant centers consider reduced-intensity conditioning chemotherapy for patients over 60 years old. Conditioning chemotherapy serves several main purposes: (1) reduce disease burden as much as possible; (2) clear out the cellular components of the host bone marrow, and (3) suppress the host immune system to minimize graft rejection. Reduced-intensity conditioning regimens are associated with lower rates of treatment-related mortality but higher rates of relapsed-related mortality compared with conventional myeloablative conditioning regimens, such as busulfan-cyclophosphamide or cyclophosphamide–total body irradiation, where the reverse is true.[69] Retrospective studies have generally indicated similar OS rates when comparing reduced-intensity versus myeloablative chemotherapy.[70] The major caveats for applying this data to clinical practice, however, include the inherent selection bias of choosing various treatment approaches based on patient and disease characteristics and the short-term follow-up data. The decision to use reduced-intensity versus myeloablative conditioning regimens should be carefully considered based on age, comorbidities (eg, hematopoietic cell transplantation comorbidity index), donor type, graft source, and disease biology.[70,71] A randomized controlled US study (BMT Clinical Trials Network 0901) was closed early in 2014 due to preliminary analysis indicating superior relapse reduction of myeloablative regimens compared with reduced intensity regimens.[70] The study has not been published but was recently presented at the American Society of Hematology annual meeting in 2015 (Bart Scott, MD and colleagues late-breaking abstract) so the OS design and quality of the data have not been fully evaluated. In the meantime, in appropriate patients, a conventional myeloablative regimen or the most intense reduced-intensity regimen should be considered.[70] In this case, the patient received one of the more intense reduced-intensity regimens (fludarabine and melphalan).

Long-term survival in remission after HLA-matched related or unrelated donor sources for IPSS intermediate-2 and high-risk groups are approximately 40% and 30%, respectively.[72] For those patients with high-risk cytogenetics (complex or monosomy karyotype), long-term survival is 10% or less.[73] In this current era of nearly complete genetic characterization of hematologic malignancies, more sensitive, convenient markers of disease may be followed to monitor residual disease or early relapse. Studies are ongoing to define the use of disease-related genetic markers after allogeneic BMT. If a genetic marker persists, would a postallogeneic BMT maneuver improve survival and prevent disease relapse? Such maneuvers might include early donor leukocyte infusions, tapering of immunosuppressive agents, small molecule inhibitors, and/or other targeted interventions. DNMT and FLT3 inhibitors are being investigated as maintenance therapy postallogeneic BMT in cases of very high-risk disease characteristics and minimal residual disease detection.[74–81] In this case, the patient's DNMT3A p.R635L mutation may be followed in his blood after transplant and DNMT inhibitors may be beneficial to reduce his risk for disease relapse.

SUMMARY AND FUTURE CONSIDERATIONS

In summary, in the time span of approximately 10 years, 3 FDA-approved drugs are available for MDS and several groups have genetically characterized MDS to a greater extent than previously. The genetic data will aid in diagnosis of MDS with equivocal pathologic data and, in time, enhance utilization of novel and existing drugs (singly or in combination) and treatment after postallogeneic BMT. An important question is, could there be a role for earlier treatment with DNMT inhibitors for select CCUS and low-risk MDS phases if a convenient oral formulation allows for chronic, less toxic dosing? The necessity to eradicate the disease versus stabilization of a disease so that it never transforms into something much worse, such has high-risk MDS and AML, should also be reconsidered. DNMT inhibitors fail to induce complete remission in the vast majorly of patients yet those with hematologic responses experience survival benefit and longer time to AML transformation. Novel, less toxic biologic and targeted therapies are needed in MDS, such as those that target mutations in isocitrate dehydrogenase 1/2 and spliceosome genes. Antibody-based therapies, such as those that target CD33 and PD1, are also being actively investigated in clinical trials. Having better tools, such as more cost-effective massive parallel sequencing and newer strategies for gene editing (clustered regularly interspaced short palindromic repeats-Caspase 9 [CRISPR-Cas9]), will help advance MDS basic, translational, and clinical research. For example, many of the genetic mutations in MDS result in states of haploinsufficiency for the genes affected. Therefore, to better recapitulate the human disease in mouse models, one wildtype allele and one mutant allele should be maintained in mouse bone marrow cells. These models provide important tools for basic research and preclinical drug testing. In addition, first-in-human studies using CRISPR/Cas9 are now under way in other human diseases to correct specific gene defects. Research progress in MDS has occurred at an exciting pace. As I illustrate in this article, there is still an art to taking care of MDS patients because no two cases are exactly the same and there are mimickers of MDS. With recent advances in research, hopefully there will be substantial improvements in quality of life and survival of patients with MDS in the next 10 years.

REFERENCES

1. Ma X. Epidemiology of myelodysplastic syndromes. Am J Med 2012;125(7 Suppl):S2–5.

2. Gangat N, Patnaik MM, Tefferi A. Myelodysplastic syndromes: contemporary review and how we treat. Am J Hematol 2016;91(1):76–89.

3. Hartsock RJ, Smith EB, Petty CS, et al. Normal variations with aging of the amount of hematopoietic tissue in bone marrow from the anterior iliac crest. A study made from 177 cases of sudden death examined by necropsy. Am J Clin Pathol 1965; 43:326–31.

4. Brunning RD. WHO Classification of Tumours of Haematopoietic and Lymphoid Tissue, Introduction and overview of the classification of the myeloid neoplasms. In: Swerdlow S, Campo E, Harris NL, editors. Geneva (Switzerland): World Health Organization; 2008. p. 88–93.

5. Haase D, Germing U, Schanz J, et al. New insights into the prognostic impact of the karyotype in MDS and correlation with subtypes: evidence from a core dataset of 2124 patients. Blood 2007;110(13):4385–95.

6. Schanz J, Tuchler H, Sole F, et al. New comprehensive cytogenetic scoring system for primary myelodysplastic syndromes (MDS) and oligoblastic acute myeloid leukemia after MDS derived from an international database merge. J Clin Oncol 2012;30(8):820–9.

7. Cazzola M, Della Porta MG, Malcovati L. The genetic basis of myelodysplasia and its clinical relevance. Blood 2013;122(25):4021–34.

8. Bejar R, Ebert BL. The genetic basis of myelodysplastic syndromes. Hematol Oncol Clin North Am 2010;24(2):295–315.

9. Papaemmanuil E, Gerstung M, Malcovati L, et al. Clinical and biological implications of driver mutations in myelodysplastic syndromes. Blood 2013;122(22): 3616–27 [quiz: 3699].

10. Genovese G, Kahler AK, Handsaker RE, et al. Clonal hematopoiesis and blood-cancer risk inferred from blood DNA sequence. N Engl J Med 2014;371(26): 2477–87.

11. Jaiswal S, Fontanillas P, Flannick J, et al. Age-related clonal hematopoiesis associated with adverse outcomes. N Engl J Med 2014;371(26):2488–98.

12. Xie M, Lu C, Wang J, et al. Age-related mutations associated with clonal hematopoietic expansion and malignancies. Nat Med 2014;20(12):1472–8.

13. McKerrell T, Park N, Moreno T, et al. Leukemia-associated somatic mutations drive distinct patterns of age-related clonal hemopoiesis. Cell Rep 2015;10(8):1239–45.

14. Greenberg P, Cox C, LeBeau MM, et al. International scoring system for evaluating prognosis in myelodysplastic syndromes. Blood 1997;89(6):2079–88.

15. Greenberg PL, Tuechler H, Schanz J, et al. Revised international prognostic scoring system for myelodysplastic syndromes. Blood 2012;120(12):2454–65.

16. Greenberg P, Cox C, LeBeau MM, et al. International scoring system for evaluating prognosis in myelodysplastic syndromes. Blood 1997;89(6):2079–88.

17. Malcovati L, Porta MG, Pascutto C, et al. Prognostic factors and life expectancy in myelodysplastic syndromes classified according to WHO criteria: a basis for clinical decision making. J Clin Oncol 2005;23(30):7594–603.

18. Kantarjian H, O'Brien S, Ravandi F, et al. Proposal for a new risk model in myelodysplastic syndrome that accounts for events not considered in the original International Prognostic Scoring System. Cancer 2008;113(6):1351–61.

19. Garcia-Manero G, Shan J, Faderl S, et al. A prognostic score for patients with lower risk myelodysplastic syndrome. Leukemia 2008;22(3):538–43.

20. Komrokji R, Ramadan H, Al Ali N, et al. Validation of the lower-risk MD Anderson Prognostic Scoring System for patients with myelodysplastic syndrome. Clin Lymphoma Myeloma Leuk 2015;15(Suppl):S60–3.

21. Valcarcel D, Sanz G, Ortega M, et al. Use of newer prognostic indices for patients with myelodysplastic syndromes in the low and intermediate-1 risk categories: a population-based study. Lancet Haematol 2015;2(6):e260–6.

22. Fenaux P, Mufti GJ, Hellstrom-Lindberg E, et al. Efficacy of azacitidine compared with that of conventional care regimens in the treatment of higher-risk myelodysplastic syndromes: a randomised, open-label, phase III study. Lancet Oncol 2009;10(3):223–32.

23. Lyons RM, Cosgriff TM, Modi SS, et al. Hematologic response to three alternative dosing schedules of azacitidine in patients with myelodysplastic syndromes. J Clin Oncol 2009;27(11):1850–6.

24. Hellstrom-Lindberg E, Gulbrandsen N, Lindberg G, et al. A validated decision model for treating the anaemia of myelodysplastic syndromes with erythropoietin + granulocyte colony-stimulating factor: significant effects on quality of life. Br J Haematol 2003;120(6):1037–46.

25. Park S, Grabar S, Kelaidi C, et al. Predictive factors of response and survival in myelodysplastic syndrome treated with erythropoietin and G-CSF: the GFM experience. Blood 2008;111(2):574–82.

26. Bejar R, Lord A, Stevenson K, et al. TET2 mutations predict response to hypomethylating agents in myelodysplastic syndrome patients. Blood 2014;124(17):2705–12.

27. Itzykson R, Kosmider O, Cluzeau T, et al. Impact of TET2 mutations on response rate to azacitidine in myelodysplastic syndromes and low blast count acute myeloid leukemias. Leukemia 2011;25(7):1147–52.

28. Metzeler KH, Walker A, Geyer S, et al. DNMT3A mutations and response to the hypomethylating agent decitabine in acute myeloid leukemia. Leukemia 2012; 26(5):1106–7.

29. Traina F, Visconte V, Elson P, et al. Impact of molecular mutations on treatment response to DNMT inhibitors in myelodysplasia and related neoplasms. Leukemia 2014;28(1):78–87.

30. Kantarjian H, Issa JP, Rosenfeld CS, et al. Decitabine improves patient outcomes in myelodysplastic syndromes: results of a phase III randomized study. Cancer 2006;106(8):1794–803.

31. Lubbert M, Suciu S, Baila L, et al. Low-dose decitabine versus best supportive care in elderly patients with intermediate- or high-risk myelodysplastic syndrome (MDS) ineligible for intensive chemotherapy: final results of the randomized phase III study of the European Organisation for Research and Treatment of Cancer Leukemia Group and the German MDS Study Group. J Clin Oncol 2011; 29(15):1987–96.

32. Lubbert M, Suciu S, Hagemeijer A, et al. Decitabine improves progression-free survival in older high-risk MDS patients with multiple autosomal monosomies: results of a subgroup analysis of the randomized phase III study 06011 of the EORTC Leukemia Cooperative Group and German MDS Study Group. Ann Hematol 2016;95(2):191–9.

33. Saunthararajah Y, Sekeres M, Advani A, et al. Evaluation of noncytotoxic DNMT1-depleting therapy in patients with myelodysplastic syndromes. J Clin Invest 2015; 125(3):1043–55.

34. Kantarjian HM, Issa JP. Decitabine dosing schedules. Semin Hematol 2005;42(3 Suppl 2):S17–22.

35. Santos FP, Kantarjian H, Garcia-Manero G, et al. Decitabine in the treatment of myelodysplastic syndromes. Expert Rev Anticancer Ther 2010;10(1):9–22.

36. Hollenbach PW, Nguyen AN, Brady H, et al. A comparison of azacitidine and decitabine activities in acute myeloid leukemia cell lines. PLoS One 2010;5(2):e9001.

37. Lee YG, Kim I, Yoon SS, et al. Comparative analysis between azacitidine and decitabine for the treatment of myelodysplastic syndromes. Br J Haematol 2013;161(3):339–47.

38. Lin SJ, Schranz J, Teutsch SM. Aspergillosis case-fatality rate: systematic review of the literature. Clin Infect Dis 2001;32(3):358–66.

39. Duong VH, Lin K, Reljic T, et al. Poor outcome of patients with myelodysplastic syndrome after azacitidine treatment failure. Clin Lymphoma Myeloma Leuk 2013;13(6):711–5.

40. Prebet T, Gore SD, Esterni B, et al. Outcome of high-risk myelodysplastic syndrome after azacitidine treatment failure. J Clin Oncol 2011;29(24):3322–7.

41. Prebet T, Thepot S, Gore SD, et al. Outcome of patients with low-risk myelodysplasia after azacitidine treatment failure. Haematologica 2013;98(2):e18–9.

42. Pedersen-Bjergaard J, Andersen MT, Andersen MK. Genetic pathways in the pathogenesis of therapy-related myelodysplasia and acute myeloid leukemia. Hematology Am Soc Hematol Educ Program 2007;392–7.

43. Pedersen-Bjergaard J, Pedersen M, Roulston D, et al. Different genetic pathways in leukemogenesis for patients presenting with therapy-related myelodysplasia and therapy-related acute myeloid leukemia. Blood 1995;86(9):3542–52.

44. Pedersen-Bjergaard J. Insights into leukemogenesis from therapy-related leukemia. N Engl J Med 2005;352(15):1591–4.

45. Qian Z, Joslin JM, Tennant TR, et al. Cytogenetic and genetic pathways in therapy-related acute myeloid leukemia. Chem Biol Interact 2010;184(1–2):50–7.

46. Ok CY, Hasserjian RP, Fox PS, et al. Application of the international prognostic scoring system-revised in therapy-related myelodysplastic syndromes and oligoblastic acute myeloid leukemia. Leukemia 2014;28(1):185–9.

47. Quintas-Cardama A, Daver N, Kim H, et al. A prognostic model of therapy-related myelodysplastic syndrome for predicting survival and transformation to acute myeloid leukemia. Clin Lymphoma Myeloma Leuk 2014;14(5):401–10.

48. Bernasconi P, Klersy C, Boni M, et al. Incidence and prognostic significance of karyotype abnormalities in de novo primary myelodysplastic syndromes: a study on 331 patients from a single institution. Leukemia 2005;19(8):1424–31.

49. Patnaik MM, Hanson CA, Hodnefield JM, et al. Monosomal karyotype in myelodysplastic syndromes, with or without monosomy 7 or 5, is prognostically worse than an otherwise complex karyotype. Leukemia 2011;25(2):266–70.

50. Kobayashi H, Matsuyama T, Ueda M, et al. Predictive factors of response and survival following chemotherapy treatment in acute myeloid leukemia progression from myelodysplastic syndrome. Intern Med 2009;48(18):1629–33.

51. Kayser S, Zucknick M, Dohner K, et al. Monosomal karyotype in adult acute myeloid leukemia: prognostic impact and outcome after different treatment strategies. Blood 2012;119(2):551–8.

52. Valcarcel D, Adema V, Sole F, et al. Complex, not monosomal, karyotype is the cytogenetic marker of poorest prognosis in patients with primary myelodysplastic syndrome. J Clin Oncol 2013;31(7):916–22.

53. van Gelder M, de Wreede LC, Schetelig J, et al. Monosomal karyotype predicts poor survival after allogeneic stem cell transplantation in chromosome 7 abnormal myelodysplastic syndrome and secondary acute myeloid leukemia. Leukemia 2013;27(4):879–88.

54. Wudhikarn K, Van Rheeden R, Leopold C, et al. Outcome of allogeneic stem cell transplantation in myelodysplastic syndrome patients: prognostic implication of monosomal karyotype. Eur J Haematol 2012;89(4):294–301.

55. Koenecke C, Gohring G, de Wreede LC, et al. Impact of the revised International Prognostic Scoring System, cytogenetics and monosomal karyotype on outcome after allogeneic stem cell transplantation for myelodysplastic syndromes and secondary acute myeloid leukemia evolving from myelodysplastic syndromes: a retrospective multicenter study of the European Society of Blood and Marrow Transplantation. Haematologica 2015;100(3):400–8.

56. Ustun C, Trottier BJ, Sachs Z, et al. Monosomal karyotype at the time of diagnosis or transplantation predicts outcomes of allogeneic hematopoietic cell transplantation in myelodysplastic syndrome. Biol Blood Marrow Transplant 2015;21(5):866–72.

57. Shih AH, Chung SS, Dolezal EK, et al. Mutational analysis of therapy-related mye-lodysplastic syndromes and acute myelogenous leukemia. Haematologica 2013; 98(6):908–12.

58. Ok CY, Patel KP, Garcia-Manero G, et al. Mutational profiling of therapy-related myelodysplastic syndromes and acute myeloid leukemia by next generation sequencing, a comparison with de novo diseases. Leuk Res 2015;39(3):348–54.

59. Cerquozzi S, Tefferi A. Blast transformation and fibrotic progression in polycy-themia vera and essential thrombocythemia: a literature review of incidence and risk factors. Blood Cancer J 2015;5:e366.

60. Mesa RA, Li CY, Ketterling RP, et al. Leukemic transformation in myelofibrosis with myeloid metaplasia: a single-institution experience with 91 cases. Blood 2005; 105(3):973–7.

61. Bjorkholm M, Hultcrantz M, Derolf AR. Leukemic transformation in myeloprolifer-ative neoplasms: therapy-related or unrelated? Best Pract Res Clin Haematol 2014;27(2):141–53.

62. Yakoub-Agha I, Deeg J. Are hypomethylating agents replacing induction-type chemotherapy before allogeneic stem cell transplantation in patients with myelo-dysplastic syndrome? Biol Blood Marrow Transplant 2014;20(12):1885–90.

63. Krug U, Rollig C, Koschmieder A, et al. Complete remission and early death after intensive chemotherapy in patients aged 60 years or older with acute myeloid leukaemia: a web-based application for prediction of outcomes. Lancet 2010; 376(9757):2000–8.

64. Pastore F, Dufour A, Benthaus T, et al. Combined molecular and clinical prog-nostic index for relapse and survival in cytogenetically normal acute myeloid leu-kemia. J Clin Oncol 2014;32(15):1586–94.

65. Walter RB, Othus M, Borthakur G, et al. Prediction of early death after induction ther-apy for newly diagnosed acute myeloid leukemia with pretreatment risk scores: a novel paradigm for treatment assignment. J Clin Oncol 2011;29(33):4417–23.

66. Cutler CS, Lee SJ, Greenberg P, et al. A decision analysis of allogeneic bone marrow transplantation for the myelodysplastic syndromes: delayed transplanta-tion for low-risk myelodysplasia is associated with improved outcome. Blood 2004;104(2):579–85.

67. Ahn JS, Kim YK, Min YH, et al. Azacitidine Pre-Treatment Followed by Reduced-Intensity Stem Cell Transplantation in Patients with Higher-Risk Myelodysplastic Syndrome. Acta Haematol 2015;134(1):40–8.

68. Kim DY, Lee JH, Park YH, et al. Feasibility of hypomethylating agents followed by allogeneic hematopoietic cell transplantation in patients with myelodysplastic syndrome. Bone Marrow Transplant 2012;47(3):374–9.

69. Deeg HJ. Hematopoietic cell transplantation for myelodysplastic syndrome. Am Soc Clin Oncol Educ Book 2015;e375–80.

70. Reshef R, Porter DL. Reduced-intensity conditioned allogeneic SCT in adults with AML. Bone Marrow Transplant 2015;50(6):759–69.

71. Sorror ML, Maris MB, Storb R, et al. Hematopoietic cell transplantation (HCT)-specific comorbidity index: a new tool for risk assessment before allogeneic HCT. Blood 2005;106(8):2912–9.

72. Appelbaum FR, Anderson J. Allogeneic bone marrow transplantation for myelo-dysplastic syndrome: outcomes analysis according to IPSS score. Leukemia 1998;12(Suppl 1):S25–9.

73. Deeg HJ, Scott BL, Fang M, et al. Five-group cytogenetic risk classification, monosomal karyotype, and outcome after hematopoietic cell transplantation for MDS or acute leukemia evolving from MDS. Blood 2012;120(7):1398–408.

74. Pusic I, Choi J, Fiala MA, et al. Maintenance therapy with decitabine after alloge-neic stem cell transplantation for acute myelogenous leukemia and myelodys-plastic syndrome. Biol Blood Marrow Transplant 2015;21(10):1761–9.
75. Jabbour E, Giralt S, Kantarjian H, et al. Low-dose azacitidine after allogeneic stem cell transplantation for acute leukemia. Cancer 2009;115(9):1899–905.
76. Griffin PT, Komrokji RS, De Castro CM, et al. A multicenter, phase II study of main-tenance azacitidine in older patients with acute myeloid leukemia in complete remission after induction chemotherapy. Am J Hematol 2015;90(9):796–9.
77. de Lima M, Giralt S, Thall PF, et al. Maintenance therapy with low-dose azacitidine after allogeneic hematopoietic stem cell transplantation for recurrent acute mye-logenous leukemia or myelodysplastic syndrome: a dose and schedule finding study. Cancer 2010;116(23):5420–31.
78. Winkler J, Rech D, Kallert S, et al. Sorafenib induces sustained molecular remis-sion in FLT3-ITD positive AML with relapse after second allogeneic stem cell transplantation without exacerbation of acute GVHD: a case report. Leuk Res 2010;34(10):e270–2.
79. Tarlock K, Chang B, Cooper T, et al. Sorafenib treatment following hematopoietic stem cell transplant in pediatric FLT3/ITD acute myeloid leukemia. Pediatr Blood Cancer 2015;62(6):1048–54.
80. Sharma M, Ravandi F, Bayraktar UD, et al. Treatment of FLT3-ITD-positive acute myeloid leukemia relapsing after allogeneic stem cell transplantation with sorafe-nib. Biol Blood Marrow Transplant 2011;17(12):1874–7.
81. Schiller GJ, Tuttle P, Desai P. Allogeneic hematopoietic stem cell transplantation in FLT3-ITD-positive acute myelogenous leukemia: the role for FLT3 tyrosine ki-nase inhibitors post-transplantation. Biol Blood Marrow Transplant 2016;22(6): 982–90.

Autoimmune Hemolytic Anemia

Howard A. Liebman, MA, MD*, Ilene C. Weitz, MS, MD

KEYWORDS

- Anemia • Hemolysis • Autoantibodies

KEY POINTS

- Autoimmune hemolytic anemia results from antibody-mediated destruction of red blood cells.
- It can be a primary disorder or associated with other immune and nonimmune disorders.
- In most cases, immune modulation is required for treatment.

INTRODUCTION

Autoimmune hemolytic anemia (AIHA) is an acquired heterogeneous autoimmune disorder characterized by the development of antibodies directed against antigens on autologous erythrocytes. It is a relatively rare disorder, with an estimated incidence of 1 to 3 cases in 100,000 persons per year.[1] Depending upon the type and concentration of the autoantibody, erythrocyte destruction can occur by extravascular red blood cell phagocytosis in the spleen, liver, and bone marrow, or by intravascular complement-mediated lysis of the erythrocyte.

The heterogeneity of the disorder is exemplified by the different types of autoantibodies associated with hemolysis and the differing clinical presentations. There are generally 4 serologic forms of the disease.[2–8] Most common are hemolytic anemias mediated by immunoglobulin G (IgG, termed warm) autoantibodies that bind to red cells at 37°C. The red cell destruction occurs extravascularly by erythrocyte phagocytosis mediated by antibody binding to tissue macrophage Fc receptors.[2–4] Warm antibody hemolytic anemia accounts for 65% to 70% of autoimmune hemolytic anemias. Depending on the IgG antibody subtype (IgG1, IgG3) and concentration, the antibodies may also fix complement to the red blood cell, resulting in both intravascular hemolysis and additional extravascular phagocytosis medicated by complement C3b receptors.

Jane Anne Nohl Division of Hematology, Department of Medicine, Keck School of Medicine, University of Southern California, Los Angeles, CA, USA
* Corresponding author. Jane Anne Nohl Division of Hematology, USC Norris Cancer Hospital, 1441 Eastlake Avenue, Suite 3466, Los Angeles, CA 90033.
E-mail address: liebman@usc.edu

Med Clin N Am 101 (2017) 351–359
http://dx.doi.org/10.1016/j.mcna.2016.09.007
medical.theclinics.com

Cold agglutinin hemolysis is associated with the development of IgM autoantibodies that can agglutinate red cell at cold temperatures.[2,3,5] In patients with cold agglutinin antibodies of higher thermal binding; the IgM autoantibodies rapidly fix complement-inducing intravascular lysis of red blood cell. Approximately 20% to 25% of AIHAs result from cold agglutinin antibodies. He IgM antibodies can be either polyclonal or monoclonal as observed in some patients with plasmacytoid lymphocytic lymphomas such as Waldenstrom macroglobulinemia. An additional 8% of patients with AIHA have both warm IgG and cold IgM antibodies and are termed mixed autoantibody hemolytic anemias.[6]

A rare form of cold-induced intravascular hemolysis results from the formation of IgG autoantibodies that bind to erythrocytes in the cold, but activate complement lysis when the cells are warmed to 37°C.[2,7] These IgG autoantibodies, termed Donath-Landsteiner antibodies, were historically described in paroxysmal cold hemoglobinuria (PCH) in patients with secondary syphilis. It is now most frequently described in children and adults following viral infections. Cases of PCH may account for 1% to 3% of acquired AIHAs.

The fourth serologic form of the disorder is the warm AIHA-direct antiglobulin (Coombs)-negative patient.[8] These patients most often have either a low affinity or low concentration (<200 immunoglobulin G (IgG)/erythrocyte) autoantibody that requires specialized laboratory studies to detect, but is still capable of mediating hemolysis. Smaller subsets of these patients have an IgA- or monomeric IgM-mediated hemolysis. In addition, AIHA can develop following the administration of certain drugs.[9–11] A listing of the more commonly reported drugs associated with AIHA is given in **Table 1**.

Autoimmune hemolytic anemia can occur as a primary (idiopathic) disorder or occur in association with other immune or nonimmune disorders (secondary AIHA). Secondary forms of AIHA may account for 40% to 50% of all patients with AIHA (**Box 1**).[12,13] The presence of another medical disorder can complicate the management of patients with AIHA. Therapy is often tailored with consideration of its effect on the associated illness. Also, the diagnosis of AIHA may precede the recognition of another underlying disorder consistent with secondary AIHA. A list of the common disorders associated with secondary AIHA is given in **Table 2**.

CLINICAL PRESENTATION AND DIAGNOSIS

Patients with AIHA can have a highly variable clinical presentation.[14] Patients may describe symptoms related to their anemia such as fatigue, weakness, dyspnea

Table 1
Serologic types of autoimmune hemolytic anemia

Form	Incidence	Antibody	Treatment
Warm antibody	65%–70%	IgG	Steroids, rituximab, splenectomy, azathioprine, cyclophosphamide
Cold antibody	20%–25%	IgM	Rituximab, cyclophosphamide, cold avoidance
Paroxysmal cold hemoglobinuria	1%–3%	IgG	Steroids, rituximab, cold avoidance
Coombs negative	~5%	Low titer IgG, monomeric IgM, IgA	Steroids, rituximab, cyclophosphamide, splenectomy, azathioprine

Box 1
Secondary forms of autoimmune hemolytic anemia

Autoimmune Disorders

Lupus erythematosus (SLE)

Rheumatoid arthritis (RA)

Antiphospholipid syndrome

Inflammatory bowel disease (Crohn disease and ulcerative colitis)

Primary biliary cirrhosis

Autoimmune thyroid disease

Evan syndrome

Immunodeficiency disorders

Common variable immunodeficiency (CVID)

Autoimmune lymphoproliferative syndrome (ALPS)

IgA deficiency

Post-transplant (solid organ and autologous bone marrow transplant)

Lymphoproliferative

Chronic lymphocytic leukemia (CLL)

Non-Hodgkin lymphoma (NHL)

Hodgkin lymphoma

Angioimmunoblastic lymphadenopathy

Waldenstrom macroglobulinemia

Infections

Epstein Barr virus

Cytomegalovirus

Human immunodeficiency virus

Hepatitis C

Mycoplasma pneumonia

Rare: Varicella, Rubella, Parvo B19

Table 2
Drugs frequently reported to be associated with autoimmune hemolytic anemia (>10 reports)

Drug	Mechanism
Penicillins	Membrane absorption–haptene
Cephalosporin-first generation	Nonimmune protein absorption
Cephalosporin second -third generation	Immune complex
Alpha methyl dopaimmune hemolytic anemia	Drug-dependent autoantibodies
Fludarabine	Drug-dependent autoantibodies
Oxaliplatinum	Drug-dependent autoantibodies

with exertion, palpitations, and dizziness. Onset of symptoms can be insidious or appear to be acute. With more fulminant hemolysis, patients will display pallor, jaundice, and dark urine. In addition, patients may have splenomegaly, hepatomegaly, and adenopathy. Patients with intravascular hemolysis such as with cold agglutinin hemolysis or paroxysmal cold hemoglobinuria may describe gross hemoglobinuria.

Patients with primary and, in particular, secondary AIHA may describe additional symptoms including weight loss, joint pain, abdominal pain, chest pain with or without coughing, and fever. Symptoms of respiratory distress and chest pain should also alert the clinician to the possibility of pulmonary embolism, since patients with AIHA are at increased risk of thromboembolic complications.[15,16]

The laboratory evaluation of patients with AIHA will usually show a variable level of hemoglobin and hematocrit depending upon the degree of active hemolysis and bone marrow compensation. The mean corpuscular volume (MCV) may be elevated due to an increased reticulocyte count. The reticulocyte index is usually greater that 3%, but a reticulocyte count with a reticulocyte index of no more than 2% can occur early in the presentation in 15% to 40% of patients.[17,18] In the majority of patients, the reticulocyte count will increase with the initiation of corticosteroid treatment, but a prolonged reticulocytopenia can occur in 5% to 10% of patients. Mild leukocytosis can be seen, but in rare cases, neutropenia may occur. This can occur in combination with severe thrombocytopenia as an aspect of Evan syndrome.[19]

The peripheral blood smear usually shows moderate poikilocytosis and anisocytosis, polychromasia, and in warm antibody hemolysis, variable numbers of spherocytes. Occasionally, nucleated red blood cells and rare erythrophagocytosis by macrophages and neutrophils are seen on the peripheral blood smear.

Further evidence of active hemolysis is evident by increases in total and indirect bilirubin as well as increases in serum lactic dehydrogenase (LDH). Haptoglobin will significantly decrease to less than 25 mg/dL in 85% of patients.[20] However, the presence of increased indirect bilirubin, increase serum LDH, and a low haptoglobin in a patient with anemia does not definitively confirm the diagnosis of a hemolytic anemia. Similar findings can be seen with the ineffective hematopoiesis observed with severe pernicious anemia. Review of the blood smear and determination of the reticulocyte count are essential in making the correct diagnosis.

In addition to the clinical and laboratory evidence of hemolysis, serologic evidence of erythrocyte autoantibodies is essential for the diagnosis of AIHA.[2–6] The diagnosis requires detection of an autoantibody on the erythrocyte membrane. Determination of the presence of an autoantibody on the patient's red blood cell (RBC) is made by the direct antiglobulin (direct Coombs or DAT) test. DAT positivity indicates that there has been in vivo binding of either IgG, complement C3b, or both to the patient's red cells. The identification of the erythrocyte antigens targeted by the autoantibody can subsequently be determined by eluting the antibody from the RBC and testing against a panel of control erythrocytes. The patient's serum can be tested for unbound autoantibody (indirect antiglobulin test) against control erythrocytes. However, in patients who have previously been transfused, consideration must be given to the possibility that the bound antibody could be an alloantibody. Of note, there are several clinical disorders that can result in a positive DAT without evidence of hemolysis such as liver disease or human immunodeficiency virus.[21] Therefore the DAT results must be assessed in combination with patient clinical finding and additional laboratory studies to definitively confirm a diagnosis of AIHA.

The presence of complement C3b alone on the DAT may suggest that hemolysis has resulted from the presence of a cold agglutinin or Donath-Landsteiner IgG. The blood bank can perform specific study to determine if hemolysis is due to these autoantibodies. In patients with acquired hemolytic anemia with blood smears consistent with AIHA, but a negative DAT, more specialized studies are needed to determine if hemolysis is due to a low concentration or low affinity IgG, an IgA, or monomeric IgM.[8]

TREATMENT

The correct serologic diagnosis of a patient with AIHA is essential before initiating therapy. The therapeutic approach to warm hemolytic anemia is significantly different from patients with cold agglutinin hemolysis. In patients with secondary AIHA, consideration must be given to the effect of treatment on the associated disorder. Other comorbidities such as diabetes, atherosclerotic and coronary vascular disease, renal disease, the presence of venous thrombosis, and other cytopenias may require modifications in or additions to the therapeutic approach to the AIHA.

Corticosteroids

Corticosteroids are the primary therapeutic agent for the treatment of warm antibody AIHA. However, there are no prospective trials on the optimal use of corticosteroids in patients with AIHA. An analysis of 6 studies, comprising 301 patients with warm AIHA, evaluated the initial use of corticosteroids for the treatment of AIHA.[22] Most patients were initially treated with prednisone 1 mg to 1.5/kg/d until hemoglobin stabilized and then were often treated with lower doses (<10 mg/d) for 3 to 6 months. A good response was reported in 248 (82%) patients. However, only 15% to 20% of patients achieved a long-term remission upon withdrawal of corticosteroids.[22–24] Long-term outcome data from patients with AIHA treated with corticosteroids alone are sadly lacking since up to 50% of patients require longer-term low-dose corticosteroid maintenance.[22–24]

Standard doses of corticosteroids are often less effective in some patients with secondary AIHA.[25–27] This can be particularly true for patients with chronic lymphocytic leukemia (CLL) and AIHA. In refractory CLL patients, the use of high-dose methylprednisolone or pulse dexamethasone appears to be more effective, often combined with cyclophosphamide and rituximab.[25–27] Standard doses of prednisone are relatively ineffective in cold agglutinin hemolytic anemia. However, pulse doses of dexamethasone (40 mg/d for 4 days), as used in multiple myeloma, can be effective in patients with cold agglutinin disease, but are usually combined with either rituximab or cyclophosphamide.

Splenectomy

Prior to the advent of corticosteroid therapy, splenectomy was the only effective treatment for warm antibody AIHA. In an early study of 34 patients with primary AIHA, 27 patients (79%) were treated with a splenectomy.[28] Although the subsequent long-term outcome of the splenectomized patients was not reported, 18 of the 34 (53%) primary AIHA patients died of their disease.[28] Splenectomy is not effective in cold antibody hemolytic anemia.

Most contemporary reports on the use of splenectomy for the treatment of AIHA report a 40% to 80% initial response, with up to a 20% long-term remission.[29–31] The advent of laparoscopic splenectomy combined with postsurgical antibiotic and thrombotic prophylaxis has significantly reduced surgery-related morbidity and mortality.[32] However, a long-term increased risk of overwhelming sepsis remains even with appropriate immunizations.[24,33] The risk of severe infection is approximately 3% to 7%, with a nearly 50% mortality.[33,34] In addition, a long-term increased risk of venous thromboembolism has been observed in patients treated for immune thrombocytopenia with splenectomy.[24,35]

Immunosuppressive Drugs

It was only 3 years after Robert Schwartz and William Dameshek demonstrated the ability of 6-mercaptopurine to induce immune tolerance in rabbits that the drug was found to be effective in the treatment of AIHA.[36,37] The drug and its prodrug, azathioprine, remain among the most effective second-line treatments for steroid refractory and steroid-dependent patients with warm antibody AIHA. The reported responses are 40% to 60%, with 10% to 20% of patients obtaining a complete response.[30,38] The usual treatment dose azathioprine is 2 to 3 mg/kg/d (100–250 mg). The drug's major benefit is in its ability to allow a reduction in corticosteroid dosing.[30,38] The long-term use of azathioprine appears to be well tolerated by most patients.

Cyclophosphamide has also been shown to be an effective therapy in both warm antibody and cold agglutinin AIHA.[16,30,38,39] Initial responses in warm antibody AIHA range from 40% to 60%, but durable response occurs in only 20% to 30% treated patients. Treatment doses range from daily low dose oral (50 mg to 100 mg/d) to high-dose intravenous doses (50 mg/kg for 4 days). Combination treatment with rituximab and corticosteroids appears to be most effective in treating warm and cold agglutinin AIHA associated with lymphoproliferative malignancies.[27] Toxicities of cyclophosphamide treatment include nausea, bone marrow suppression with neutropenia frequently observed, male and female sterility, hemorrhagic cystitis, and long-term use bladder fibrosis. Treatment-related myelodysplasia and leukemia are rare, but significant late complications.

Patients who fail to respond to standard second-line therapy cytotoxic agents such as azathioprine or cyclophosphamide may respond to treatment with other immune-modulating agents such as cyclosporine, mycophenolate mofetil, or sirolimus.[30,38–43] However, the few case reports that document responses to these second-line therapies provide few long-term outcome data on responding patients.

Anti-CD20 Therapy (Rituximab)

The development by recombinant technology of humanized monoclonal antibodies directed against the CD20 antigen on human B lymphocytes provided a new means by which circulating and tissue antibody-producing B lymphocytes could be selectively depleted. The first of these antibodies, rituximab, was initially shown to be an effective therapy alone or in combination for the treatment of B cell lymphomas.[44] Subsequently it has found use in the treatment of a variety of antibody-mediated immunopathic disorders including warm antibody and cold agglutinin AIHA.[45–49] In a recent meta-analysis of encompassing 402 patients, the overall response rate (ORR) was 73% (97% confidence interval [CI]: 64%–81%).[49] Complete responses were reported in 37% (95% CI: 26%–49%). The ORR for warm AIHA alone in 154 patients was 79% (95% CI: 60%–90%), and the ORR for 109 patients with cold agglutinin AIHA was 57% (95% CI: 47%–66%). Complete response rate for warm AIHA was 42% (95% CI: 27%–58%) and 21% (95% CI: 6%–51%) for cold agglutinin AIHA. There was no statistical difference in response between patients with primary AIHA (67%, 95% CI: 49%–81%, 161 patients) and secondary AIHA (72%, 95% CI: 60%–82%, 66 patients). Durability of response could not be determined in this meta-analysis.[49] Overall, most frequent toxicities reported were related to drug infusion. However, rituximab treatment in hematologic malignancies and other disorders has been associated with the development of late neutropenia, reactivation of herpes viruses, hepatitis B with fulminant liver failure, and progressive multifocal leukoencephalopathy due to JC virus activation.

A recent single-center report on 60 patients with warm AIHA evaluated the efficacy of 34 courses of rituximab in 25 patients.[16] This center used 2 treatment regimens; 15 patients were treated with the 375 mg/m^2 weekly for 4 weeks regimen as used in lymphoma treatment. Ten patients were treated with 1000 mg given twice 2 weeks apart. The latter regimen is similar to that employed in the treatment of rheumatoid arthritis. The overall complete and partial responses were observed in 20 of 25 (80%) patients. Half (10 patients) of the responders relapsed after a mean of 14 plus or minus 8 months.[16] In total, 9 of the 10 relapsed patients received a second course, with the same pattern of response. There was no difference between the 2 rituximab dosing regimens and response or toxicity.[50]

In 4 patients, treatment was associated with late-onset neutropenia, with febrile presentation in 1 patient. Two patients developed hypogammaglobulinemia with no reported symptomatic infections or febrile complications.[16]

SUMMARY

Autoimmune hemolytic anemia is a rare autoimmune disorder in which erythrocytes are targeted for rapid destruction by autoantibodies. The diagnosis includes, in addition to a detailed history (including all medications and supplements taken by the patient) and physical examination, review of the complete blood count with reticulocyte count, expert review of the peripheral blood smear by a hematologist or pathologist, and laboratory studies that include evaluation of total and indirect bilirubin, LDH, and haptoglobin. Finally a complete serologic examination by the blood bank will confirm the present of the autoantibody and therefore, define the subtype of AIHA. Treatment should be undertaken by an experienced hematologist working in close consultation with the blood bank.

REFERENCES

1. Bottiger LE, Westerholm B. Acquired haemolytic anaemia. Acta Med Scand 1973;193:223–6.
2. Engelfriet CC, Overbeeke MAM, von dem borne AEG. Autoimmune hemolytic anemia. Semin Hematol 1992;29:3–12.
3. Quist E, Koepsell S. Autoimmune hemolytic anemia and red blood cell autoantibodies. Arch Pathol Lab Med 2015;139:1455–8.
4. Nailk R. Warm autoimmune hemolytic anemia. Hematol Oncol Clin North Am 2015;29:445–53.
5. Berentsen S, Randen U, Tjonnfjord GE. Cold agglutinin-mediated hemolytic anemia. Hematol Oncol Clin North Am 2015;29:455–71.
6. Shulman IA, Branch DR, Nelson JM, et al. Autoimmune hemolytic anemia with both cold and warm autoantibodies. JAMA 1985;253:1746–8.
7. Shanbhag S, Spivak J. Paroxysmal cold haemoglobinuria. Hematol Oncol Clin North Am 2015;29:473–8.
8. Segel GB, Lichtman MA. Direct antiglobulin ("Coombs") test-negative autoimmune hemolytic anemia. Blood Cells Mol Dis 2014;52:152–60.
9. Arndt PA, Garratty G. The changing spectrum of drug-induced immune hemolytic anemia. Semin Hematol 2005;42:137–44.
10. Salama A. Drug-induced immune hemolytic anemia. Expert Opin Drug Saf 2009; 8:73–9.

11. Garbe E, Andersohn F, Bronder E, et al. Drug induced immune haemolytic anaemia in the Berlin case-control surveillance study. Br J Haematol 2011;154: 644–53.
12. Dacie JV, Worlledge SM. Auto-immune hemolytic anemia. In: Brown EB, Morre CV, editors. Progress in hematology VI. New York: Grune & Stratton; 1969. p. 82.
13. Sokol RJ, Booker DJ, Stamps R. The pathology of autoimmune haemolytic anaemia. J Clin Pathol 1992;45:1047–52.
14. Pirofsky B. Clinical aspects of autoimmune hemolytic anemia. Semin Hematol 1976;13:251–65.
15. Pullarkat V, Ngo M, Iqbal S, et al. Detection of lupus anticoagulant identifies patients with autoimmune hemolytic anemia at increased risk for venous thrombosis. Br J Haematol 2002;118:1166–9.
16. Roumier M, Loustau V, Guillaud C, et al. Characteristics and outcome of warm autoimmune hemolytic anemia in adults: new insights based on a single-center experience with 60 patients. Am J Hematol 2014;89:E150–5.
17. Conely CL, Lippman SM, Ness PM, et al. Al. Autoimmune hemolytic anemia with reticulocytopenia and erythroid marrow. N Engl J Med 1982;306:281–6.
18. Liesveld JL, Rowe JM, Lichtman MA. Variability of the erythropoietic response in autoimmune hemolytic anemia: analysis of 109 cases. Blood 1987;69:820–8.
19. Evans RS, Takahashi K, Duane RT, et al. Primary thrombocytopenic purpura and acquired hemolytic anemia. Evidence for a common etiology. Arch Intern Med 1951;87:48–65.
20. Marchand A, Galen RS, Van Lente F. The predictive value of serum haptoglobin in hemolytic disease. JAMA 1980;243:1909–11.
21. Lai M, Visconti E, D'Onofrio G, et al. Lower hemoglobin levels in human immunodeficiency virus-infected patients with a positive direct antiglobulin test (DAT): relationship with DAT strength and clinical stages. Transfusion 2006;46:1237–43.
22. Petz LD, Garratty G. Immune hemolytic anemias. 2nd edition. Philadelphia: Churchill Livingstone; 2004.
23. Murphy S, LoBuglio AF. Drug therapy of autoimmune hemolytic anemia. Semin Hematol 1976;13:323–48.
24. Zanella A, Barcellini W. Treatment of autoimmune hemolytic anemias. Haematologica 2014;99:1547–54.
25. Ozsoylu F. Megadose methylprednisolone for treatment of patients with Evan's syndrome. Pediatr Hematol Oncol 2004;21:739–40.
26. Meyer O, Stahl D, Beckhove P, et al. Pulse high-dose dexamethasone in chronic autoimmune hemolytic anaemia of warm type. Br J Haematol 1997;98:860–2.
27. Gupta N, Kavuru S, Patel D, et al. Rituximab-based chemotherapy for steroid-refractory autoimmune hemolytic anemia in chronic lymphocytic leukemia. Leukemia 2002;16(10):2092–5.
28. Crosby WH, Rappaport H. Autoimmune hemolytic anemia. Analysis of hematologic observations with particular reference to their prognostic value. A survey of 57 cases. Blood 1956;12:42–55.
29. Bowdler AS. The role of the spleen and splenectomy in autoimmune hemolytic anemia. Semin Hematol 1976;13:335–85.
30. Zupanska B, Sylwestrowicz T, Pawelski S. The results of prolonged treatment of autoimmune haemolytic anaemia. Haematologica 1981;14:425–33.
31. Crowther M, Chan YL, Garbett IK, et al. Evidence-based focused review of treatment of idiopathic warm immune hemolytic anemia in adults. Blood 2011;118: 4036–40.

32. Casaccia M, Torelli IP, Squarcia S, et al. Laparoscopic splenectomy for hematologic diseases: a preliminary analysis performed on the Italian registry of laparoscopic surgery of the spleen. Surg Endosc 2006;20:1214–20.
33. Bisharat N, Omari H, Lavi I, et al. Risk of infection and death among postsplenectomy patients. J Infect 2001;43:182–6.
34. Kyaw MH, Holmes EM, Toolis F, et al. Evaluation of severe infection and survival after splenectomy. Am J Med 2006;119:276.e1-7.
35. Boyle S, White R, Brunson A, et al. Splenectomy and the incidence of venous thromboembolism and sepsis in patients with immune thrombocytopenia. Blood 2013;121:4782–90.
36. Schwartz R, Dameshek W. Drug-induced immune tolerance. Nature 1959;183: 1682–3.
37. Schwartz R, Dameshek W. Treatment of autoimmune hemolytic anemia with 6-mercaptopurine and thioguanine. Blood 1962;19:483–500.
38. Barcellini W. Current treatment strategies in autoimmune hemolytic disorders. Expert Rev Hematol 2015;8:681–91.
39. Moyo VM, Smith D, Brodsky I, et al. High-dose cyclophosphamide for refractory autoimmune hemolytic anemia. Blood 2002;100:704–6.
40. Hershko C, Sonneblick M, Ashkenazi J. Control of steroid-resistant autoimmune hemolytic anaemia by cyclosporine. Br J Haematol 1990;76:436–7.
41. Emilia G, Messora C, Longo G, et al. Long-term salvage treatment by cyclosporin in refractory haematologic disorders. Br J Haematol 1996;93:341–4.
42. Howard J, Hoffbrand AV, Prentice HG, et al. Mycophenolate mofetil for treatment of refractory auto-immune haemolytic anaemia and auto-immune thrombocytopenia. Br J Haematol 2002;117:712–5.
43. Miano M, Calvillo M, Palmisani E, et al. Sirolimus for the treatment of multiresistant autoimmune haemolytic in children. Br J Haematol 2014;167:571–4.
44. Feugier P. A review of rituximab: the first anti-CD20 monoclonal antibody used in the treatment of B non-Hodgkin's lymphomas. Future Oncol 2015;11:1327–41.
45. Norbert A, Kingreen D, Seltsam A, et al. Treatment of refractory autoimmune haemolytic anaemia with anti-CD20 rituximab. Br J Haematol 2001;114:244–5.
46. Perrotta S, Locatelle F, Manna AL, et al. Anti-CD20 monoclonal antibody (rituximab) for life-threatening autoimmune haemolytic anaemia in a patient with systemic lupus erythematosus. Br J Haematol 2002;116:465–7.
47. Berentsen S, Ulvestad E, Gjertsen BT, et al. Rituximabn for primary chronic cold agglutinin disease: a prospective study of 37 courses of therapy in 37 patients. Blood 2004;103:2925–8.
48. Barcellini W, Zaja F, Zaninoni A, et al. Low-dose rituximab in adult patients with idiopathic autoimmune hemolytic anemia: clinical efficacy and biologic studies. Blood 2012;119:3691–7.
49. Reynaud Q, Durieu I, Dutertre M, et al. Efficacy and safety of rituximab in autoimmune hemolytic anemia: A meta-analysis of 21 studies. Autoimmun Rev 2015;14:304–13.
50. Birgens H, Frederiksen H, Hasselbalch HC, et al. A phase III randomized trial comparing glucocorticoid monotherapy versus glucocorticoid and rituximab in patients with autoimmune haemolytic anaemia. Br J Haematol 2013;163(3): 393–9.

Congenital Hemolytic Anemia

Kristina Haley, DO, MCR

KEYWORDS

- Hemolysis • Jaundice • Aplastic crisis • Splenectomy

KEY POINTS

- Congenital hemolytic anemia typically presents in childhood, but more milder forms can result in a delayed presentation until adulthood.
- The congenital hemolytic anemias can be broadly classified as red blood cell (RBC) membrane disorders, RBC enzyme disorders, or hemoglobinopathies.
- Congenital hemolytic anemias cause a baseline level of anemia, which can be exacerbated by episodes of hyperhemolysis or aplasia and result in symptomatic transfusion dependent anemia.
- Complications of congenital hemolytic anemia, such as gallstones, are common in adolescents and young adults.
- Splenectomy is an effective treatment for some congenital hemolytic anemias but is not necessary in all of the congenital hemolytic anemias.

INTRODUCTION

Red blood cells (RBCs) are biconcave discs with a diameter of 7.5 μm.[1] RBCs are efficient vehicles for oxygen exchange, and their function depends upon healthy hemoglobin and an easily deformed shape. RBCs depend upon anaerobic metabolism in order to maintain their shape, prevent oxidative damage, and maintain hemoglobin in its functional form. The average lifespan of an RBC is 100 to 120 days.[2] Premature destruction of red blood cells due to acquired or congenital abnormalities in hemoglobin, RBC membrane proteins, or in enzymes critical for RBC metabolism results in hemolytic anemia.[2] While there are several different types of hemolytic anemias, they are all characterized by similar features. RBCs have a shortened lifespan, and there is typically a compensatory increase in erythrocytosis. Patients are variably symptomatic from the anemia, and the anemia may worsen depending upon the clinical scenario.

Conflict of Interest: The author has served on advisory boards for Baxalta and CSL Behring on topics unrelated to hemolytic anemia.
Department of Pediatrics, Division of Pediatric Hematology/Oncology, Oregon Health & Science University, 3181 Southwest Sam Jackson Park Road, Mail Code CDRCP, Portland, OR 97239, USA
E-mail address: haley@ohsu.edu

Hemolytic anemias are broadly classified into 2 groups: immune and nonimmune. In this article, the focus will be on congenital nonimmune hemolytic anemias.

The congenital hemolytic anemias are further divided into 3 categories: (1) disorders of the RBC membrane, (2) disorders of RBC enzymes, and (3) abnormal hemoglobin structures (**Table 1**). The most common of these disorders are hereditary spherocytosis, glucose-6-phosphate dehydrogenase (G6PD) deficiency, and alpha and beta hemoglobinopathies, respectively.[3] Although each of these anemias mediates hemolysis through different mechanisms, their clinical presentations and laboratory features are similar.

CLINICAL PRESENTATION

The congenital hemolytic anemias typically present in infancy or in early childhood. There may be a family history of hemolytic anemia that draws attention to the condition, or the infant may have significant hyperbilirubinemia out of proportion to what is expected in the newborn period. Alternatively, the patient may present at times of increased hemolysis with anemia, hyperbilirubinemia, and reticulocytosis. At baseline, the symptoms may be so limited that they go undetected. Patients may not present until adulthood in mild forms of congenital hemolytic anemia, but severe forms present in childhood. In an adult with a direct antiglobulin test-negative hemolytic anemia, a congenital hemolytic anemia should be considered.[4] The patients, regardless of age, present with pallor, anemia, jaundice, indirect hyperbilirubinemia, splenomegaly (not universally), and reticulocytosis.

Baseline

At baseline, the congenital hemolytic anemias often result in a mild-to-moderate chronic level of hemolysis that is well compensated by an increased reticulocytosis, and only mild-to-moderate anemia results. In each of the congenital hemolytic anemias presented, more severe forms can be present but are rare. In those instances, the chronic hemolysis occurs at a faster rate, and more significant anemia can develop.

Hemolytic Event

Although each of the congenital hemolytic anemias result in a baseline steady state that is largely asymptomatic, stresses such as infection, drugs, or toxins can result in increased rates of hemolysis and subsequent severe, transfusion-dependent anemias. In RBC membrane defects, increased hemolysis can occur, with illness likely due to increased splenomegaly and thus increased RBC destruction. The RBC enzyme disorders result in increased hemolysis with drug exposure, illness, or with certain foods as a result of increased oxidative stress.

Table 1		
Types of congenital hemolytic anemia		
Membrane and Cytoskeleton Defects	**Enzyme Defects**	**Hemoglobin Defects**
1. Hereditary spherocytosis (HS) 2. Hereditary elliptocytosis (HE) 3. Hereditary pyropoikilocytosis (HPP)	1. Glucose 6 phosphate dehydrogenase (G-6-PD) deficiency 2. Pyruvate kinase (PK) deficiency	1. Sickle cell disease 2. Alpha thalassemia 3. Beta thalassemia 4. Unstable hemoglobin

Aplastic Event

In each of the congenital hemolytic anemias, baseline hemolysis is counteracted by increased reticulocytosis. Transient bone marrow aplasia can result in a halt in reticulocyte production and a worsening of the baseline anemia. As opposed to the clinical features of a hemolytic event, in which pallor and jaundice are present, in an aplastic event, jaundice is typically absent while pallor persists.[1] The classic viral infection to cause a transient aplastic event in patients with congenital hemolytic anemia is Parvovirus B19. Parvovirus B19 preferentially infects erythroid precursors, resulting in their death. Patients can have severe, life-threatening anemia, particularly those with lower steady-state hemoglobin.[5,6] A patient with congenital hemolytic anemia who has a fever should be evaluated with a complete blood cell count (CBC) and reticulocyte count. The aplastic event typically lasts 10 to 14 days.[1]

Complications

Aside from worsening anemia caused by increased hemolysis or transient aplasia, patients with congenital hemolytic anemia are also at risk for gallstone formation. Increased breakdown of hemoglobin results in a higher concentration of bilirubin in the biliary tract and subsequent development of gallstones.[7] Coinheritance of Gilbert syndrome increases the risk of gallstone formation significantly.[1] There is some information suggesting that patients with chronic hemolysis are at increased risk for thrombotic complications, particularly patients with hemoglobinopathies. The pathophysiology is related to increased thrombin and fibrin generation, as well as increased tissue factor activity and platelet activation.[8] The risk of thrombosis is increased following splenectomy.[9] Asplenic patients are also at risk for infectious complications, particularly with encapsulated bacteria.[9] Patients who receive chronic or frequent transfusions are at risk for iron overload.

LABORATORY FEATURES

The hallmark laboratory features of hemolysis include anemia, reticulocytosis, and elevated unconjugated (indirect) bilirubin (**Box 1**). The anemia is most often normocytic; however, macrocytic anemia can also be seen when the reticulocytosis is brisk. Reticulocytes have an average mean corpuscular volume[10] of 150 femtoliter, which can elevate the overall Mean Corpuscular Volume if the reticulocytes are present in high numbers.[11] In some congenital hemolytic anemias, the reticulocyte response is adequate to maintain a normal to near-normal hemoglobin, and anemia is only present during times of increased hemolysis or times of bone marrow aplasia.[11] The

---

Box 1
Laboratory features of congenital hemolytic anemias

Anemia

Reticulocytosis

Hyperbilirubinemia (indirect)

Elevated LDH

Decreased haptoglobin

Elevated MCHC (hereditary spherocytosis)

DAT negative

reticulocyte count in congenital hemolytic anemia typically exceeds 2%. The mean corpuscular hemoglobin concentration (MCHC) is typically elevated in hereditary spherocytosis. The peripheral blood smear should be evaluated for abnormalities in red cell shapes and red cell inclusions (**Table 2**). Although most congenital hemolytic anemias result in a normocytic anemia, the thalassemias are typically microcytic, with a more significant microcytosis than what is expected for the degree of anemia. Apart from the RBC indices and reticulocyte counts, the indirect bilirubin may be elevated. In hemolytic anemias, the Lactate Dehydrogenase is often increased, and the hapto-globin is decreased.

DIFFERENTIAL DIAGNOSIS

In a patient presenting with signs or symptoms of hemolysis, the congenital hemolytic anemias should be considered, as some may result in only minor hemolysis until a sufficient stressor results in increased hemolysis that cannot be compensated by reticulocytosis. Alternatively, an aplastic event, such as infection with Parvovirus B19, may result in significant anemia without evidence of significant infection. Thus, the congenital hemolytic anemias should be considered in someone presenting with severe anemia and an insufficient reticulocyte response. In addition to the congenital hemolytic anemias, in a patient presenting with signs or symptoms of hemolysis (pallor, jaundice, fatigue, anemia, hyperbilirubinemia, elevated LDH, or decreased haptoglobin), the differential diagnosis includes

- Autoimmune hemolytic anemia
- Drug-induced immune hemolytic anemia
- Hemolytic uremic syndrome
- Infection-associated immune hemolytic anemia
- Malaria
- Malignant hypertension
- Mechanical valve hemolytic anemia
- Microangiopathic hemolytic anemia
- Pre-eclampsia or eclampsia
- Thrombotic thrombocytopenic purpura
- Transfusion reaction

MEMBRANOPATHIES

The RBC membrane consists of an outer lipid bilayer and an inner spectrin-based cytoskeleton. The 2 layers are connected via several linker proteins. An RBC membrane defect is typically suspected in a patient with hemolytic anemia when review of the peripheral smear demonstrates RBCs that are not of the typical biconcave shape. Membranopathies are the result of qualitative abnormalities or quantitative deficiencies of the RBC cytoskeletal proteins.[12] The 3 most common RBC membranopathies are hereditary spherocytosis (HS), hereditary elliptocytosis (HE), and hereditary pyropoikilocytosis (HPP), with HS being the most common.

Hereditary Spherocytosis

Pathophysiology
HS results from mutations in proteins involved in maintaining the vertical interactions between the lipid bilayer and the spectrin-based cytoskeleton. Deficiency or dysfunction of band 3, protein 4.2, ankyrin, and α- and β-spectrin proteins results in the formation of spherocytic RBCs secondary to a reduction in the surface-to-volume ratio of

Table 2
Peripheral blood smear findings in congenital hemolytic anemias

	Polychromasia	Spherocytes	Elliptocytes	Basophilic Stippling	Heinz Bodies	Microcytosis	Sickle-Shaped RBC
Hereditary Spherocytosis	X	X					
Hereditary elliptocytosis	X		X				
G-6-PD deficiency	X				X		
Pyruvate kinase deficiency	X						
Alpha thalassemia	X			X	X	X	
Beta thalassemia	X			X		X	
Sickle cell anemia	X						X

the RBC.[12] Combination defects may result in more severe hemolytic anemia than partial or singular defects. The spherocytes that result from mutations in the genes encoding these proteins have reduced deformability and are selectively retained and damaged in the spleen. In the spleen, the RBCs lose additional surface area and are typically destroyed. HS RBCs are particularly sensitive to osmotic changes, and osmotic fragility is the hallmark of HS.[1]

Epidemiology

HS is predominantly found in patients of northern European ancestry, although it has been reported in all ethnic groups.[1] It affects about 1 in 2000 people in northern Europe and North America.[1] Autosomal-dominant inheritance is present in about 75% of cases, and is primarily associated with mutations in ankyrin, band 2, or β-spectrin. For the remaining 25% of cases, spontaneous mutations and autosomal-recessive inheritance have been described.

Diagnosis

HS is diagnosed through a combination of clinical history, family history, physical examination, and laboratory data. For patients with a known family history, typical physical findings (splenomegaly, jaundice), and typical laboratory features (spherocytes on peripheral blood smear, reticulocytosis, and negative direct antiglobulin test), more specific diagnostic testing is often not necessary. When the diagnosis is not straightforward or there are inconsistencies in the history, further testing is needed. The osmotic fragility test evaluates the RBC sensitivity to changes in sodium chloride concentrations, thereby taking advantage of the reduced surface area-to-volume ratio in spherocytes, resulting in impaired resilience to changes in osmolality. The osmotic fragility test has been considered the gold standard diagnostic test for HS, but it is falsely negative in about 25% of patients.[13] Further, patients with autoimmune hemolytic anemia (AIHA) can have a positive osmotic fragility test.[1] The 2011 update to the guidelines for the diagnosis and management of hereditary spherocytosis recommend the eosin-5-maleimide (EMA) binding test as the appropriate screening test.[12] The EMA binding test employs flow cytometry in order to assess extent of EMA binding to transmembrane proteins, which are deficient in hereditary spherocytosis.

Disease severity

The clinical presentation and severity of HS vary widely and are classified as mild, moderate, and severe (some authors note a fourth category of moderately severe).[1] The clinical severity within a family, however, is fairly consistent. Approximately 20% to 30% of patients have mild disease. In these patients, the only laboratory abnormalities may be spherocytes (with an elevated MCHC) and reticulocytosis. The increased reticulocyte count is often able to overcome the hemolysis and allow for maintenance of a normal hemoglobin. Patients with mild disease may not come to attention until adulthood when a relative (often son or daughter with neonatal jaundice) is diagnosed, if they develop splenomegaly as a complication of an illness, or if they develop cholelithiasis secondary to chronic hemolysis.

Patients with moderate disease, approximately 60% to 70% of patients, typically are diagnosed with HS in childhood when they present with anemia. In moderate disease, there is baseline anemia with hemoglobin ranging from 8 to 10 g/dL. At baseline, the patient may experience intermittent fatigue. Splenomegaly is common in patients with moderate and severe disease. Although splenomegaly is common, splenic rupture is not more common than the general population and not in and of itself an indication for splenectomy. The remaining patients have severe (or moderately severe) disease. In these patients, reticulocytosis is not able to keep up with hemolysis, and severe anemia develops. Patients frequently need regular transfusions in order to maintain their hemoglobin.

Clinical presentation

The baseline clinical picture of a patient with HS is that he or she is generally well with likely mild-to-moderate pallor. Chronic hemolysis, however, may lead to the formation of gallstones. In a retrospective review of pediatric patients with HS, 27% of patients developed gallstones at an average age of 10 years.[14] Overall in HS, gallstones are present in 21% to 63% of patients.[15] The hereditary spherocytosis management guidelines note that it is not clear if regular screening for asymptomatic gallstones is needed.[12] This is based on the idea that it is also not known if it is necessary to remove asymptomatic gallstones. However, consensus guidelines indicate that patients with symptomatic gallstones should undergo cholecystectomy.[12]

Treatment

Splenectomy is an effective therapy for hereditary spherocytosis, and it significantly reduces hemolysis.[12] Splenectomy effectively eliminates symptoms in patients with mild disease and decreases symptoms in patients with moderate or severe disease.[12] Current recommendations indicate that splenectomy should be performed in childhood in patients with severe HS, should be considered in those with moderate HS, and is typically not necessary in patients with mild HS. Splenectomy is associated with a lifelong risk of overwhelming infection, and patients should be vaccinated prior to splenectomy. Adults with HS who underwent splenectomy in childhood may need catch-up vaccines based on newly available vaccines and should be reminded of their lifelong risk for infectious complications. In addition to infectious complications, there is an increased risk of thrombosis following splenectomy. Current guidelines do not suggest extended thrombosis prophylaxis.[12] The 2011 HS management guidelines indicate that laparoscopic splenectomy is preferred over open splenectomy and that a cholecystectomy should be performed simultaneously if there are symptomatic gallstones.[12]

Hereditary Elliptocytosis

Although HS is the most common membranopathy, several other RBC membrane defects can result in hemolytic anemia. The second most common membrane disorder is hereditary elliptocytosis (HE). The RBCs in HE are elliptical or oval in shape. HE results from defects in horizontal protein connections in the RBC membrane. HE affects 3 to 5 individuals per 10,000 population.[16] HE is a heterogeneous disorder, and most patients are asymptomatic. However, the neonatal presentation can be dramatic, with jaundice, hemolytic anemia, and hydrops fetalis.[17] HE is inherited in an autosomal-dominant fashion, and patients with a heterozygous mutation are generally asymptomatic. Patients with homozygous mutations or compound heterozygous mutations can have significant symptoms. A variant form of HE is hereditary pyropoikilocytosis (HPP),[17] which is characterized by elliptocytoes, microspherocytes, and RBC fragments on peripheral smear. Patients with severe HE should be considered for splenectomy. Patients with HE and HPP have incomplete response to splenectomy, and some degree of hemolysis persists after splenectomy.[3]

ENZYMOPATHIES

RBCs are dependent upon the production of adenosine triphosphate (ATP) through glycolysis, and ATP is the only source of energy for the RBCs. Defects in the glycolytic pathway enzymes may lead to hemolysis. The group of enzymopathies, glycolytic pathway enzyme deficiencies, is termed the congenital nonspherocytic hemolytic anemias (CNSHAs) as these deficiencies have no characteristic morphology on blood smear. The 2 most common are (G6PD) deficiency and pyruvate kinase deficiency (PKD).

Glucose-6-Phosphate Dehydrogenase Deficiency

Pathophysiology

G6PD deficiency is the most common RBC enzymopathy.[2] G6PD plays a critical role in the production of nicotinamide adenine dinucleotide phosphate (NADPH), and NADPH plays a critical role in preventing oxidative damage to proteins within cells which RBCs are particularly sensitive. The mechanism of hemolysis in G6PD deficiency is as follows:

1. An oxidative agent causes conversion of glutathione to glutathione disulfide
2. Because G6PD deficient cells do not efficiently make glutathione, the glutathione is rapidly depleted
3. Once glutathione is depleted, the sulfhydryl groups of hemoglobin are oxidized
4. Oxidized hemoglobin precipitates and damages the RBC membrane
5. RBC hemolysis

This series of events is most often triggered by drugs that can oxidize NADPH.[18] Fava beans also cause hemolysis in G6PD. Infections additionally can trigger hemolysis in patients with G6PD deficiency. G6PD decreases exponentially as RBCs age. Thus, reticulocytes have more G6PD than older RBCs, which can affect diagnostic evaluations.

Epidemiology

The G6PD gene is located on the X chromosome, and thus the deficiency is an X-linked disorder. Males are more likely affected, although there are symptomatic females as a result of X inactivation. G6PD is a common disorder, affecting more than 400 million people worldwide.[19] It is most prevalent in areas of high malaria infection, as G6PD deficiency is protective from severe malaria infection.[19]

Disease severity

The World Health Organization (WHO) groups G6PD deficiency into 5 categories. G6PD enzyme activity of less than 10% is considered severe deficiency. Two forms of severe deficiency exist: severe deficiency with chronic hemolytic anemia and severe deficiency with intermittent hemolysis. Enzyme activity between 10% and 60% is defined as mild deficiency, and hemolysis occurs with stressors only. There is also a nondeficient variant that results in activity of 60% to 100% and is not associated with clinical symptoms or hemolysis. Increased enzyme activity (>100% activity) is also not associated with clinical symptoms or hemolysis.[19] Most patients with G6PD deficiency are typically not anemic or jaundiced at baseline, and hemolytic events are triggered by stressors such as a medication, fava beans, or infection.

Diagnosis

The specific laboratory features of G6PD include peripheral smear findings (anisocytosis, poikilocytosis, and bite cells). There is significant reticulocytosis, which can falsely elevate G6PD activity because of the high G6PD content of reticulocytes. In patients presenting with a hemolytic event and a significantly elevated reticulocytosis, the diagnosis can be missed due to falsely high G6PD levels. Once the hemolytic event is resolved and the reticulocyte count decreased, G6PD levels should be repeated if they were previously normal. With supravital staining, Heinz bodies can be seen within RBCs, which are precipitates of denatured hemoglobin. Enzyme activity can be measured, and this is the most common way to diagnose G6PD deficiency.[19] Genetic testing is also available, but not all genetic variants in the G6PD gene are associated with clinically significant deficiency. Thus, it is important to correlate genetic findings to the clinical picture.[19]

Clinical presentation

For the majority of patients, even those with severe deficiency, there is no anemia or jaundice at baseline, and patients are asymptomatic. However, oxidative stressors can result in severe hemolysis that may require transfusion support. The offending agent causes hemolysis of the oldest, most G6PD-deficient RBCs. And, despite ongoing exposure to a drug or ongoing infection, hemolysis typically slows or stops as the younger RBCs are able to sustain the oxidative damage.[20] A variety of medications can result in an oxidative stress and subsequent hemolysis in patients with G6PD deficiency. Some of the most common agents include primaquine and sulfa drugs. Not all drugs cause the same degree of hemolysis in every patient, and some drugs only cause hemolysis at supratherapeutic concentrations. A complete list of drugs that can cause hemolysis in G6PD deficiency can be found at http://www.g6pd.org/G6PDDeficiency/SafeUnsafe.aspx.

In addition to medication-induced hemolysis, infection can also cause hemolysis in patients with G6PD deficiency, and this is the most common precipitating factor for hemolysis.[18] Patients with G6PD deficiency should be counseled on the risk of hemolysis during infections, and if signs or symptoms of anemia develop during a febrile illness, a CBC and reticulocyte count should be obtained. Ingestion of fava beans is also a cause of hemolysis in patients with G6PD deficiency, but not all patients with G6PD deficiency have hemolysis after eating fava beans.[18] For patients with severe deficiency and chronic hemolysis, there is baseline anemia and reticulocytosis, with or without jaundice.

Treatment

Treatment of patients with G6PD deficiency is aimed at avoiding triggers for hemolysis. However, if hemolysis develops, close monitoring is warranted, and packed RBC transfusion support should be provided if the patient develops symptomatic anemia. Splenectomy is generally not indicated. However, for patients with chronic hemolysis, there are reports of improvement of hemolysis following splenectomy.[21] Patients should be supplemented with folic acid during hemolytic events.

Pyruvate Kinase Deficiency

Pathophysiology

The second most common enzymopathy is pyruvate kinase (PK) deficiency. Pyruvate kinase is a critical enzyme in the Embden-Meyerhof pathway,[2] and it converts phosphenol pyruvate to lactate, thereby generating ATP. Deficiency of PK results in depletion of ATP and increased 2,3-disphosphoglycerate (2,3-DPG).[22] The mechanism of hemolysis in PK deficiency is poorly understood,[23] but it is hypothesized that decreased ATP generation contributes to ATP deficiency.[22] ATP-depleted cells are rigid due to loss of potassium and water, and rigid RBCs are more likely to get destroyed in the spleen. However, this is not a sufficient explanation, as other disorders resulting in more severe ATP deficiency are not associated with hemolysis.[22,23]

Epidemiology

PK deficiency is an autosomal-recessive trait.[22] It has a worldwide distribution, but it is most often recognized in patients of northern European decent.[22] There is also a high frequency in the Pennsylvania Amish population.[23] It is not a common disorder, with only 400 reported cases.[22] Heterozygotes are clinically asymptomatic, and symptoms are only seen in compound heterozygotes or in homozygotes.[22] Greater than 100 mutations have been reported in PK deficiency.[23]

Diagnosis

PK deficiency should be suspected in a patient with DAT-negative, nonspherocytic hemolytic anemia with normal G6PD levels. PK enzyme activity can be measured by specialized laboratories.[23] Symptomatic patients typically have PK enzyme activity between 5% and 40% of normal.[22] If a patient was recently transfused prior to assay of PK activity, the PK activity of the transfused cells may falsely elevate the level and result in a falsely negative test.[22]

Clinical presentation

The clinical course of PK deficiency is variable. Some patients have lifelong mild or fully compensated anemia, but others have lifelong transfusion-dependent anemia. Neonatal hyperbilirubinemia can be severe and require exchange transfusion.[22] Similar to other hemolytic anemias, gallstones are common.[22] The degree of hemolysis and subsequent anemia is constant, with occasional exacerbations during infections or pregnancy.[22] Iron overload is also common, especially in patients who have undergone splenectomy.[22]

Treatment

Treatment of PK deficiency is mainly supportive, with packed red cell transfusions. Splenectomy can reduce the need for transfusion in transfusion-dependent patients, although it does not eliminate hemolysis.[22] Splenectomy is only recommended in patients with severe, transfusion-dependent anemia. Response to splenectomy is similar among family members.[22] There is a characteristic significant rise in the reticulocyte count following splenectomy.[23]

HEMOGLOBINOPATHIES

Adult hemoglobin consists of 2 α-globins and 2 β-globins. Hemoglobinopathies include genetic defects in the α- or β-globin genes. Quantitative deficiencies of globin production result in the thalassemias. Qualitative deficiencies that result in a change of hemoglobin structure result in abnormal hemoglobin formation. Variants in structural hemoglobin include sickle cell anemia, hemoglobin E, hemoglobin C, and many others. The 2 types of hemoglobinopathies can exist in combination, and a patient may have both a thalassemic disorder as well as a structural defect in the hemoglobin. In this article, the focus will be on the quantitative deficiencies: the thalassemias with the focus on types that can lead to hemolysis.

THALASSEMIA

RBCs contain equal amounts of each globin chain. In the thalassemia syndromes, production of either the α- or β-globin chains is impaired and leads to a mismatch of production. α-thalassemia is caused by defects in synthesis of the α-globin. β-thalassemia is caused by defects in synthesis of the β-globin. Anemia in the thalassemia syndromes results both from hemolysis and ineffective erythropoiesis. Hemolysis is secondary to accumulation of excess globin chains. In α-thalassemia, β-tetramers precipitate in the cell and cause RBC membrane disruption and hemolysis. In β-thalassemia, α-chains precipitate in the cell and result in increased red cell destruction.

As discussed in the article on unusual anemias, laboratory abnormalities in the thalassemia syndromes are similar between α- and β-thalassemia. Microcytosis is prominent and is often more significant than expected for the degree of anemia in milder phenotypes. The degree of anemia depends upon the number of genes deleted. Reticulocytosis is prominent. Hemoglobin electrophoresis can aid in the diagnosis.

Alpha-Thalassemia

Pathophysiology

Each cell contains 4 copies of the α-globin gene, which are located on chromosome 16.[24] In α-thalassemia, at least 1 of those genes is deleted.[24] α-thalassemia occurs most commonly in patients from Africa, southeast Asia, and the Middle East. There are 4 α-thalassemia types[24]:

- Silent carrier (no hemolysis)
- α-thalassemia trait (no hemolysis)
- Hemoglobin H disease (hemolysis present)
- Hydrops fetalis (severe, in utero hemolysis)

The silent carrier state results from a single gene deletion (-α/αα) and is an asymptomatic state but with mild hypochromia and potentially slightly reduced hemoglobin.[25] α-thalassemia trait (also called α-thalassemia minor by some) is caused by a 2-gene deletion (–/αα, or -α/-α). In patients with α-thalassemia trait, there is mild anemia, hypochromia, and microcytosis. Whether the gene deletion is in the cis formation (–/αα) or the trans formation (-α/-α) has implications for genetic counseling. If 2 individuals with α-thalassemia trait in the cis formation reproduce together, there is risk that their offspring could have a 4-gene deletion.

Hemoglobin H disease results from a 3-gene deletion (–/-α). Because of the mismatch in α-globin and β-globin production, there is an excess of β-globin chains. The β-globin chains form tetramers, termed hemoglobin H. Hemoglobin H can precipitate in RBCs and damage the RBC membrane and result in hemolysis.[24] Hemoglobin H is not an effective oxygen carrier due to its high oxygen affinity. Hydrops fetalis results from a 4-gene deletion (–/–). Hydrops fetalis results in severe hemolytic anemia, which presents in utero and is fatal if not treated.[25]

Treatment

Treatment is not required for the silent carrier form of α-thalassemia nor for α-thalassemia trait.[25] It is important that iron deficiency is not presumed based on the hypochromia, microcytosis, and mild anemia and iron panels should be obtained if iron deficiency is suspected. Empiric treatment with iron is contraindicated,[25] as patients with the α-thalassemia syndromes are efficient at iron uptake and are at risk for iron overload. The clinical picture of hemoglobin H disease is variable, and transfusions are not routinely necessary.[25] Hydrops fetalis requires treatment with in utero transfusions in order to prevent fetal demise.[25]

Beta-Thalassemia

Pathophysiology

Each cell contains 2 copies of the β-globin gene, which is on chromosome 11. β-thalassemia results from either absence or partial deficiency of β-globin production.[24] β-thalassemia occurs most commonly in the Mediterranean countries, southeastern Europe, Asia, and the Middle East.[25] e β denotes normal β-globin production; β⁺ denotes insufficient β-globin production, and β° denotes absent β-globin production. The β-globin production starts in utero but is not at full capacity until 3 to 6 months of age. Thus, in contrast to the α-thalassemia syndromes, which present in utero or early in infancy if clinically relevant, the β-thalassemia syndromes typically present at around 3 to 6 months of age or beyond.[25]

Thalassemia minor results from the heterozygous state, with 1 β-globin gene being abnormal, and it is clinically asymptomatic. Laboratory findins may be slightly abnormal, with a complete blood count showing microcytosis and hypochromia with or without anemia. Thalassemia intermedia is clinically variable, with mild-to-moderate anemia and variable need for transfusions.[25] Thalassemia intermedia results from either a mild homozygous state or a mixed heterozygous state. Thalassemia major causes transfusion dependent anemia and is a result of a severe homozygous state or a mixed heterozygous state.[25]

Patients with thalassemia major or intermedia should be cared for by a hematology team familiar with the complications of thalassemia. Treatment for transfusion-dependent thalassemia, which is thalassemia major by definition, is with regular transfusions to suppress erythropoiesis, optimize oxygen delivery, and maximize growth and organ function. Patients are at risk for iron overload, and iron chelation therapy is necessary in order to prevent organ dysfunction. Hematopoietic stem cell transplant is curative, and is recommended if a donor is available.[25]

Unstable Hemoglobins

In patients with nonimmune hemolysis, reticulocytosis, and a normal hemoglobin electrophoresis, congenital unstable hemoglobinopathy should enter the differential diagnosis.[26] Unstable hemoglobins result from globin chain mutations that lead to hemoglobin variants that may undergo rapid denaturation. This results in precipitation of denatured hemoglobin within the RBC and subsequent hemolysis. Rapid denaturation can make these hemoglobins so unstable that they cannot be detected by hemoglobin electrophoresis.[26] Hemolysis occurs both at the steady state and increases with oxidative stress.[27] The clinical spectrum is highly variable: from severe hemolysis starting at birth to minor hemolysis causing no symptoms.[27] Many of the unstable hemoglobins migrate with hemoglobin A on electrophoresis. In β-globin unstable hemoglobins, hemoglobin A_2 will be elevated to between 4% and 5%.[27] Hemoglobin F may also be elevated. The heat instability test is helpful in diagnosing unstable hemoglobins.[27] Treatment is often supportive, but splenectomy is indicated in severe cases.[27]

SUMMARY

The congenital hemolytic anemias are secondary to RBC membrane defects, RBC enzyme deficiencies, or hemoglobin structure or content defects. Compensated hemolytic anemia is the most common clinical presentation, but some of the congenital hemolytic anemias can result in lifelong transfusion-dependent anemia. Alternatively, patients with congenital hemolytic anemias may come to medical attention when a physiologic stressor results in increased hemolysis and ultimately symptomatic anemia. Long-term complications include gallstones and increased risk of infection if the patient undergoes splenectomy. Splenectomy is not curative in all of the congenital hemolytic anemias. Folic acid supplementation is recommended, particularly in patients with a brisk reticulocytosis in order to support red cell production.

REFERENCES

1. Perrotta S, Gallagher PG, Mohandas N. Hereditary spherocytosis. Lancet 2008; 372(9647):1411–26.

2. Addiego J, Hurst D, Lubin B. Congenital hemolytic anemia. Pediatr Rev 1985; 6(7):201–8.
3. Gallagher PG. Diagnosis and management of rare congenital nonimmune hemolytic disease. Hematology Am Soc Hematol Educ Program 2015;2015:392–9.
4. Faughnan ME, Palda VA, Garcia-Tsao G, et al. International guidelines for the diagnosis and management of hereditary haemorrhagic telangiectasia. J Med Genet 2011;48(2):73–87.
5. Noronha SA. Acquired and congenital hemolytic anemia. Pediatr Rev 2016;37(6): 235–46.
6. Kobayashi Y, Hatta Y, Ishiwatari Y, et al. Human parvovirus B19-induced aplastic crisis in an adult patient with hereditary spherocytosis: a case report and review of the literature. BMC Res Notes 2014;7:137.
7. Tamary H, Aviner S, Freud E, et al. High incidence of early cholelithiasis detected by ultrasonography in children and young adults with hereditary spherocytosis. J Pediatr Hematol Oncol 2003;25(12):952–4.
8. Ataga KI. Hypercoagulability and thrombotic complications in hemolytic anemias. Haematologica 2009;94(11):1481–4.
9. Crary SE, Buchanan GR. Vascular complications after splenectomy for hematologic disorders. Blood 2009;114(14):2861–8.
10. Steen M, Norstrom EA, Tholander AL, et al. Functional characterization of factor V-Ile359Thr: a novel mutation associated with thrombosis. Blood 2004;103(9): 3381–7.
11. Dhaliwal G, Cornett PA, Tierney LM Jr. Hemolytic anemia. Am Fam Physician 2004;69(11):2599–606.
12. Bolton-Maggs PH, Langer JC, Iolascon A, et al. General Haematology Task Force of the British Committee for Standards in H. Guidelines for the diagnosis and management of hereditary spherocytosis–2011 update. Br J Haematol 2012;156(1):37–49.
13. Bianchi P, Fermo E, Vercellati C, et al. Diagnostic power of laboratory tests for hereditary spherocytosis: a comparison study in 150 patients grouped according to molecular and clinical characteristics. Haematologica 2012;97(4):516–23.
14. Oliveira MC, Fernandes RA, Rodrigues CL, et al. Clinical course of 63 children with hereditary spherocytosis: a retrospective study. Rev Bras Hematol Hemoter 2012;34(1):9–13.
15. Rutkow IM. Twenty years of splenectomy for hereditary spherocytosis. Arch Surg 1981;116(3):306–8.
16. Da Costa L, Galimand J, Fenneteau O, et al. Hereditary spherocytosis, elliptocytosis, and other red cell membrane disorders. Blood Rev 2013;27(4):167–78.
17. Gallagher PG, Weed SA, Tse WT, et al. Recurrent fatal hydrops fetalis associated with a nucleotide substitution in the erythrocyte beta-spectrin gene. J Clin Invest 1995;95(3):1174–82.
18. Beutler E. Glucose-6-phosphate dehydrogenase deficiency: a historical perspective. Blood 2008;111(1):16–24.
19. von Seidlein L, Auburn S, Espino F, et al. Review of key knowledge gaps in glucose-6-phosphate dehydrogenase deficiency detection with regard to the safe clinical deployment of 8-aminoquinoline treatment regimens: a workshop report. Malar J 2013;12:112.
20. Frank JE. Diagnosis and management of G6PD deficiency. Am Fam Physician 2005;72(7):1277–82.
21. Vulliamy TJ, Kaeda JS, Ait-Chafa D, et al. Clinical and haematological consequences of recurrent G6PD mutations and a single new mutation causing chronic nonspherocytic haemolytic anaemia. Br J Haematol 1998;101(4):670–5.

22. Zanella A, Bianchi P. Red cell pyruvate kinase deficiency: from genetics to clinical manifestations. Baillieres Best Pract Res Clin Haematol 2000;13(1):57–81.

23. Prchal JT, Gregg XT. Red cell enzymes. Hematol Am Soc Hematol Educ Program 2005;19–23.

24. Marengo-Rowe AJ. The thalassemias and related disorders. Proc (Bayl Univ Med Cent) 2007;20(1):27–31.

25. Kohne E. Hemoglobinopathies: clinical manifestations, diagnosis, and treatment. Dtsch Arztebl Int 2011;108(31–32):532–40.

26. Yates AM, Mortier NA, Hyde KS, et al. The diagnostic dilemma of congenital unstable hemoglobinopathies. Pediatr Blood Cancer 2010;55(7):1393–5.

27. White JM, Dacie JV. The unstable hemoglobins–molecular and clinical features. Prog Hematol 1971;7(0):69–109.

Sickle Cell Disease
A Brief Update

Sharl Azar, MD[a],*, Trisha E. Wong, MD, MS[b,c]

KEYWORDS

- Sickle cell disease • Sickle cell anemia • Hemoglobinopathy • Hydroxyurea
- Iron overload • Review

KEY POINTS

- Sickle cell disease (SCD) is a systemic disease with the potential to affect numerous organs acutely, chronically, and both (acute-on-chronic), which can lead to early morbidity and mortality.
- The acute and chronic complications of SCD can be mitigated with preventive care, such as routine surveillance studies and appropriate use of hydroxyurea.
- When interventions are needed, timely access to a medical home with expertise in SCD is important to maximize quantity and quality of life.

INTRODUCTION

Diseases impacting the production, longevity, and function of the hemoglobin molecule are diverse in their impact on an individual and population basis. This article focuses on sickle cell disease (SCD), the condition resulting from the presence of hemoglobin S (Hb S), and is not only the most common hemoglobinopathy but is also the most common heritable hematologic disease in humans.[1] Hb S earns its name from the sickle shape it imparts on the red blood cells (RBCs). Since it was first described in the early twentieth century,[2] SCD is now understood as a disease that requires a multidisciplinary approach to diagnosis and management given its

Financial Disclosure: Neither the authors nor those recognized in the Acknowledgments section have any financial relationships relevant to this article to disclose. Neither the authors nor those recognized in the Acknowledgments section received any compensation to produce this article.
Conflict of Interest: Neither the authors nor those recognized in the Acknowledgments section have any conflicts of interest to disclose.
[a] Division of Hematology and Medical Oncology, Department of Medicine, Oregon Health and Science University, 3181 Southwest Sam Jackson Park Road, Mailstop L586, Portland, OR 97239, USA; [b] Division of Hematology/Oncology, Department of Pediatrics, Oregon Health and Science University, 3181 Southwest Sam Jackson Park Road, Mailstop CDRCP, Portland, OR 97239, USA; [c] Division of Transfusion Services, Department of Pathology, Oregon Health and Science University, 3181 Southwest Sam Jackson Park Road, Mailstop HRC9, Portland, OR 97239, USA
* Corresponding author.
E-mail address: wong@ohsu.edu

fundamental impact on physical, psychological, and socioeconomic aspects. Unfortunately, such resources are absent or scarce in countries most impacted by SCD, accounting for a high morbidity and mortality rate.

An understanding of the disorder first hinges on a clear definition of terms: SCD is any condition in which the inheritance of Hb S can lead to the sickle shape of RBCs and therefore includes co-inheritance of Hb S with another qualitative or quantitative beta globin chain defect, such as in Hb C or β^+-thalassemia. However, sickle cell anemia is specifically defined as the state when Hb S is the only hemoglobin present, such as in homozygous Hb S (Hb SS) or when co-inherited with a null beta globin mutation (Hb $S\beta^0$-thalassemia). Sickle cell trait is defined as inheritance of the Hb S from one parent, but a normal Hb A gene from the other. RBCs from people with sickle cell trait do not sickle and these individuals are largely unaffected.

EPIDEMIOLOGY

Nearly 50 years after the first report of Hb S was made, an association was suggested between the presence of the genetic mutation and a favorable resistance against malaria. Comprehensive analysis of the global Hb S allele frequency compared with the distribution of malaria endemicity supports the hypothesized protective effect of those with sickle cell trait.[3]

It is thus not surprising that the highest prevalence of Hb S in the world remains in sub-Saharan Africa with the Middle East and Indian subcontinents as close seconds.[4] For each World Health Organization region, annual rates of neonates born with SCD are estimated at 230,000 in the African Region, 43,000 in the South-East Asia Region, 13,000 in the Region of the Americas, 10,000 in the Eastern Mediterranean Region, 3500 in the European Region, and 4 in the Western Pacific Region per year.[5] Although analyses of the β^S haplotypes suggest that the Hb S allele arose independently at least 5 times in Africa and the Middle East/India,[6] SCD has been reported in persons who self-identify as Hispanic, Caucasian, Native American, and Asian, presumably owing to immigration patterns.[7,8] The global burden of SCD is increasing and is expected to continue increasing for the foreseeable future.[9]

PATHOPHYSIOLOGY

Given the heterogeneity in severity of SCD, it is amazing to recognize that the disease arises from a single point mutation. This mutation occurs in the sixth codon of the β-globin gene where adenine is substituted with thymine, thereby encoding a valine in place of glutamic acid in the β-globin chain. This solitary amino acid swap confers a significant impact on the stability of the resulting hemoglobin molecule and on the function of the RBC as a whole. An in-depth review of the pathophysiology of SCD is outside the scope of this article, especially given that several excellent reviews of the topic have been recently published.[10–14]

Molecular Mechanisms

The concentration of Hb S within the RBC largely determines the extent to which the erythrocyte sickles. Indeed, as the erythrocyte concentration of Hb S nears 30 g/dL, a semisolid gel forms within the cell.[15] In a deoxygenated state, Hb S can form individual or aggregated fibers that lead to RBC elongation and rigidity.[16] This formation is driven directly by the substituted valine residue that binds to a hydrophobic pocket between a phenylalanine and leucine residue at the 85th and 88th position in the neighboring β-globin chain. In an oxygenated state, these polymers disintegrate.

The polymerization of Hb S itself reduces the affinity for oxygen and thereby stabilizes the deoxygenated form of the molecule. As such, oxygen concentration and the concentration of Hb S play a critical role in the formation and disintegration of Hb S polymers, as does the association of Hb S with other hemoglobin variants. Deoxygenated Hb S most readily polymerizes with itself and far less readily polymerizes with Hb A. It copolymerizes least effectively with fetal hemoglobin (Hb F), which likely stems from the nearly 20 surface amino acid differences between the 2 hemoglobin variants.[17] Comparatively, there is only a single residue difference between Hb S and Hb A. These findings were the rationale for seeking out therapies that increase Hb A (like RBC transfusion) and Hb F (like hydroxyurea) concentration in vivo, thus inhibiting polymerization and gel formation.

Variable propensity toward Hb S polymerization is insufficient to explain the clinical heterogeneity found among people with SCD. There is increasing evidence from studies in patients and mouse models of SCD that oxidative stress and inflammation is associated with SCD pathophysiology. Recent evidence suggests that sickle RBCs and RBC-derived microparticles initiate a cascade that activates neutrophils, monocytes, and platelets, which then secrete various cytokines and chemokines. Concurrently, chronic hemolysis liberates large amounts of cell-free hemoglobin, which then binds nitric oxide (NO), a potent vasodilator. Soluble cytokines, chemokines, and low NO levels then potentiate further inflammation, endothelial dysfunction, and eventually end-organ damage. As the role of oxidative stress and inflammation in SCD is better appreciated, pharmaceutical targets that counteract these mechanisms are currently in clinical trials, as discussed later in this article.[12,18]

Cellular Mechanisms

Although the polymerization of Hb S is the sine qua non of SCD, RBC membrane changes drive many of the clinical manifestations of the disease.[19] Changes affect both lipid and protein components of the RBC membrane and alter how sickled RBCs interact with white blood cells, platelets, and the vascular endothelium. The composition of the lipids is significantly altered as deoxygenation causes loss of membrane, evidenced by increased circulation of RBC-derived microparticles, and gives rise to the greater presence of negatively charged phosphatidyl serine on the outer lipid monolayer.[19] This critical change is thought to augment the conversion of prothrombin to thrombin and thereby increase the rate of thrombotic events in these patients.[19] At the same time, key protein changes occur on endothelial cells, including upregulation of several adhesion molecules, including E-selectin, P-selectin, and VCAM.[20] As discussed later, these molecules have recently been exploited as potential pharmaceutical targets in the mitigation of SCD symptoms. Based on these observations, sickled erythrocytes are 2 to 10 times more adherent to the endothelium than normal RBCs contributing to the vasculopathy that is observed in SCD.[21]

Membrane injury also contributes to the pathologic intravascular and extravascular hemolysis that accompanies the disease. Intravascular hemolysis is driven by further fragmentation of an already damaged membrane through shear forces generated as deformed erythrocytes pass through the microvasculature. Furthermore, clustering of membrane protein band 3 leads to the aberrant accumulation of both immunoglobulin G (IgG) and complement on the erythrocyte surface, which in turn can lead to complement-mediated RBC destruction.[22] Extravascular hemolysis is mediated by splenic and tissue macrophages and monocytes that recognize damaged RBCs and remove them from circulation.[23] As noted, the free hemoglobin that results from chronic hemolysis binds NO, further contributing to vasoconstriction and vasculopathy.

The culmination of Hb S polymerization, increased viscosity of sickle blood, increased adherence of aberrant cells to the endothelium, oxidative stress, and inflammation all give rise to one of the defining features of SCD: vaso-occlusive events. The wide variability of the triggers, including the absence of a known trigger, demonstrates that multiple mechanisms can drive them. White cell elevation, increased platelet activation, or increased von Willebrand factor release by the endothelium can all play a role.[24] Indeed, increased white cell counts in patients with SCD have been associated with increased mortality, silent brain infarcts, hemorrhagic strokes, and acute chest syndrome.[25–28] With each of these contributors, it is no surprise that patients with SCD are thought to exist in a state of chronic inflammation with elevated inflammatory biomarkers like C-reactive protein and erythrocyte sedimentation rate as well as increased inflammatory cytokines.[29]

DISEASE SEVERITY AND PROGNOSIS

SCD is truly a systemic condition, with well-described complications affecting virtually every organ (**Table 1**). However, polymerization of Hb S is insufficient to explain the clinical heterogeneity of SCD. Genotype-phenotype association studies have identified co-inherited, genetic modifiers that can modulate complications seen in SCD. The most studied is hereditary persistence of fetal hemoglobin, in which several known alleles prevent the physiologic switch from fetal to adult hemoglobin that ordinarily occurs shortly after birth. Individuals with this genotype have approximately 20% Hb F in each sickle RBC and are either asymptomatic or have mild hematologic findings for their entire life span.[30] Co-inheritance of α-thalassemia also ameliorates some complications by reducing the concentration of Hb S.[31] Newer studies have identified or validated the association between other genes and specific subphenotypes of SCD. For example, polymorphisms of *UGT1A1*, the gene that codes for UDP-glucuronosyltransferases and is thus responsible for conjugating bilirubin, is strongly associated with cholelithiasis risk in SCD.[31]

Within the past decade, the potential life span of SCD has markedly improved in large part as a result of newborn screening, immunizations, improved detection and treatment of infection, and disease-modifying medications like hydroxyurea.[35] In regions without such comprehensive care, however, death remains a reality in early childhood.

In infants and young children in the United States, mortality rates have declined in the past 20 years with the greatest impact seen in children aged zero to 3 years who had a 68% reduction in mortality.[36] Improvements in vaccination, especially with the pneumococcal vaccine, and prophylactic and therapeutic antibiotics likely account for this improved survival. Today, 94% of children with SCD in the United States will survive to adulthood.[35]

Although increased survival to adulthood is certainly progress, people with SCD die at a much younger age than race-matched peers. The overall median survival is 58 years.[37] Adolescents and young adults in the second and third decades of life suffer significant morbidity with higher rates of SCD-related complications and higher health care costs.[38] This is in part due to observations showing that these young adult patients receive fewer transfusions and are less likely to be on hydroxyurea and/or chelation therapy when eligible for such treatments as they transition from pediatric to adult care.[38] The most common cause of death is cardiac, respiratory, renal, infectious, neurologic, gastrointestinal, and hepatobiliary disease in descending order.[39] Leukocytosis remains a key predictor of poor outcome along with renal insufficiency, recurrent episodes of acute chest syndrome, low Hb F concentration, severe anemia, higher rates of hemolysis, and dactylitis before 1 year of age.[25,40,41]

Table 1
Acute and chronic complications of sickle cell disease

Clinical Feature	Description	Preventive Measures	Specific Therapeutic Measures
Acute complications			
Vaso-occlusive crisis • Pain • Dactylitis	Typically acute, localized, severe pain, but can be gradual	HU, hydration, knowledge about personal triggers	Analgesics, namely NSAIDs and opioids
Bacteria/sepsis	Bloodborne bacterial infection resulting from functional asplenia	Prophylactic antibiotics such as penicillin, vaccinations	Therapeutic antibiotics
Acute renal failure	Acute increase in serum creatinine and/or decreased GFR due to infarction of renal tissue	Annual screening for proteinuria starting at age 10, minimizing nephrotoxic drugs and agents	Renal replacement therapy, such as hemodialysis
Priapism	A sustained, unwanted painful erection lasting 4 or more hours	Exercise, masturbation, hyperhydration, and HU may prevent escalation of symptoms	Oral or intravenous hydration, analgesia, and emergent urologic consult for possible sympathomimetic injection, shunt or aspiration
Hepatobiliary complications	Cholelithiasis, cholecystitis, biliary sludge, choledocholithiasis, acute hepatic sequestration (AHS), acute intrahepatic cholestasis (AIC) due to chronic hemolysis and organ damage	Routine monitoring; early AHS and AIC symptoms may be treated with hydration, rest, and close observations	Surgical consultation for symptomatic gall bladder disease
Acute anemia • Splenic or hepatic sequestration • Aplastic crisis • Hyperhemolysis	Acute-on-chronic anemia due to sequestration, hypoproduction, or destruction	Monitor trend of CBC and reticulocyte count during illnesses and hospitalizations	Emergent consultation of SCD expert for transfusion guidelines
Acute chest syndrome	Sudden onset of lower respiratory tract disease and new pulmonary infiltrate on chest radiograph triggered by, for example, infection, fat embolus, pulmonary edema	HU, incentive spirometry, and judicious use of IV fluids during all hospitalizations	IV cephalosporin, PO macrolide antibiotic, supplemental oxygen, and possible transfusion

(continued on next page)

Table 1
(continued)

Clinical Feature	Description	Preventive Measures	Specific Therapeutic Measures
Acute stroke	Focal neurologic or acute altered mental status due to intracerebral ischemia or, less commonly, hemorrhage	TCD annually for children; chronic transfusions for those with elevated risk identified on TCD; HU for those with normal MRI and TCD after 1 y of transfusions	Chronic transfusions indefinitely
Multisystem organ failure	Severe and life-threatening complication characterized by failure of the lungs, liver, and/or kidneys	Routine health care to maintain organ health, rapid diagnosis, and treatment to prevent death	Exchange transfusion
Acute ocular conditions	Trauma, infection, vaso-occlusive episodes leading to occlusion of the eye vasculature, or progression of proliferative sickle retinopathy	Annual or bi-annual dilated fundal examinations by an ophthalmologist starting at age 10 years	Immediate referral to eye specialist capable of performing a dilated eye examination to assess visual acuity, intraocular pressure, and the peripheral retina
Chronic complications			
Chronic pain	Severe pain that can be either localized or systemic	Treatment of pain-related depression, anxiety, or insomnia	Analgesics, namely NSAIDs and opioids
Vascular necrosis	Compromised blood supply leading to bone death most commonly at the hip joint	Routine monitoring of pain with early imaging as needed	Analgesics with physical therapy and orthopedic support; joint replacement
Leg ulcers	Skin and soft tissue erosion that can give way to cellulitis or osteomyelitis from diminished blood flow	Regular physical examination, pressure-release devices in bed-bound patients	Debridement, wet to dry dressings, systemic or local antibiotics for culture-proven bacterial infection

Pulmonary hypertension	Restriction of the pulmonary arteries leading to an increased mean pulmonary arterial pressure	Consider diagnostic testing for patients with exercise intolerance, fatigue, peripheral edema, or chest pain	Supplemental oxygen, diuretics, HU, chronic transfusion therapy, pulmonary vasodilator therapy in symptomatic patients
Renal complications	Development of proteinuria, nephrotic syndrome, and hypertension due to vaso-occlusive events at the renal microvasculature	Regular assessment of creatinine, GFR, and screening for proteinuria and microalbuminuria	ACE inhibitor or ARB for proteinuria, transfusion therapy or EPO infusions for anemia, dialysis in ESRD
Stuttering/recurrent priapism	Multiple unwanted, painful erections lasting less than 4 h combined with prolonged priapism	HU, pseudoephedrine, chronic blood transfusions	Analgesia, urology consult, self-injection of an alpha agonist
Ophthalmologic complications	Development of proliferative sickle retinopathy or vitreous hemorrhage	Dilated fundal examinations starting at age 10 y and every 1–2 y thereafter	Consult to ophthalmology for consideration of laser therapy
Fertility complications	Development of hypogonadism, sperm abnormalities, erectile dysfunction	Iron chelation if iron overloaded	Hormone therapy

Abbreviations: ACE, angiotensin-converting enzyme; AHS, acute hepatic sequestration; AIC, acute intrahepatic cholestasis; ARB, angiotensin receptor blockers; CBC, complete blood count; EPO, erythropoietin; ESRD, end-stage renal disease; GFR, glomerular filtration rate; HU, hydroxyurea; IV, intravenous; NSAID, nonsteroidal anti-inflammatory; PO, per os; SCD, sickle cell disease; TCD, transcranial Doppler.
Data from Refs.[32–34]

MANAGEMENT

Ideally, people with SCD are served through a multidisciplinary, comprehensive clinic where symptom management and tracking can be combined with patient and family education and empowerment.[42] However, in reality, such centers are rarely available to patients, even in developed countries. Regardless, it is of utmost importance that patients are educated on infection prevention, pain management, and early detection of complications and that a clinician with expertise in sickle cell be available for consultation in-person or by telephone. Genetic counseling and psychosocial support are pivotal at all stages of development and into adulthood. At the same time, routine clinical visits allow for the acquisition of baseline laboratories that can help differentiate crisis events.

Infection Prevention

Functional asplenia can occur at an early age, putting patients at risk for infection by encapsulated organisms. As a result, maintaining updated immunizations and routine prophylactic penicillin for all children younger than 5 years is paramount to prevent poor outcomes associated with these infections. All people with SCD should be vaccinated against *Streptococcus pneumoniae*, *Neisseria meningitidis*, and *Haemophilus influenzae* type B, as well as for hepatitis B virus and seasonal influenza in addition to all other standard vaccines.[43–45] It is equally important to educate patients of all ages and their families to seek medical care should they develop signs of infection, for example, for any temperature higher than 101.3°F or 38.5°C due to the risk for bacterial infections.[32]

Red Blood Cell Transfusions

Given the integral role that Hb S concentration plays in the development of vaso-occlusive events and vasculopathy in SCD, RBC transfusions have potential to improve quality and quantity of life. Transfusions work to raise Hb A concentration and reduce the concentration of Hb S through dilution by donor RBCs.[46] The administration of a transfusion also suppresses endogenous erythropoietin production and subsequently reduces the formation of new RBCs containing Hb S.[47]

Indications for transfusion are summarized in **Table 2**. In general, RBCs can be given acutely as first-line treatment for life-threatening complications or as part of a chronic transfusion program, where RBCs are transfused at regularly scheduled intervals based on symptoms or laboratory tests to prevent initial occurrence or recurrence of complications. Although never prospectively studied, a common goal in prophylactic transfusions is to maintain a percent Hb S of less than 30% of the total hemoglobin while at the same time achieving an overall hemoglobin concentration that increases oxygen carrying capacity without putting the patient at risk for hyperviscosity.[48] Alternatively, especially when transfusing a compound heterozygous hemoglobinopathy such as Hb SC disease, a goal can be to achieve Hb A of greater than 70%. Determination of the frequency of transfusions is then dependent on close observation of the patient's total hemoglobin concentration, percent Hb S, and reticulocyte count, as well as the serum ferritin given the risk for iron overload from frequent transfusions.

Once the decision has been made to instate a prophylactic transfusion regimen, RBCs can be delivered as either a simple transfusion or an exchange transfusion. The former involves delivery of one or more units of RBCs without removing any of the patient's own blood. This method of transfusion can be used when the goal is to improve oxygen carrying capacity or during acute episodes of anemia when the

Table 2
Indications for transfusion therapy in sickle cell disease

Clinical Complication	Transfusion Method
Established indications[a]	
Acute ischemic stroke	Simple or exchange transfusion[b]
Primary stroke prevention following elevated velocities on transcranial Doppler studies	Chronic simple or exchange transfusion[c]
Secondary stroke prevention	Chronic simple or exchange transfusion[c]
Acute chest syndrome	Simple or exchange transfusion
Acute anemia • Acute splenic sequestration • Acute hepatic sequestration • Acute aplastic crisis	Simple transfusion
Acute multiorgan failure	Simple or exchange transfusion[b]
Acute intrahepatic cholestasis	Simple or exchange transfusion[b]
Before general anesthesia[d]	Simple or exchange transfusion[b]
Acute sickle or obstetric complication during pregnancy	Simple or exchange transfusion[b]
Controversial indications	
Recurrent acute chest syndrome	Chronic simple or exchange transfusion[c]
Recurrent vaso-occlusive episodes	Chronic simple or exchange transfusion[c]
Pulmonary hypertension	Chronic simple or exchange transfusion[c]
Relative contraindications	
Uncomplicated vaso-occlusive episodes	N/A
Priapism	N/A
Recurrent splenic sequestration	N/A
Uncomplicated pregnancy	N/A
Leg ulcers	N/A
Nonsurgical avascular necrosis	N/A

Abbreviations: N/A, not applicable.

[a] Either by studies or expert consensus.

[b] Decision as to whether to do an acute simple versus exchange transfusion may depend on urgency, patient's overall hemoglobin level, availability of erythrocytapheresis, and number of available compatible red blood cell units, etc. For example, if a patient's hemoglobin level is near his or her baseline, an exchange transfusion, if available, may be best to maximize effectiveness but minimize risk of hyperviscosity.

[c] Decision as to whether to do a chronic simple versus exchange transfusion may depend on patient's iron overload status and preference.

[d] As per the Transfusion Alternatives Preoperatively in Sickle Cell Disease study, homozygous hemoglobin S (Hb SS) patients undergoing medium-risk surgeries should be transfused preoperatively to achieve a total hemoglobin level of ~10 g/dL to minimize risk of adverse risks, namely acute chest syndrome.[50]

Data from Refs.[32,48–50]

risk of posttransfusion hyperviscosity is low. By contrast, for a patient whose hemoglobin is near their baseline, a simple transfusion may not dilute Hb S to any clinically significant extent and may put the patient at risk of hyperviscosity.[48]

Exchange transfusion relies on the removal of the patient's blood and replacing it with allogeneic RBCs. This intervention more rapidly reduces the concentration of Hb S toward a typical goal of less than 30% of the total hemoglobin. In the setting of a critically ill patient, exchange transfusion is always preferred over a simple transfusion, as it more efficiently removes Hb S.[51,52] For patients on a chronic transfusion regimen, such as those undergoing primary or secondary stroke prophylaxis, exchange transfusion may be preferred to mitigate iron overload and hyperviscosity. A total exchange of the patient's blood volume can be done either manually or by erythrocytapheresis, with the latter being a more effective approach to exchanging larger blood volumes and thus more rapidly reducing the concentration of Hb S.[53] However, erythrocytapheresis requires specialized personnel and equipment, more units of compatible RBCs, and requires a dialysis catheter or 2 large-bore peripheral intravenous (IV) lines.

Although RBC transfusions are life-saving, there are associated risks. Complications more specific to SCD include high rates of alloimmunization and iron overload. Of SCD patients who have been transfused, 6% to 85% are alloimmunized.[32,54] Alloantibodies to the Rh antigens (namely C and E) and Kell are most frequent.[48,54] Multiple factors have been proposed to explain this high rate of alloimmunization, including frequent transfusions, disparate blood group genetics between donors and recipients, chronic inflammation, co-inheritance of a yet-unidentified immunoregulatory element, or an entity intrinsic to the β^S-globin gene itself.[55,56] As alloimmunized patients tend to have poorer outcomes,[57] extended phenotype matching for C, c, E, e, and Kell is often used to decrease the rate of alloimmunization.[58–60] However, extended phenotype matching has not abrogated alloimmunization completely,[55,61] so many transfusion and donor blood centers obtain RBC or Rh genotyping for patients with SCD and potential donors.[62] Ongoing research will determine whether molecular matching further reduces alloimmunization when weighed against the resultant increased difficulty in finding such highly matched units.

Iron Chelation

With each unit of RBCs introducing 200 to 250 mg of elemental iron into the body, the risk for iron overload is high and can give rise to significant morbidity through the development of hepatic, cardiac, or endocrine impairment. This emphasizes the importance of iron chelation therapy as an adjunct to any transfusion-based treatment regimen. Few studies have investigated the mortality and morbidity of long-term iron chelation in people with SCD[63]; however, data substantiate that iron chelation ameliorates complications induced by otherwise untreated elevated iron stores.[64–66]

In chronically transfused patients, liver iron stores should be quantified regularly. Serum ferritin is a rough estimation of body iron stores and is typically obtained quarterly. Accuracy of ferritin in estimating iron stores is confounded by chronic inflammation, which, as previously discussed, is commonly found in patients with SCD. Liver biopsy is the gold-standard method to quantitate iron burden, but is invasive and therefore giving way to newer, noninvasive techniques such as quantitative R2* or T2* MRI and, although very limited in its availability, superconducting quantum interference device (SQUID, also known as a ferrometer).[67–69] Chelation therapy can be considered when liver iron concentration is ≥ 7 mg Fe/g dry weight as measured by liver biopsy or quantitative MRI.[48] Serum ferritin can be used to monitor effectiveness of chelation. Based on cardiac MRI studies, myocardial iron loading appears to happen at higher serum iron concentrations than in thalassemia.[70]

Three iron chelators are currently commercially available in the United States: deferoxamine, deferiprone, and deferasirox. No head-to-head trial compares the efficacy and safety of these 3 drugs in SCD. As a result, local experience, availability and cost of each chelator, age of the patient, drug side effects, patient comorbidities, and preference largely inform the decision of what agent to initiate. Although it is typically well tolerated, deferoxamine requires a daily subcutaneous infusion that can be difficult for patients to manage long-term. As such, deferiprone and deferasirox are often preferred long-term by patients despite both having black box warnings in the United States about potentially fatal adverse effects.[71,72]

Hydroxyurea

Once it was observed that fetal hemoglobin ameliorates SCD severity, pharmacologic drivers of Hb F have been sought. Hydroxyurea induces Hb F by recruiting a population of erythroid precursors that can continue γ-chain synthesis into adulthood and that otherwise remain quiescent in the marrow unless conscripted in times of RBC expansion.[73] The Multicenter Study of Hydroxyurea (MSH) was the seminal randomized control trial of hydroxyurea that demonstrated a reduction of vaso-occlusive events by nearly 50%.[74] It also showed an increase in total hemoglobin and Hb F and a reduction in the incidence of acute chest syndrome, transfusion requirement, and mortality when compared with those on placebo.[74–77] Additional studies have confirmed the tolerance of the medication and demonstrated its safety when taken over many years.[75,76,78]

Although hydroxyurea initially entered clinical trials because it increased Hb F, ongoing research suggests that it minimizes complications of SCD through multiple mechanisms. The medication augments the release of NO, which in turn, upregulates genes, such as BCL11A, which synchronize fetal hemoglobin transcription.[79,80] By increasing circulating NO, hydroxyurea can improve pulmonary blood flow and reduce the risk of pulmonary hypertension in SCD.[81–83] The medication can also directly increase the expression of the secretion-associated and ras-related signaling protein (SAR1), which further activates expression of γ-globin genes.[84] By increasing the mean corpuscular volume of RBCs, hydroxyurea improves cellular deformability and rheology.[42] Last, hydroxyurea is also thought to reduce chronic inflammation and thrombosis risk through reductions in neutrophil and platelet counts and decreased RBC adhesion molecule expression.[74,85]

Hydroxyurea is indicated for adult patients with SCD who have 3 or more pain episodes within a 12-month period. However, efficacy and safety data are reassuring for its use in adults with history of substantial pain, acute chest syndrome, or symptomatic anemia and is thus generally recommended for these indications despite a lack of an indication approved by the Food and Drug Administration (FDA).[32,86] Although a chronic RBC transfusion program is indicated following a stroke, some sources suggest that hydroxyurea is acceptable when chronic transfusions cannot be used.[86,87]

Although current evidence does not suggest one implantation protocol over another, it is highly recommended that a standard protocol be followed to ensure efficacy and safety.[32] One protocol based on expert consensus recommends starting adults at 15 mg/kg (rounding to the closest 500-mg capsule) after fertility counseling and baseline laboratory tests (complete blood count [CBC] with differential, quantitative Hb F measurement, comprehensive metabolic profile, and pregnancy test for women) have been obtained and increasing as tolerated to a maximum tolerated dose.[32] A CBC with differential and reticulocyte count should be obtained every 4 weeks while adjusting the dose or every 2 to 3 months once on a stable dose. Every protocol should include criteria for when to hold hydroxyurea, such as for an absolute neutrophil count of less than 2000/µL or platelet count less than 80,000/µL. If hydroxyurea is held for toxicities, the drug should be restarted once the patient is back to baseline at a lower dose than previous (such as 20% or 5 mg/kg less). Maximum dose is typically 35 mg/kg, but minimum effective dose or fixed-dose strategies have been used depending on patient characteristics and access to medical care.[32,88,89] A clinical response may be evident only after 3 to 6 months of daily adherence, so a repeat quantitative Hg F measurement may be obtained then, but hydroxyurea should be continued even if Hb F does not increase.[32] Hydroxyurea should be continued during hospitalization and illnesses.[32] Especially for adolescents and young adults, adherence should be discussed at every appointment and various strategies discussed to maximize adherence, including use of alarm clocks and medication apps on mobile devices, for example.[90,91]

Cytopenias are the most common side effect with use of hydroxyurea but are generally mild and readily reversible. Other reported side effects include gastrointestinal disturbances, skin and nail changes, and leg ulcers, although the causative association remains unproven. Greater concerns surround the potential genotoxicity of hydroxyurea, including birth defects, infertility, and cancer. MSH long-term follow-up studies and in vivo and ex vivo studies have not substantiated these concerns to date.[86,92-95]

Hematopoietic Stem Cell Transplantation

Although RBC transfusions and hydroxyurea play an important role in the treatment of SCD, their primary impact is a reduction in morbidity and mortality. The only potential cure for the disease is hematopoietic stem cell transplantation (HSCT), but this more aggressive intervention comes with risks and barriers to its use, particularly for adult patients.

Pediatric trials using HLA-matched siblings as donors show promising results.[96,97] and trials using matched, unrelated donors are under way. Although the data for HSCT in adults with SCD is more limited, 2 series that evaluated patients older than 16 show good outcomes with overall disease-free survival at 93% and 97%, with a median time to follow-up of 3.4 years in both studies.[97,98] Despite these outcomes, the risk of graft-versus-host disease and failure to engraft is relatively high, and must be weighed against the risk of untransplanted SCD.[96] New studies, including large consortium studies such as the Centre for International Blood and Marrow Transplant Research, are looking to the increasing role of reduced intensity conditioning regimens and haploidentical donors.[99-103]

Selection of the appropriate patient population to undergo HSCT has not been well defined. Until it has, HSCT is not feasible for most people with SCD.

Treatments in Development

Although hydroxyurea is the cornerstone of treatment for SCD and remains the only FDA-approved medication for its management, drugs aiming to target several other key elements of the complex pathophysiology of the disease are actively being investigated in human today.

As RBC and white cell adhesion to the vascular endothelium in an inflammatory state plays an important role in sponsoring SCD complications, several pipeline agents aim to impact this effect by targeting P-selectin and E-selectin–mediated adhesion.[104-106] The pan-selectin inhibitor, Rivipansel, demonstrated a reduction in the mean time to vaso-occlusive event resolution by 28%, as well as an 83% reduction in mean cumulative IV opioid analgesic use. A phase 3 study is currently under way.[107] A phase 1 single-center, double-blind, placebo-controlled study of a humanized monoclonal antibody specifically targeting P-selectin demonstrated an effective blockade of P-selectin for 1 month and was well tolerated, leading to the design of a phase 2 trial.[108] Increasing interest has recently focused on targets of the MEK and ERK pathways, which can impact the recruitment and activation of adhesion molecules.[87,88]

Targeting RBC adhesion in an entirely different manner is the investigational copolymer, Vepoloxamer, which aims to modulate RBC membrane surface tension by targeting hydrophobic domains exposed on injured RBC membranes. In early-phase studies, this agent decreased the duration of vaso-occlusive events especially in children or patients who were also being treated with hydroxyurea. A phase 3 clinical trial was recently completed.[109]

The propensity of Hb S to depolymerize in the oxygenated state makes hemoglobin oxygen affinity an attractive target. GBT440 is an investigational agent that reversibly binds to the α-globin chain and augments hemoglobin affinity for oxygen, an ability already native to Hb F.[110] A phase 1/2 study demonstrates reduced RBC hemolysis, improved anemia, and a significant reduction in circulating sickle cells in the peripheral blood of patients.[111]

Beyond these approaches, the holy grail of SCD treatment for the past 3 decades steadfastly remains gene correction therapy with the aim of introducing normal β-globin genes via a vector into hematopoietic stem cells. Current studies are cautiously evaluating the efficacy of a lentiviral vector in adults (NCT02247843 and NCT02186418). With the application of precision genome-editing tools, like clustered regularly interspaced short palindromic repeats or transcription activator-like effector nucleases, the application of gene therapy may become even more precise.[112]

Ultimately, with greater understanding of the complex mechanisms that underlie a disease so deceivingly driven by only a single point mutation, there is good reason to be hopeful for the development of new means by which to reduce the significant morbidity and mortality of SCD.

ACKNOWLEDGMENTS

The authors thank Ted Wun, MD, for reviewing the article and providing his insightful recommendations.

REFERENCES

1. Kohne E. Hemoglobinopathies: clinical manifestations, diagnosis, and treatment. Dtsch Arztebl Int 2011;108(31–32):532–40.
2. Serjeant GR. One hundred years of sickle cell disease. Br J Haematol 2010; 151(5):425–9.
3. Rees DC, Williams TN, Gladwin MT. Sickle-cell disease. Lancet 2010;376(9757): 2018–31.
4. Hassell KL. Population estimates of sickle cell disease in the U.S. Am J Prev Med 2010;38(4 Suppl):S512–21.
5. Piel FB. The present and future global burden of the inherited disorders of hemoglobin. Hematol Oncol Clin North Am 2016;30(2):327–41.
6. Gabriel A, Przybylski J. Sickle-cell anemia: A look at global haplotype distribution. Nature Education 2010;3(3):2. Available at: http://www.nature.com/scitable/topicpage/sickle-cell-anemia-a-look-at-global-8756219. Accessed August 18, 2016.
7. Shafer FE, Lorey F, Cunningham GC, et al. Newborn screening for sickle cell disease: 4 years of experience from California's newborn screening program. J Pediatr Hematol Oncol 1996;18(1):36–41.
8. Rogers ZR, Powars DR, Kinney TR, et al. Nonblack patients with sickle cell disease have African beta S gene cluster haplotypes. JAMA 1989;261(20):2991–4.
9. Piel FB, Hay SI, Gupta S, et al. Global burden of sickle cell anaemia in children under five, 2010-2050: modelling based on demographics, excess mortality, and interventions. PLoS Med 2013;10(7):e1001484.

10. Hay D, Atoyebi W. Update on sickle cell disease. Br J Hosp Med (Lond) 2016; 77(4):C55–9.
11. Gordeuk VR, Castro OL, Machado RF. Pathophysiology and treatment of pulmonary hypertension in sickle cell disease. Blood 2016;127(7):820–8.
12. Zhang D, Xu C, Manwani D, et al. Neutrophils, platelets, and inflammatory pathways at the nexus of sickle cell disease pathophysiology. Blood 2016;127(7): 801–9.
13. Paradowski K. Pathophysiology and perioperative management of sickle cell disease. J Perioper Pract 2015;25(6):101–4.
14. Wang W, Lukens J. Sickle cell anemia and other sickling syndromes. Wintrobe's clinical hematology. Philadelphia (PA): Lippincott Williams & Wilkins; 2009. p. 1038–82.
15. Dong C, Chadwick RS, Schechter AN. Influence of sickle hemoglobin polymerization and membrane properties on deformability of sickle erythrocytes in the microcirculation. Biophys J 1992;63(3):774–83.
16. Magdoff-Fairchild B, Swerdlow PH, Bertles JF. Intermolecular organization of deoxygenated sickle haemoglobin determined by x-ray diffraction. Nature 1972;239(5369):217–9.
17. Noguchi CT, Rodgers GP, Serjeant G, et al. Levels of fetal hemoglobin necessary for treatment of sickle cell disease. N Engl J Med 1988;318(2):96–9.
18. Silva DG, Belini Junior E, de Almeida EA, et al. Oxidative stress in sickle cell disease: an overview of erythrocyte redox metabolism and current antioxidant therapeutic strategies. Free Radic Biol Med 2013;65:1101–9.
19. Setty BN, Kulkarni S, Rao AK, et al. Fetal hemoglobin in sickle cell disease: relationship to erythrocyte phosphatidylserine exposure and coagulation activation. Blood 2000;96(3):1119–24.
20. Hebbel RP, Osarogiagbon R, Kaul D. The endothelial biology of sickle cell disease: inflammation and a chronic vasculopathy. Microcirculation 2004;11(2):129–51.
21. Hebbel RP, Yamada O, Moldow CF, et al. Abnormal adherence of sickle erythrocytes to cultured vascular endothelium: possible mechanism for microvascular occlusion in sickle cell disease. J Clin Invest 1980;65(1):154–60.
22. Test ST, Woolworth VS. Defective regulation of complement by the sickle erythrocyte: evidence for a defect in control of membrane attack complex formation. Blood 1994;83(3):842–52.
23. Kato GJ, Gladwin MT, Steinberg MH. Deconstructing sickle cell disease: reappraisal of the role of hemolysis in the development of clinical subphenotypes. Blood Rev 2007;21(1):37–47.
24. Conran N, Franco-Penteado CF, Costa FF. Newer aspects of the pathophysiology of sickle cell disease vaso-occlusion. Hemoglobin 2009;33(1):1–16.
25. Platt OS, Brambilla DJ, Rosse WF, et al. Mortality in sickle cell disease. Life expectancy and risk factors for early death. N Engl J Med 1994;330(23):1639–44.
26. Kinney TR, Sleeper LA, Wang WC, et al. Silent cerebral infarcts in sickle cell anemia: a risk factor analysis. The cooperative study of sickle cell disease. Pediatrics 1999;103(3):640–5.
27. Castro O, Brambilla DJ, Thorington B, et al. The acute chest syndrome in sickle cell disease: incidence and risk factors. The cooperative study of sickle cell disease. Blood 1994;84(2):643–9.
28. Ohene-Frempong K, Weiner SJ, Sleeper LA, et al. Cerebrovascular accidents in sickle cell disease: rates and risk factors. Blood 1998;91(1):288–94.
29. Rees DC, Gibson JS. Biomarkers in sickle cell disease. Br J Haematol 2012; 156(4):433–45.

30. Ngo DA, Aygun B, Akinsheye I, et al. Fetal haemoglobin levels and haematological characteristics of compound heterozygotes for haemoglobin S and deletional hereditary persistence of fetal haemoglobin. Br J Haematol 2012;156(2):259–64.
31. Steinberg MH, Sebastiani P. Genetic modifiers of sickle cell disease. Am J Hematol 2012;87(8):795–803.
32. National Heart, Lung, and Blood Institute. Evidence-based management of sickle cell disease: expert panel report. 2014. Available at: http://www.nhlbi.nih.gov/health-pro/guidelines/sickle-cell-disease-guidelines/. Accessed July 13, 2016.
33. Ware RE, Davis BR, Schultz WH, et al. Hydroxycarbamide versus chronic transfusion for maintenance of transcranial Doppler flow velocities in children with sickle cell anaemia—TCD With Transfusions Changing to Hydroxyurea (TWiTCH): a multicentre, open-label, phase 3, non-inferiority trial. Lancet 2016;387(10019):661–70.
34. Smith-Whitley K. Reproductive issues in sickle cell disease. Blood 2014;124(24):3538–43.
35. Quinn CT, Rogers ZR, McCavit TL, et al. Improved survival of children and adolescents with sickle cell disease. Blood 2010;115(17):3447–52.
36. Yanni E, Grosse SD, Yang Q, et al. Trends in pediatric sickle cell disease-related mortality in the United States, 1983-2002. J Pediatr 2009;154(4):541–5.
37. Elmariah H, Garrett ME, De Castro LM, et al. Factors associated with survival in a contemporary adult sickle cell disease cohort. Am J Hematol 2014;89(5):530–5.
38. Blinder MA, Vekeman F, Sasane M, et al. Age-related treatment patterns in sickle cell disease patients and the associated sickle cell complications and healthcare costs. Pediatr Blood Cancer 2013;60(5):828–35.
39. Hamideh D, Alvarez O. Sickle cell disease related mortality in the United States (1999-2009). Pediatr Blood Cancer 2013;60(9):1482–6.
40. Sebastiani P, Nolan VG, Baldwin CT, et al. A network model to predict the risk of death in sickle cell disease. Blood 2007;110(7):2727–35.
41. Miller ST, Sleeper LA, Pegelow CH, et al. Prediction of adverse outcomes in children with sickle cell disease. N Engl J Med 2000;342(2):83–9.
42. Claster S, Vichinsky EP. Managing sickle cell disease. Br Med J 2003;327(7424):1151.
43. Wong WY, Overturf GD, Powars DR. Infection caused by *Streptococcus pneumoniae* in children with sickle cell disease: epidemiology, immunologic mechanisms, prophylaxis, and vaccination. Clin Infect Dis 1992;14(5):1124–36.
44. Vernacchio L, Neufeld EJ, MacDonald K, et al. Combined schedule of 7-valent pneumococcal conjugate vaccine followed by 23-valent pneumococcal vaccine in children and young adults with sickle cell disease. J Pediatr 1998;133(2):275–8.
45. Marcinak JF, Frank AL, Labotka RL, et al. Immunogenicity of *Haemophilus influenzae* type b polysaccharide-diphtheria toxoid conjugate vaccine in 3- to 17-month-old infants with sickle cell diseases. J Pediatr 1991;118(1):69–71.
46. Nifong TP, Domen RE. Oxygen saturation and hemoglobin A content in patients with sickle cell disease undergoing erythrocytapheresis. Ther Apher 2002;6(5):390–3.
47. Wayne AS, Kevy SV, Nathan DG. Transfusion management of sickle cell disease. Blood 1993;81(5):1109–23.
48. Chou ST, Fasano RM. Management of patients with sickle cell disease using transfusion therapy: guidelines and complications. Hematol Oncol Clin North Am 2016;30(3):591–608.

49. DeBaun MR, Gordon M, McKinstry RC, et al. Controlled trial of transfusions for silent cerebral infarcts in sickle cell anemia. N Engl J Med 2014;371(8):699–710.

50. Howard J, Malfroy M, Llewelyn C, et al. The transfusion alternatives preoperatively in sickle cell disease (TAPS) study: a randomised, controlled, multicentre clinical trial. Lancet 2013;381(9870):930–8.

51. Hulbert ML, Scothorn DJ, Panepinto JA, et al. Exchange blood transfusion compared with simple transfusion for first overt stroke is associated with a lower risk of subsequent stroke: a retrospective cohort study of 137 children with sickle cell anemia. J Pediatr 2006;149(5):710–2.

52. Hassell KL, Eckman JR, Lane PA. Acute multiorgan failure syndrome: a potentially catastrophic complication of severe sickle cell pain episodes. Am J Med 1994;96(2):155–62.

53. Singer ST, Quirolo K, Nishi K, et al. Erythrocytapheresis for chronically transfused children with sickle cell disease: an effective method for maintaining a low hemoglobin S level and reducing iron overload. J Clin Apher 1999;14(3):122–5.

54. Rosse WF, Gallagher D, Kinney TR, et al. Transfusion and alloimmunization in sickle cell disease. The Cooperative Study of Sickle Cell Disease. Blood 1990; 76(7):1431–7.

55. Chou ST, Jackson T, Vege S, et al. High prevalence of red blood cell alloimmunization in sickle cell disease despite transfusion from Rh-matched minority donors. Blood 2013;122(6):1062–71.

56. Hendrickson JE, Zimring JC. Factors that regulate RBC alloimmunization: lessons from animal models, in AABB audioconference. Bethesda (MD): AABB; 2013.

57. Nickel RS, Hendrickson JE, Fasano RM, et al. Impact of red blood cell alloimmunization on sickle cell disease mortality: a case series. Transfusion 2016;56(1): 107–14.

58. Tahhan HR, Holbrook CT, Braddy LR, et al. Antigen-matched donor blood in the transfusion management of patients with sickle cell disease. Transfusion 1994; 34(7):562–9.

59. Vichinsky EP, Earles A, Johnson RA, et al. Alloimmunization in sickle cell anemia and transfusion of racially unmatched blood. N Engl J Med 1990;322(23):1617–21.

60. Vichinsky EP, Luban NL, Wright E, et al. Prospective RBC phenotype matching in a stroke-prevention trial in sickle cell anemia: a multicenter transfusion trial. Transfusion 2001;41(9):1086–92.

61. O'Suoji C, Liem RI, Mack AK, et al. Alloimmunization in sickle cell anemia in the era of extended red cell typing. Pediatr Blood Cancer 2013;60(9):1487–91.

62. Fasano RM, Chou ST. Red blood cell antigen genotyping for sickle cell disease, thalassemia, and other transfusion complications. Transfus Med Rev 2016; 30(4):197–201.

63. Maggio A. Light and shadows in the iron chelation treatment of haematological diseases. Br J Haematol 2007;138(4):407–21.

64. Brittenham GM. Iron-chelating therapy for transfusional iron overload. N Engl J Med 2011;364(2):146–56.

65. Lucania G, Vitrano A, Filosa A, et al. Chelation treatment in sickle-cell-anaemia: much ado about nothing? Br J Haematol 2011;154(5):545–55.

66. Jordan L, Adams-Graves P, Kanter-Washko J, et al. Multicenter COMPACT study of COMplications in patients with sickle cell disease and utilization of iron chelation therapy. Curr Med Res Opin 2015;31(3):513–23.

67. Harmatz P, Butensky E, Quirolo K, et al. Severity of iron overload in patients with sickle cell disease receiving chronic red blood cell transfusion therapy. Blood 2000;96(1):76–9.

68. Brittenham GM, Cohen AR, McLaren CE, et al. Hepatic iron stores and plasma ferritin concentration in patients with sickle cell anemia and thalassemia major. Am J Hematol 1993;42(1):81–5.
69. Fung E, Fischer R, Pakbaz Z, et al. The New SQUID biosusceptometer at Oakland: first year of experience. Neurol Clin Neurophysiol 2004;2004:5.
70. Badawy SM, Liem RI, Rigsby CK, et al. Assessing cardiac and liver iron overload in chronically transfused patients with sickle cell disease. Br J Haematol 2016. [Epub ahead of print].
71. Ferriprox [package insert]. 2011. Available at: http://www.accessdata.fda.gov/drugsatfda_docs/label/2011/021825lbl.pdf. Accessed August 19, 2016.
72. Jadenu [package insert]. 2016. Available at: https://www.pharma.us.novartis.com/sites/www.pharma.us.novartis.com/files/jadenu.pdf. Accessed August 19, 2016.
73. Xu J, Zimmer DB. Differential regulation of A gamma and G gamma fetal hemoglobin mRNA levels by hydroxyurea and butyrate. Exp Hematol 1998;26(3): 265–72.
74. Charache S, Terrin ML, Moore RD, et al. Effect of hydroxyurea on the frequency of painful crises in sickle cell anemia. Investigators of the multicenter study of hydroxyurea in sickle cell anemia. N Engl J Med 1995;332(20):1317–22.
75. Steinberg MH, McCarthy WF, Castro O, et al. The risks and benefits of long-term use of hydroxyurea in sickle cell anemia: a 17.5 year follow-up. Am J Hematol 2010;85(6):403–8.
76. Voskaridou E, Christoulas D, Bilalis A, et al. The effect of prolonged administration of hydroxyurea on morbidity and mortality in adult patients with sickle cell syndromes: results of a 17-year, single-center trial (LaSHS). Blood 2010; 115(12):2354–63.
77. Le PQ, Gulbis B, Dedeken L, et al. Survival among children and adults with sickle cell disease in Belgium: benefit from hydroxyurea treatment. Pediatr Blood Cancer 2015;62(11):1956–61.
78. Gilmore A, Cho G, Howard J, et al. Feasibility and benefit of hydroxycarbamide as a long-term treatment for sickle cell disease patients: results from the North West London sickle cell disease registry. Am J Hematol 2011;86(11):958–61.
79. Costa FC, da Cunha AF, Fattori A, et al. Gene expression profiles of erythroid precursors characterise several mechanisms of the action of hydroxycarbamide in sickle cell anaemia. Br J Haematol 2007;136(2):333–42.
80. Flanagan JM, Steward S, Howard TA, et al. Hydroxycarbamide alters erythroid gene expression in children with sickle cell anaemia. Br J Haematol 2012; 157(2):240–8.
81. Cokic VP, Smith RD, Beleslin-Cokic BB, et al. Hydroxyurea induces fetal hemoglobin by the nitric oxide-dependent activation of soluble guanylyl cyclase. J Clin Invest 2003;111(2):231–9.
82. Gladwin MT, Shelhamer JH, Ognibene FP, et al. Nitric oxide donor properties of hydroxyurea in patients with sickle cell disease. Br J Haematol 2002;116(2):436–44.
83. Nahavandi M, Tavakkoli F, Wyche MQ, et al. Nitric oxide and cyclic GMP levels in sickle cell patients receiving hydroxyurea. Br J Haematol 2002;119(3):855–7.
84. Zhu J, Chin K, Aerbajinai W, et al. Hydroxyurea-inducible SAR1 gene acts through the Gialpha/JNK/Jun pathway to regulate gamma-globin expression. Blood 2014;124(7):1146–56.
85. Styles LA, Lubin B, Vichinsky E, et al. Decrease of very late activation antigen-4 and CD36 on reticulocytes in sickle cell patients treated with hydroxyurea. Blood 1997;89(7):2554–9.

86. Wong TE, Brandow AM, Lim W, et al. Update on the use of hydroxyurea therapy in sickle cell disease. Blood 2014;124(26):3850–7 [quiz: 4004].

87. Bernaudin F, Verlhac S, Arnaud C, et al. Long-term treatment follow-up of children with sickle cell disease monitored with abnormal transcranial Doppler velocities. Blood 2016;127(14):1814–22.

88. Jain DL, Sarathi V, Desai S, et al. Low fixed-dose hydroxyurea in severely affected Indian children with sickle cell disease. Hemoglobin 2012;36(4):323–32.

89. Wang WC, Ware RE, Miller ST, et al. Hydroxycarbamide in very young children with sickle-cell anaemia: a multicentre, randomised, controlled trial (BABY HUG). Lancet 2011;377(9778):1663–72.

90. Badawy SM, Thompson AA, Liem RI. Technology access and smartphone app preferences for medication adherence in adolescents and young adults with sickle cell disease. Pediatr Blood Cancer 2016;63(5):848–52.

91. Walsh KE, Cutrona SL, Kavanagh PL, et al. Medication adherence among pediatric patients with sickle cell disease: a systematic review. Pediatrics 2014; 134(6):1175–83.

92. McGann PT, Flanagan JM, Howard TA, et al. Genotoxicity associated with hydroxyurea exposure in infants with sickle cell anemia: results from the BABY-HUG phase III clinical trial. Pediatr Blood Cancer 2012;59(2):254–7.

93. McGann PT, Howard TA, Flanagan JM, et al. Chromosome damage and repair in children with sickle cell anaemia and long-term hydroxycarbamide exposure. Br J Haematol 2011;154(1):134–40.

94. Ballas SK, McCarthy WF, Guo N, et al. Exposure to hydroxyurea and pregnancy outcomes in patients with sickle cell anemia. J Natl Med Assoc 2009;101(10):1046–51.

95. Berthaut I, Guignedoux G, Kirsch-Noir F, et al. Influence of sickle cell disease and treatment with hydroxyurea on sperm parameters and fertility of human males. Haematologica 2008;93(7):988–93.

96. Shenoy S. Hematopoietic stem-cell transplantation for sickle cell disease: current evidence and opinions. Ther Adv Hematol 2013;4(5):335–44.

97. Hsieh MM, Fitzhugh CD, Weitzel RP, et al. Nonmyeloablative HLA-matched sibling allogeneic hematopoietic stem cell transplantation for severe sickle cell phenotype. JAMA 2014;312(1):48–56.

98. Kuentz M, Robin M, Dhedin N, et al. Is there still a place for myeloablative regimen to transplant young adults with sickle cell disease? Blood 2011; 118(16):4491–2 [author reply: 4492–3].

99. Amado RG, Schiller GJ. Nonmyeloablative approaches to the treatment of sickle hemoglobinopathies. Semin Oncol 2000;27(2 Suppl 5):82–9.

100. Iannone R, Casella JF, Fuchs EJ, et al. Results of minimally toxic nonmyeloablative transplantation in patients with sickle cell anemia and beta-thalassemia. Biol Blood Marrow Transplant 2003;9(8):519–28.

101. Horan JT, Liesveld JL, Fenton P, et al. Hematopoietic stem cell transplantation for multiply transfused patients with sickle cell disease and thalassemia after low-dose total body irradiation, fludarabine, and rabbit anti-thymocyte globulin. Bone Marrow Transplant 2005;35(2):171–7.

102. Bolanos-Meade J, Fuchs EJ, Luznik L, et al. HLA-haploidentical bone marrow transplantation with posttransplant cyclophosphamide expands the donor pool for patients with sickle cell disease. Blood 2012;120(22):4285–91.

103. Dallas MH, Triplett B, Shook DR, et al. Long-term outcome and evaluation of organ function in pediatric patients undergoing haploidentical and matched related hematopoietic cell transplantation for sickle cell disease. Biol Blood Marrow Transplant 2013;19(5):820–30.

104. Zennadi R, Chien A, Xu K, et al. Sickle red cells induce adhesion of lymphocytes and monocytes to endothelium. Blood 2008;112(8):3474–83.

105. Chang J, Patton JT, Sarkar A, et al. GMI-1070, a novel pan-selectin antagonist, reverses acute vascular occlusions in sickle cell mice. Blood 2010;116(10): 1779–86.

106. Matsui NM, Borsig L, Rosen SD, et al. P-selectin mediates the adhesion of sickle erythrocytes to the endothelium. Blood 2001;98(6):1955–62.

107. Telen MJ, Wun T, McCavit TL, et al. Randomized phase 2 study of GMI-1070 in SCD: reduction in time to resolution of vaso-occlusive events and decreased opioid use. Blood 2015;125(17):2656–64.

108. Mandarino D, et al. Placebo-controlled, double-blind, first-in-human, ascending single dose and multiple dose, healthy subject study of intravenous-administered SelG1, a humanized anti-P-selectin antibody in development for sickle cell disease. Blood 2013;122(21):970.

109. Orringer EP, Casella JF, Ataga KI, et al. Purified poloxamer 188 for treatment of acute vaso-occlusive crisis of sickle cell disease: a randomized controlled trial. JAMA 2001;286(17):2099–106.

110. Oksenberg D, Dufu K, Patel MP, et al. GBT440 increases haemoglobin oxygen affinity, reduces sickling and prolongs RBC half-life in a murine model of sickle cell disease. Br J Haematol 2016;175:141–53.

111. Lehrer-Graiwer J, Howard J, Hemmaway CJ, et al. GBT440, a potent anti-sickling hemoglobin modifier reduces hemolysis, improves anemia and nearly eliminates sickle cells in peripheral blood of patients with sickle cell disease. Blood 2015;126(23):542.

112. Cottle RN, Lee CM, Bao G. Treating hemoglobinopathies using gene-correction approaches: promises and challenges. Hum Genet 2016;135(9):993–1010.

Syndromes of Thrombotic Microangiopathy

Joseph J. Shatzel, MD[a], Jason A. Taylor, MD, PhD[b],*

KEYWORDS

- Thrombotic thrombocytopenic purpura (TTP) • Hemolytic uremic syndrome (HUS)
- Microangiopathic hemolytic anemia (MAHA)
- Atypical hemolytic uremic syndrome (aHUS)
- Pregnancy induced microangiopathic hemolytic anemia
- Transplant induced microangiopathic hemolytic anemia

KEY POINTS

- The presence of thrombocytopenia and microangiopathic hemolytic anemia should prompt an acute work-up for thrombotic thrombocytopenic purpura (TTP) and consideration of immediate initiation of plasma exchange.
- Congenital TTP or atypical hemolytic uremic syndrome (HUS) should be considered in patients with recurrent episodes of TTP/HUS that do not have appropriate ADAMTS13 (a disintegrinlike and metalloprotease with thrombospondin type 1 Motifs 13) levels or detectable inhibitors.
- Eculizumab has been shown to be effective in improving renal function in atypical HUS.

INTRODUCTION

Thrombotic thrombocytopenic purpura (TTP) is a rare hematologic disorder (annual incidence of 11.3 cases per 1 million population), characterized by microangiopathic hemolytic anemia, thrombocytopenia, and varying levels of end-organ damage, including renal insufficiency, neurologic phenomena including stroke, and fever.[1–4] However, only a minority of patients with TTP present with all of the aforementioned features, often making the initial diagnosis challenging. There is no acute test to rule TTP in or out with enough speed and accuracy to safely guide initial therapy. Therefore the diagnosis is mostly a clinical one, based on the presence of thrombocytopenia and the characteristic findings of microangiopathic hemolysis on evaluation of the

[a] Division of Hematology and Medical Oncology, Knight Cancer Institute, Oregon Health & Science University, 3181 Southwest Sam Jackson Park Road, Portland, OR 97239, USA; [b] Division of Hematology and Medical Oncology, The Hemophilia Center, Portland VA Medical Center, Knight Cancer Institute, Oregon Health & Science University, 3181 Southwest Sam Jackson Park Road, L586, Portland, OR 97239, USA
* Corresponding author.
E-mail address: taylojas@ohsu.edu

Med Clin N Am 101 (2017) 395–415
http://dx.doi.org/10.1016/j.mcna.2016.09.010
0025-7125/17/Published by Elsevier Inc.

patient's blood smear, including the presence of schistocytosis, increased serum levels of lactate dehydrogenase (LDH), and decreased levels of haptoglobin with no other obvious cause.[5] The LDH level is often extremely increased and is a prognostic factor in TTP.[6] Other features, such as fever and neurologic sequela, are often absent or nonspecific, and cannot be relied on for routine diagnosis.[7] Thrombocytopenia may range from a mild decrease in platelet number to platelets being undetectable. The findings of thrombocytopenia with a normal prothrombin time helps eliminate disseminated intravascular coagulation (DIC) from the differential.[8]

TTP and the hemolytic uremic syndrome (HUS) have a spectrum of presentations and therapies, each unique to its specific pathophysiology. This article outlines the varying types of TTP/HUS by category, describing the current literature on their pathophysiology and therapy.

Classical Thrombotic Thrombocytopenic Purpura

Clinical presentation

Many patients with TTP first have a prodrome of a flulike or diarrheal illness. Patients can present with a variety of conditions ranging from general malaise to sudden death. The disease can strike at any age, although it predominantly occurs between 20 and 50 years of age, with women affected more than men in a 2:1 ratio.[9]

The classic reported pentad of fever, mental status changes, renal insufficiency, thrombocytopenia, and microangiopathic hemolytic anemia is only seen in a minority of patients.[10] As described later, the pentad can range in severity from mild to severe.

Neurologic

Neurologic complaints are present in more than half of patients on presentation and range from mild confusion to a stroke like syndrome.[11] In mild cases these symptoms must only be elicited through direct questioning. Patients often complain of tiredness, confusion, and headaches. Seizures were present in 9% of patients in one series, and may be recurrent.[11] Up to a quarter of patients develop transient focal neurologic defects, which may wax and wane over several hours.[11] MRI can show reversible posterior leukoencephalopathy.[12]

Hematologic

The initial diagnosis of TTP and other thrombotic microangiopathies (TMs) depends on the hematologic picture. By definition of the syndrome, patients are thrombocytopenic, because of the spontaneous aggregation of platelets and their deposition on damaged endothelial surfaces. The platelet count may range from 80,000/μL in mild cases of TTP to less than 1000/μL in severe cases. The median platelet count is generally 10,000 to 30,000/μL.[13] In mild cases of TTP, the thrombocytopenia is mistakenly ascribed to other causes and diagnosis is delayed. The platelet function is impaired because of continual platelet activation. Even though a seemingly adequate number of platelets are circulating, they are unable to support hemostasis, often leading to clinically significant bleeding with platelet counts that are not dramatically decreased.

The hematocrit in TTP is low because of hemolysis. Patients have clinical testing consistent with intravascular hemolysis: high reticulocyte counts, LDH level, and indirect bilirubin with low haptoglobin. Direct antibody (Coombs) test is negative. Review of the peripheral smear is diagnostic for microangiopathic hemolytic anemia. Clinicians should carefully examine the smear for red cell fragments. In very ill patients, rare schistocytes are often present, but in TTP and other TMs there is at least 1 red cell fragment per high-powered field. The presence of microangiopathic hemolytic anemia is the *sine qua non* for diagnosis of any TM. The LDH level is strikingly increased, often more than 2 to 4 times normal. The source of the LDH is not only lysed red cells. On fractionation, LDH fraction 5 and 4 are increased, suggesting damage beyond just the red cells.[14]

The patient's coagulation status can otherwise be normal. The markers of DIC, such as Fibrin Degradation Products (FDPs) and D-dimers, may be absent or present in only low titers (ie, 1–2 ng/dL).[15]

Renal
Patients with TTP often present with renal insufficiency and, unlike HUS, rarely renal failure. The creatinine level is usually only mildly to moderately increased. Often the urinalysis shows hemoglobinuria and mild proteinuria.[10,11]

Gastrointestinal
The most common gastrointestinal complaints are nausea, abdominal pain, and diarrhea, which are present in more than half of patients on presentation.[10] Patients rarely present with ileus and frank bowel necrosis from ischemia.[16] Very rarely pancreatitis caused by microvascular occlusion and small bowel infarction is also seen.[17]

Pulmonary
Although not classically described, patients occasionally present with pulmonary infiltrates and/or respiratory insufficiency consistent with acute respiratory distress syndrome.[18]

Cardiac
Patients often have signs of cardiac ischemia, including arrhythmias caused by myocardial microinfarctions.[19] Many patients who die of TTP have sudden death, suggesting that cardiac ischemia/infarction may play a prominent role in fatal cases.[20]

Pathogenesis
In the early 1980s the presence of ultralarge von Willebrand multimers in the plasma of patients with TTP was discovered, and a dysfunction of von Willebrand multimer cleavage was theorized to be the driver behind the syndrome.[21] These ultralarge von Willebrand multimers are secreted by endothelial cells, and anchored to their surface by P-selectin. Platelets adhere through glycoprotein (Gp) Ib and the GpIIb/GpIIIa complex to the A1 and A3 domains of the monomeric von Willebrand subunits. When these subunits polymerize unopposed in TTP, these very long von Willebrand multimers have increased avidity for platelets, forming large, occlusive thrombi.[7] In the mid-1990s it was discovered that a disintegrin-like and metalloprotease with thrombospondin type 1 motifs 13 (ADAMTS13) was responsible for regulating the length and, therefore, the thrombogenic potential of these von Willebrand multimers, by cleaving the peptide bonds in the A2 domain.[22–25]

Many patients with the classic form of TTP have an inhibitor against ADAMTS13, particularly in idiopathic cases, in which an inhibitor can be detected in 70% to 80% of cases.[3,7,26,27] Most commonly an immunoglobulin (Ig) G4 antibody, these inhibitors can block the proteolytic function of ADAMTS13, and increase the clearance of ADAMTS13 among other potential inhibitory functions.[28] Very low levels of ADAMTS13 caused by an inhibitory antibody is a negative prognostic factor.[29]

Although ADAMTS13 and associated inhibitor levels can be obtained, therapy should not be delayed while waiting for results due to high mortality. Untreated TTP is rapidly fatal. Mortality in the pre–plasma exchange era ranged from 95% to 100%.[30] Plasma exchange therapy is now the cornerstone of TTP treatment and has reduced mortality to less than 20%.[3,31–33] Plasma infusion is beneficial,[34] but plasma exchange has been shown to be superior.[31] Patients should immediately receive plasma exchange with 1 to 1.5 plasma volumes. If there is a delay in plasma exchange, then plasma should be infused at the rate of 1 unit every 4 to 6 hours until exchange. The American Society of Apheresis recommends daily therapy until platelet count greater than 150,000/μL for 2 consecutive days, a normal or near-normal LDH level, and stable or improving neurologic deficits are achieved.[35] Plasma exchange is presumed to work by replacing the deficient ADAMTS13 and removing inhibitory autoantibodies.[36] Glucocorticoid therapy should also be considered in the upfront management of TTP.[32] Prednisone 1 mg/kg/d, 1 to 2 mg/kg of methylprednisolone per day or 1 g of methylprednisolone initially for several days, may be given to patents presumed to have TTP.[3,32,37–39] There are prospective clinical trial data to suggest that high-dose steroids result in higher clinical remission rates.[39] Steroids should be tapered once the patient goes into remission.

The reported incidence of patients who do not respond to or relapse after the combination of plasma exchange and corticosteroids is high, and has been reported to be between 10% and 40%.[37] Several adjunctive treatment options exist for refractory or relapsed TTP in addition to plasma exchange and corticosteroids. Rituximab, a monoclonal antibody to CD20-positive B cells, has reported efficacy in several case series and is recommended by many investigators as the initial therapy of choice for refractory or relapsed disease.[40] Often given at a dose of 375 mg/m^2 once a week for 4 weeks, care must be taken if dosing the drug with plasma exchange because approximately 65% is removed with the exchange.[41] High response rates from rituximab have been reported in some series of refractory or severely relapsed TTP.[42] Other, less commonly used, therapeutic options for relapsed or refractory TTP that has progressed despite the use of steroids and/or rituximab include twice-daily plasma exchange,[43] cyclosporine,[44] cyclophosphamide, and vincristine,[45] or rarely splenectomy.[46] Emerging novel therapies for TTP are discussed in the end of the article.

CONGENITAL THROMBOTIC THROMBOCYTOPENIC PURPURA

Congenital TTP, also known as Upshaw-Schulman syndrome, is rare, and likely accounts for no more than 5% of cases of TTP with more than 100 cases reported to date.[13] Patients may present with classic TTP symptoms and have low levels of ADAMTS13, but no detectable inhibitor. Both Upshaw and Schulman described relapsing cases of TTP in the 1960 and 1970s, leading to speculation over congenital defects producing the disease phenotype.[47] In 2001 the mechanism was elucidated by Levy and colleagues[24] who showed mutations in ADAMTS13 that lead to significantly decreased von Willebrand factor–cleaving protease activity. The disease is transmitted in an autosomal dominant fashion, with more than 75 reported mutations to date.[48] Because of the rarity of the disease, no definitive correlation between genotype and disease phenotype or severity can be drawn.[48] The disease has a varying phenotype, and may present either in infancy or adulthood.[48] In infancy, congenital TTP may present as neonatal jaundice, or later in childhood with more typical symptoms.[49,50] Adult patients may be asymptomatic despite significantly low levels of ADAMTS13 activity, but can develop the disease phenotype after certain triggering events, including febrile illness, infections, vaccinations, alcohol use, and pregnancy.[34,51,52]

Congenital TTP should be considered in patients with clinical TTP who have a significantly low ADAMTS13 activity level, without a detectable inhibitor. Genetic testing is available and may be considered in direct relatives of the patient if a confirmatory mutation is discovered.[13]

Treatment of congenital TTP should be tailored to the patient's phenotype. Although plasma exchange may be used in the acute setting, plasma infusion (10–15 mL/kg) or infusion of a factor VIII concentrate containing ADAMTS13 can be given as needed, every 10 to 20 days, to achieve sustained hematologic response. The ultimate frequency of treatments depends on the patient's phenotype.[13] Some patients require very sparse plasma transfusions to maintain normal platelet and LDH values.

HEMOLYTIC UREMIC SYNDROME

Classically, HUS comprises the triad of renal failure, microangiopathic anemia, and thrombocytopenia.[53,54] Two major forms are recognized: a typical form, which occurs most commonly in young children with an antecedent bloody diarrheal illness, and the atypical, often compliment-mediated, form. Frank renal dysfunction is more common in HUS than in TTP.

Typical Hemolytic Uremic Syndrome

The term HUS was first proposed in 1955, but it was not until 1975 that the first associated organism, *Shigella dysenteriae* type 1, was described.[55,56] In 1983 it was discovered during an outbreak of hemorrhagic colitis that *Escherichia coli* O157:H7 was an associated pathogen as well.[57] It has since been found that multiple *E coli* strains produce the causative agent, Shiga toxin, including *E coli* O157:H7, O111:H8, O103:H2, O123, and O26.[58] Rarely HUS has been associated with other bacteria, including *Streptococcus pneumoniae*.[59] *E coli* O157:H7 is the most commonly associated pathogen in Europe and the Americas.[60] Typical HUS (also referred to as HUS D+, or diarrhea associated) generally occurs in children less than the age of 4 years, although cases in adolescents and adults may occur. Children often have a prodrome of diarrhea, which is usually bloody and often presents to medical attention because of symptoms of renal failure.[61,62] Thrombocytopenia is normally in the 50,000/µL range, with extrarenal involvement being common. Neurologic involvement can be seen in 40% of patients, with seizure being the predominant feature. Increased liver function tests are also seen in 40% of patients and 10% of patients also have pancreatitis.

Shiga toxin may provoke HUS through several mechanisms. It causes direct cell damage by binding to globotriaosylceramide (Gb3, also known as CD77 or ceramide trihexoside) on endothelial, renal mesangial, and epithelial cells, resulting in apoptosis.[63] Shiga toxin is also cell activating, leading to inflammatory signaling and release of von Willebrand factor from endothelial cells.[64]

The benefits of plasma exchange and anticomplement treatment are uncertain in classic HUS, and the primary treatment remains supportive.[63] Plasma exchange may be considered for severe cases or those with prominent extrarenal manifestations.[65] Hemodialysis may be required for patients with acute renal failure.[61] However, although most patients recover renal function, many patients have long-term renal damage.

Atypical Hemolytic Uremic Syndrome

Approximately 5% to 10% of cases of HUS are not preceded by diarrheal infection.[62,66] Dubbed atypical HUS (aHUS), in general this term has been applied to HUS without diarrheal infection. Extrarenal manifestations occur approximately 20% of the time.[67,68] Although nonspecific, inclusion criteria for clinical trials have included a serum creatinine level at or above the upper limit of the normal range, microangiopathic hemolytic anemia, thrombocytopenia, ADAMTS13 activity of 5% or more, and negative stool tests for Shiga toxin–producing infection.[69] The prognosis is worse than that of typical HUS, with mortalities as high as 25% being reported.[66,70] As described later, the disease is secondary to either genetic or autoimmune dysregulation of the alternative complement pathway. Rarely, disorders of innate anticoagulants or metabolism can also cause this syndrome.

The alternative complement pathway, unlike the classic or lectin pathways, is constitutively active because of spontaneous hydrolysis of C3, and is normally inactivated by factor H and factor I. The pathway leads to the assembly of the C5b-9 terminal complement complex (the membrane attack complex) on pathogens. The precise role of complement dysregulation in provoking HUS is not full elucidated, but it is thought that the formation of membrane attack complexes on endothelial cells as well as platelets, leading to platelet activation, is a major precipitant of the disease.[71]

Although hereditary cases of HUS had been described earlier, in 1981, 2 brothers were identified with deficiencies in the compliment regulatory protein factor H.[72] Their parents were first cousins and had normal levels of factor H. In 1998, genetic mutations specific to factor H leading to aHUS were established.[73] Since that time numerous mutations and autoimmune phenomena associated with complement-mediated HUS have been identified, as outlined here.

Complement Factor H Point Mutations

Complement factor H point mutations are the most commonly encountered mutations, accounting for 25% to 30% of cases of atypical HUS with more than 80 unique mutations identified, which are generally heterozygous.[62,66] In patients who carry the mutation, the disease may present at any age, and may not present at all in some individuals.[74] It may also present sporadically, or in familial clusters. Individuals with factor H mutations have excess lifetime cardiovascular mortality thought to be caused by atherosclerosis from chronic complement activation.[68,75] Patients with this mutation can rapidly progress to renal failure, with a high risk of relapse after renal transplant (75%–90%).[76,77] Overall, long-term survival is poor (50% at 10 years).[67]

Autoantibodies to Factor H

Autoantibodies to factor H are present in 6% to 10% of patients with atypical HUS, which generally presents in infancy or youth, almost always before age 16 years.[66,78] The clinical course is characterized by a high frequency of relapses. Progression to end-stage renal disease is observed in 20% to 35% of cases.[74] Relapsed aHUS can occur after renal transplant if autoantibodies are still present.[79]

Membrane Cofactor Protein

Membrane cofactor protein (also known as CD46) is a cofactor for complement factor I. Mutations leading to its dysregulation account for 10% to 15% of cases of aHUS.[67,80,81] Approximately 75% of mutations are heterozygous.[62] Clinical signs of aHUS often develop in childhood, with a fairly good renal prognosis and a low rate of relapse after renal transplant.[66]

Complement Factor B and C3 Convertase

Complement factor B and C3 convertase gain-of-function mutations have been reported in 1% to 2% and 4% to 10% of patients with aHUS respectively.[82,83] Patients with factor B mutations have a high rate of renal failure and relapse after transplant.[66]

Factor I

Factor I mutations occur in 3% to 10% of patients with aHUS.[84] The disease generally manifests in childhood and progresses to renal failure more than 50% of the time.[85] Recurrence after renal transplant is common, occurring in 45% to 80% of patients.[66]

Work-up of aHUS can be challenging. Patients who display laboratory signs of microangiopathic hemolysis and organ dysfunction, particularly renal failure, may be considered for a work-up to rule out the presence of Shiga toxin, including stool polymerase chain reaction, culture, and serologic testing including IgM against common Shiga toxin serotypes. The presence of a preceding diarrheal illness or current systemic infection should be investigated. If the patient later turns out to have intact levels of ADAMTS13, complement genotyping can be obtained from a variety of laboratories along with testing for factor H antibodies. This work-up should be considered in patients who fit the criteria, particularly those who developed aHUS at a young age, during pregnancy or postpartum, with recurrent episodes, or those with a positive family history.

Initial therapy for aHUS is plasma exchange but the effectiveness of this intervention is debatable, and may be varied based on the underlying complement defect.[67] At least 1 meta-analysis suggests that outcomes with plasma exchange may be similar to those of supportive care.[86] Nevertheless, guidelines suggest initiating plasma exchange within 24 hours with 1 to 2 plasma volumes per day or an infusion of 20 to 30 mL/kg of body weight.[87,88] Some reports suggest individuals with complement factor H mutations resulting in complete factor H deficiency can be treated with scheduled plasma infusion.[89] Patients with anti–factor H antibodies require immunosuppressive therapy in addition to plasma exchange.[78]

The compliment C5 inhibitor eculizumab has been shown to be effective in improving renal function in both native and transplanted kidneys in patients with complement-mediated aHUS.[90] The drug may also be effective as initial therapy in patients with antibodies to factor H.[91] Eculizumab should be started when aHUS is suspected, and, once therapy is started and the diagnosis is confirmed, patients need to stay on the drug because relapses can occur when the agent is stopped.[92] The hematologic changes respond rapidly but renal function improves over months. Eculizumab is associated with severe meningococcal infections, and thus vaccination against *Neisseria meningitidis*, *S pneumoniae*, and *Haemophilus influenzae* type b is recommended.

METABOLISM-MEDIATED MICROANGIOPATHY

Genetic disorders of cobalamin (vitamin B_{12}) can cause thrombotic microangiopathy, which most often presents in infancy but has been reported in a sole adult who did not respond to eculizumab.[93–95] The disorder generally results from homozygous mutations in the methylmalonic aciduria and homocystinuria type C protein (*MMACHC*) gene. Parenteral hydroxocobalamin is the main treatment of infants, whereas hydroxocobalamin, betaine, and folinic acid reportedly provided response in an adult patient. Neurologic sequel and renal disease are common in infants with this disease.[63]

COAGULATION-MEDIATED MICROANGIOPATHY

Mutations in the genes encoding plasminogen, thrombomodulin, protein kinase C–associated protein, and diacylglycerol kinase ε (DGKE), have all been reported in patients with thrombotic microangiopathy.[96–99] Thrombomodulin mutations may inhibit the ability of factor I to inhibit C3b, which leads to excessive complement activation.[66] DGKE mutations may result in protein kinase C activation, leading to upregulation of von Willebrand factor and tissue factor producing the disease state. The benefits of plasma infusion/exchange in these patients have been inconsistent, and many patients progress to end-stage renal disease.[63,100]

DRUG-RELATED THROMBOTIC MICROANGIOPATHY

Thrombotic microangiopathic syndromes have been associated with an extensive variety of drugs.[101,102] First recognized in the 1980s in a patient who developed kidney injury and microangiopathic hemolysis after taking quinine, it was later determined to be secondary to drug-dependent antibodies that cross react with multiple different cells, including platelets, neutrophils, and endothelial cells.[103–105] The second recognized drug association, and a more prevalent mechanism of drug-induced thrombotic microangiopathy, is the direct toxic tissue effects, which occur in a dose-dependent and time-dependent fashion. Common examples of offending drugs include the calcineurin inhibitors tacrolimus and cyclosporine, the antineoplastics gemcitabine and mitomycin, and others drugs including but not limited to quetiapine, sunitinib, bevacizumab, and clopidogrel. A good understanding of the mechanisms behind how these drugs produce microangiopathic hemolysis is lacking, as well as data on the safety of repeat exposure with many of these drugs. However, both gemcitabine and quetiapine have been shown to produce recurrent HUS with repeat exposure.[106,107]

Calcineurin inhibitors likely have directly toxic effects leading to endothelial dysfunction and increased platelet aggregation, possibly through the inhibition of prostacyclin.[63] Cyclosporine-associated or tacrolimus-associated microangiopathic hemolysis occurs within days of drug initiation, manifesting as a decreasing platelet count, decreasing hematocrit, and increasing serum LDH level.[102,108] Patients on calcineurin inhibitors for renal allografts often develop graft failure if HUS-like syndromes develop.[109] Some cases have been fatal but often the TTP/HUS resolves with decreasing the dose of the calcineurin inhibitor or changing to another agent.

Mitomycin C has a predilection for provoking TTP/HUS, with a frequency of 10% when a dose of more than 60 mg daily was used.[110] However, the most commonly used antineoplastic drug causing TTP/HUS is gemcitabine, with a reported incidence of between 0.015% and 4%.[110–114] As with mitomycin, the appearance of the TTP/HUS syndrome associated with gemcitabine can be delayed, and the condition often is fatal. Severe hypertension routinely precedes the clinical appearance of the TTP/HUS.[115] The use of plasma exchange is controversial.[116,117] There are increasing case reports of using eculizumab.[118–120]

TTP/HUS has been reported with other drugs, including the thienopyridines, ticlopidine and clopidogrel.[121,122] The frequency of ticlopidine-associated TTP may be as high as 1:1600 and, because this drug was often prescribed for patients with vascular disease, these patients may be initially misdiagnosed as having recurrent strokes or angina.[111,112] The frequency of TTP using clopidogrel is significantly less (0.0001%) but because it is widely prescribed it is the second most common cause of drug-induced TTP.[85] Almost all cases of clopidogrel-induced TTP occur within 2 weeks of starting the drug.

Plasma exchange is generally started as acute therapy for drug-induced TTP, because the underlying cause may not be known initially, although there are limited data on the benefits of this treatment. Supportive care and drug avoidance may be equally effective.[63]

STEM CELL TRANSPLANT–RELATED THROMBOTIC MICROANGIOPATHY

Allogeneic and autologous bone marrow transplant can be complicated by a thrombotic microangiopathic syndrome. The reported incidence varies widely in the literature from 0% to 74%, which is likely a reflection of poor understanding of the disease and a lack of standard definitions.[101,123,124] Rates are significantly higher with allogeneic transplant.[87,88] Risk factors include high-dose chemotherapy, radiation, unrelated donor, HLA mismatch, exposure to calcineurin inhibitors, graft-versus-host disease, and systemic infections.[125,126] The pathogenesis is thought to be secondary to direct endothelial damage and subsequent release of cytokines, whereas ADAMTS13 levels are generally unchanged.[127] Complement dysregulation in transplant-associated thrombotic microangiopathy has been suggested as well.[128,129] Mortalities are high, with reported rates up to 100%.[130]

Patients may present with fulminant multiorgan failure, which occurs early after transplant (eg, within 20–60 days), has multi–organ system involvement, is often fatal, and has been associated with severe cytomegalovirus (CMV) infection.[131] TTP/HUS can be directly caused by cyclosporine/tacrolimus. TTP/HUS that is associated with the conditioning regimen used in the transplant protocol can occur 6 months or more after total body irradiation, and is associated with primary renal involvement. In addition, patients with systemic CMV infections may present with a TTP/HUS syndrome related to vascular infection with CMV.[131]

The best management of hematopoietic stem cell transplant–related TTP/HUS is uncertain. Patients on calcineurin inhibitors should have doses of cyclosporine or tacrolimus decreased if taking calcineurin inhibitors. Although plasma exchange is often tried, patients with conditioning-related TTP/HUS or those with TTP/HUS and concomitant acute graft-versus-host disease typically do not respond.[132,133] Small series have evaluated the roles of eculizumab,[134] rituximab,[135] and vincristine,[136] and there are single reports of defibrotide[137] and pravastatin,[138] with varying results.

PREGNANCY RELATED THROMBOTIC SYNDROMES

Most pregnant women are young healthy individuals; however, rarely, severe thrombocytopenic syndromes can complicate pregnancy. Four syndromes in particular should be considered in pregnant individuals who present with thrombocytopenia: the HELLP (hemolysis, elevated liver tests, low platelet level) syndrome, fatty liver of pregnancy, classic TTP, and atypical HUS.[139–141] The salient points of each illness are outlined here.

The HELLP syndrome is classified as a variant of preeclampsia, which is generally defined as the presence of new-onset hypertension after 20 weeks of gestation along with proteinuria.[139,142–144] The pathogenesis of preeclampsia is not fully understood, but it may involve placental interactions leading to systemic hypertension.[145] Classically, HELLP syndrome occurs after 28 weeks of gestation in a patent with preeclampsia but can occur as early as 22 weeks in patients with the antiphospholipid antibody syndrome.[146] HELLP syndrome is classified as the presence of preeclampsia along with any of the following: blood pressure greater than 160/110 mm Hg, platelet count less than 100,000/μL, impaired liver function or severe right upper quadrant abdominal pain, creatinine level greater than 1.1 mg/dL, pulmonary edema, or cerebral or visual disturbances.[139,142] The first sign of HELLP is often a decrease in the platelet count followed by abnormal liver function tests. Signs of microangiopathic hemolysis are often present with abundant schistocytes on the smear along with increased LDH level, although this is not required for diagnosis. HELLP is fairly common compared with other causes of microangiopathic hemolytic anemia and may occur in approximately 0.5% to 1% of all pregnancies, and up to 20% of pregnancies with severe preeclampsia.[147,148] HELLP syndrome can result in multiple maternal and fetal complications, including DIC, renal dysfunction, hepatic infarction or capsular rupture, cerebral hemorrhage, and maternal death.[149] HELLP can produce fetal cytopenias, with up to 50% of cases having some level of fetal thrombocytopenia, unlike TTP, which does not.[150]

Delivery of the child is the cornerstone of therapy for HELLP syndrome.[151] For pregnancies of less than 34 weeks' gestation, expectant observation and therapy with dexamethasone have been trialed without promising results.[152,153] Randomized trials have failed to show a direct benefit for steroids.[152,154] Rare reports of plasma exchange have suggested a benefit.[155] Relapses are common with second pregnancies with about a quarter of women with HELLP having a recurrence with a later pregnancy.[156]

HELLP is common compared with other causes of pregnancy-associated microangiopathic hemolysis, which are rare, and are often difficult to distinguish from HELLP because of overlap in their presentation. Classic TTP, with an ADAMST13 level less than 5%, can occur anytime during pregnancy.[157–159] The incidence of TTP in pregnancy is theorized to be about 1 in 25,000, which is a much higher rate than occurs in the general population.[160–162] There seems to be a unique presentation of TTP that occurs in the second trimester at 20 to 22 weeks.[163] The fetus is uninvolved with no evidence of infarction or thrombocytopenia if the mother survives. The pregnancy seems to promote the TTP and relapses can occur with subsequent pregnancies, with some investigators citing up to a 20% relapse rate.[164,165] Patients with congenital TTP have extremely high relapse rates with pregnancy, and prophylactic plasma therapy should be initiated as soon as possible.[166] Acute therapy for pregnancy-associated TTP does not differ from that of classic TTP, with immediate initiation of plasma exchange. Immediate delivery of the child is not mandated unless HELLP syndrome is present, and pregnancies can be carried to term.[162] Delivery is necessary in patients who do not respond to plasma exchange.[13]

aHUS can also occur during pregnancy, even up to 28 weeks postpartum. Genetic complement defects are often found on evaluation, with patients often presenting in their second pregnancies.[167] This form of hemolytic uremic syndrome can be severe, with up to 75% of patients developing end-stage renal disease.[168] Effective treatment of atypical HUS with eculizumab during pregnancy has been reported, and there are data to suggest its safety during pregnancy.[168,169]

A cause of thrombocytopenia in pregnancy is acute fatty liver of pregnancy, which often occurs late in pregnancy or postpartum and is associated with preeclampsia in 50% of cases.[170–172] Patients usually present with nonspecific symptoms of nausea and vomiting but can progress to fulminant liver failure.[173] Thrombocytopenia may develop early in the course but in the later stages DIC may develop with very low fibrinogen levels.[174] Mortalities without therapy can be as high as 90%, but are reported near 18% with modern therapy.[175] Low glucose and high ammonia levels can help distinguish fatty liver from other pregnancy complications.[159] Treatment consists of prompt delivery of the child and aggressive supportive care.

UPCOMING THERAPIES

Although TTP/HUS has been a known entity for decades, alternative therapies to plasmapheresis and immunosuppression have been slow to be developed. Recently, promising therapeutic have begun to be tested in human trials.

Recombinant ADAMTS13

Recombinant versions of the ADAMTS13 metalloprotease have been developed and in vitro studies as well as animal models have suggested that recombinant ADAMTS13 can overcome inhibitors in sufficient quantities and restore cleavage of von Willebrand multimers.[176,177] A phase 1 trial of recombinant ADAMTS13 for the treatment of congenital TTP has recently been completed with favorable results.[178]

Caplacizumab

Caplacizumab is a monoclonal antibody to the A1 region of von Willebrand factor, which specifically inhibits its interaction with platelet glycoprotein Ib.[179] A recent phase 2 trial comparing caplacizumab with placebo found faster resolution of TTP episodes (in terms of time to platelet count reconstitution), at the cost of an increased rate of bleeding.[180]

Bortezomib

The proteasome inhibitor bortezomib has shown efficacy as an immunosuppressant in refractory cases of TTP in some case reports and case series.[181–183]

SUMMARY

The body of knowledge concerning TTP/HUS has expanded greatly despite the diseases' rarity. Although new therapies have arisen and others are under investigation, outcomes remain subpar in some forms of TTP/HUS, highlighting the need for further development. This article highlights the need for specialty hematologists to assist in the work-up and management of TTP/HUS given the diseases' complexity and potential mortality.

REFERENCES

1. George JN. How I treat patients with thrombotic thrombocytopenic purpura-hemolytic uremic syndrome. Blood 2000;96(4):1223–9.
2. Murrin RJ, Murray JA. Thrombotic thrombocytopenic purpura: aetiology, pathophysiology and treatment. Blood Rev 2006;20(1):51–60.
3. George JN. Clinical practice. Thrombotic thrombocytopenic purpura. N Engl J Med 2006;354(18):1927–35.
4. Frawley N, Ng AP, Nicholls K, et al. Thrombotic thrombocytopenic purpura is associated with a high relapse rate after plasma exchange: a single-centre experience. Intern Med J 2009;39(1):19–24.
5. Allford SL, Hunt BJ, Rose P, et al. Guidelines on the diagnosis and management of the thrombotic microangiopathic haemolytic anaemias. Br J Haematol 2003; 120(4):556–73.
6. Patton JF, Manning KR, Case D, et al. Serum lactate dehydrogenase and platelet count predict survival in thrombotic thrombocytopenic purpura. Am J Hematol 1994;47(2):94–9.
7. Rizzo C, Rizzo S, Scire E, et al. Thrombotic thrombocytopenic purpura: a review of the literature in the light of our experience with plasma exchange. Blood Transfus 2012;10(4):521–32.
8. Park YA, Waldrum MR, Marques MB. Platelet count and prothrombin time help distinguish thrombotic thrombocytopenic purpura-hemolytic uremic syndrome from disseminated intravascular coagulation in adults. Am J Clin Pathol 2010; 133(3):460–5.
9. Terrell DR, Williams LA, Vesely SK, et al. The incidence of thrombotic thrombocytopenic purpura-hemolytic uremic syndrome: all patients, idiopathic patients, and patients with severe ADAMTS-13 deficiency. J Thromb Haemost 2005;3(7): 1432–6.
10. George JN. How I treat patients with thrombotic thrombocytopenic purpura: 2010. Blood 2010;116(20):4060–9.

11. Vesely SK, George JN, Lämmle B, et al. ADAMTS13 activity in thrombotic thrombocytopenic purpura–hemolytic uremic syndrome: relation to presenting features and clinical outcomes in a prospective cohort of 142 patients. Blood 2003;102(1):60–8.

12. Aridon P, Ragonese P, Mazzola MA, et al. Reversible posterior leukoencephalopathy syndrome in a patient with thrombotic thrombocytopenic purpura. Neurol Sci 2011;32(3):469–72.

13. Scully M, Hunt BJ, Benjamin S, et al. Guidelines on the diagnosis and management of thrombotic thrombocytopenic purpura and other thrombotic microangiopathies. Br J Haematol 2012;158(3):323–35.

14. Cohen JA, Brecher ME, Bandarenko N. Cellular source of serum lactate dehydrogenase elevation in patients with thrombotic thrombocytopenic purpura. J Clin Apher 1998;13(1):16–9.

15. Neame PB, Hirsh J, Browman G, et al. Thrombotic thrombocytopenic purpura: a syndrome of intravascular platelet consumption. Can Med Assoc J 1976; 114(12):1108–12.

16. See JR, Sabagh T, Barde CJ. Thrombotic thrombocytopenic purpura: a case presenting with acute ischemic colitis. Case Rep Hematol 2013;2013:592930.

17. Gotlieb VK, erma V, Jacob R, et al. Thrombotic thrombocytopenic purpura induced pancreatitis– a rare complication. Blood 2010;116(21):4683.

18. Chang JC, Aly ES. Acute respiratory distress syndrome as a major clinical manifestation of thrombotic thrombocytopenic purpura. Am J Med Sci 2001;321(2): 124–8.

19. Gandhi K, Aronow WS, Desai H, et al. Cardiovascular manifestations in patients with thrombotic thrombocytopenic purpura: a single-center experience. Clin Cardiol 2010;33(4):213–6.

20. Bell MD, Barnhart JS Jr, Martin JM. Thrombotic thrombocytopenic purpura causing sudden, unexpected death–a series of eight patients. J Forensic Sci 1990;35(3):601–13.

21. Moake JL, Rudy CK, Troll JH, et al. Unusually large plasma factor VIII:von Willebrand factor multimers in chronic relapsing thrombotic thrombocytopenic purpura. N Engl J Med 1982;307(23):1432–5.

22. Tsai HM. Physiologic cleavage of von Willebrand factor by a plasma protease is dependent on its conformation and requires calcium ion. Blood 1996;87(10): 4235–44.

23. Furlan M, Robles R, Lammle B. Partial purification and characterization of a protease from human plasma cleaving von Willebrand factor to fragments produced by in vivo proteolysis. Blood 1996;87(10):4223–34.

24. Levy GG, Nichols WC, Lian EC, et al. Mutations in a member of the ADAMTS gene family cause thrombotic thrombocytopenic purpura. Nature 2001; 413(6855):488–94.

25. Zheng X, Chung D, Takayama TK, et al. Structure of von Willebrand factor-cleaving protease (ADAMTS13), a metalloprotease involved in thrombotic thrombocytopenic purpura. J Biol Chem 2001;276(44):41059–63.

26. Furlan M. von Willebrand factor-cleaving protease in thrombotic thrombocytopenic purpura and hemolytic-uremic syndrome. Adv Nephrol Necker Hosp 2000;30:71–81.

27. Sadler JE. Von Willebrand factor, ADAMTS13, and thrombotic thrombocytopenic purpura. Blood 2008;112(1):11–8.

28. Ferrari S, Mudde GC, Rieger M, et al. IgG subclass distribution of anti-ADAMTS13 antibodies in patients with acquired thrombotic thrombocytopenic purpura. J Thromb Haemost 2009;7(10):1703–10.
29. Coppo P, Wolf M, Veyradier A, et al. Prognostic value of inhibitory anti-ADAMTS13 antibodies in adult-acquired thrombotic thrombocytopenic purpura. Br J Haematol 2006;132(1):66–74.
30. Tsai H-M. Current concepts in thrombotic thrombocytopenic purpura. Annu Rev Med 2006;57:419–36.
31. Rock GA, Shumak KH, Buskard NA, et al. Comparison of plasma exchange with plasma infusion in the treatment of thrombotic thrombocytopenic purpura. Canadian Apheresis Study Group. N Engl J Med 1991;325(6):393–7.
32. Bell WR, Braine HG, Ness PM, et al. Improved survival in thrombotic thrombocytopenic purpura-hemolytic uremic syndrome. Clinical experience in 108 patients. N Engl J Med 1991;325(6):398–403.
33. Kaplan BS, Trachtman H. Improve survival with plasma exchange thrombotic thrombopenic purpura-hemolytic uremic syndrome. Am J Med 2001;110(2): 156–7.
34. Furlan M, Robles R, Solenthaler M, et al. Acquired deficiency of von Willebrand factor-cleaving protease in a patient with thrombotic thrombocytopenic purpura. Blood 1998;91(8):2839–46.
35. Sarode R, Bandarenko N, Brecher ME, et al. Thrombotic thrombocytopenic purpura: 2012 American Society for Apheresis (ASFA) consensus conference on classification, diagnosis, management, and future research. J Clin Apher 2014;29(3):148–67.
36. Zheng XL, Kaufman RM, Goodnough LT, et al. Effect of plasma exchange on plasma ADAMTS13 metalloprotease activity, inhibitor level, and clinical outcome in patients with idiopathic and nonidiopathic thrombotic thrombocytopenic purpura. Blood 2004;103(11):4043–9.
37. Sayani FA, Abrams CS. How I treat refractory thrombotic thrombocytopenic purpura. Blood 2015;125(25):3860–7.
38. Toyoshige M, Zaitsu Y, Okafuji K, et al. Successful treatment of thrombotic thrombocytopenic purpura with high-dose corticosteroid. Am J Hematol 1992; 41(1):69.
39. Balduini CL, Gugliotta L, Luppi M, et al. High versus standard dose methylprednisolone in the acute phase of idiopathic thrombotic thrombocytopenic purpura: a randomized study. Ann Hematol 2010;89(6):591–6.
40. Lim W, Vesely SK, George JN. The role of rituximab in the management of patients with acquired thrombotic thrombocytopenic purpura. Blood 2015; 125(10):1526–31.
41. McDonald V, Manns K, Mackie IJ, et al. Rituximab pharmacokinetics during the management of acute idiopathic thrombotic thrombocytopenic purpura. J Thromb Haemost 2010;8(6):1201–8.
42. Fakhouri F, Vernant JP, Veyradier A, et al. Efficiency of curative and prophylactic treatment with rituximab in ADAMTS13-deficient thrombotic thrombocytopenic purpura: a study of 11 cases. Blood 2005;106(6):1932–7.
43. Nguyen L, Li X, Duvall D, et al. Twice-daily plasma exchange for patients with refractory thrombotic thrombocytopenic purpura: the experience of the Oklahoma Registry, 1989 through 2006. Transfusion 2008;48(2):349–57.
44. Cataland SR, Jin M, Lin S, et al. Cyclosporin and plasma exchange in thrombotic thrombocytopenic purpura: long-term follow-up with serial analysis of ADAMTS13 activity. Br J Haematol 2007;139(3):486–93.

45. Beloncle F, Buffet M, Coindre JP, et al. Splenectomy and/or cyclophosphamide as salvage therapies in thrombotic thrombocytopenic purpura: the French TMA Reference Center experience. Transfusion 2012;52(11):2436–44.

46. Dubois L, Gray DK. Case series: splenectomy: does it still play a role in the management of thrombotic thrombocytopenic purpura? Can J Surg 2010;53(5): 349–55.

47. Upshaw JD Jr. Congenital deficiency of a factor in normal plasma that reverses microangiopathic hemolysis and thrombocytopenia. N Engl J Med 1978; 298(24):1350–2.

48. Lotta LA, Garagiola I, Palla R, et al. ADAMTS13 mutations and polymorphisms in congenital thrombotic thrombocytopenic purpura. Hum Mutat 2010;31(1):11–9.

49. Schiff DE, Roberts WD, Willert J, et al. Thrombocytopenia and severe hyperbilirubinemia in the neonatal period secondary to congenital thrombotic thrombocytopenic purpura and ADAMTS13 deficiency. J Pediatr Hematol Oncol 2004; 26(8):535–8.

50. Scully M, Gattens M, Khair K, et al. The use of intermediate purity factor VIII concentrate BPL 8Y as prophylaxis and treatment in congenital thrombotic thrombocytopenic purpura. Br J Haematol 2006;135(1):101–4.

51. Furlan M, Robles R, Solenthaler M, et al. Deficient activity of von Willebrand factor-cleaving protease in chronic relapsing thrombotic thrombocytopenic purpura. Blood 1997;89(9):3097–103.

52. Schneppenheim R, Budde U, Oyen F, et al. von Willebrand factor cleaving protease and ADAMTS13 mutations in childhood TTP. Blood 2003;101(5):1845–50.

53. Copelovitch L, Kaplan BS. The thrombotic microangiopathies. Pediatr Nephrol 2008;23(10):1761–7.

54. Razzaq S. Hemolytic uremic syndrome: an emerging health risk. Am Fam Physician 2006;74(6):991–6.

55. Gasser C, Gautier E, Steck A, et al. Hemolytic-uremic syndrome: bilateral necrosis of the renal cortex in acute acquired hemolytic anemia. Schweiz Med Wochenschr 1955;85(38–39):905–9 [in German].

56. Rahaman MM, JamiulAlam AK, Islam MR, et al. Shiga bacillus dysentery associated with marked leukocytosis and erythrocyte fragmentation. Johns Hopkins Med J 1975;136(2):65–70.

57. Riley LW, Remis RS, Helgerson SD, et al. Hemorrhagic colitis associated with a rare Escherichia coli serotype. N Engl J Med 1983;308(12):681–5.

58. Noris M, Remuzzi G. Hemolytic uremic syndrome. J Am Soc Nephrol 2005; 16(4):1035–50.

59. Constantinescu AR, Bitzan M, Weiss LS, et al. Non-enteropathic hemolytic uremic syndrome: causes and short-term course. Am J Kidney Dis 2004;43(6): 976–82.

60. Tarr PI, Gordon CA, Chandler WL. Shiga-toxin-producing Escherichia coli and haemolytic uraemic syndrome. Lancet 2005;365(9464):1073–86.

61. Karpac CA, Li X, Terrell DR, et al. Sporadic bloody diarrhoea-associated thrombotic thrombocytopenic purpura-haemolytic uraemic syndrome: an adult and paediatric comparison. Br J Haematol 2008;141(5):696–707.

62. Noris M, Remuzzi G. Atypical hemolytic-uremic syndrome. N Engl J Med 2009; 361(17):1676–87.

63. George JN, Nester CM. Syndromes of thrombotic microangiopathy. N Engl J Med 2014;371(7):654–66.

64. Huang J, Motto DG, Bundle DR, et al. Shiga toxin B subunits induce VWF secretion by human endothelial cells and thrombotic microangiopathy in ADAMTS13-deficient mice. Blood 2010;116(18):3653–9.

65. Dundas S, Murphy J, Soutar RL, et al. Effectiveness of therapeutic plasma exchange in the 1996 Lanarkshire Escherichia coli O157:H7 outbreak. Lancet (London, England) 1999;354(9187):1327–30.

66. Boyer O, Niaudet P. Hemolytic uremic syndrome: new developments in pathogenesis and treatment. Int J Nephrol 2011;2011:908407.

67. Caprioli J, Noris M, Brioschi S, et al. Genetics of HUS: the impact of MCP, CFH, and IF mutations on clinical presentation, response to treatment, and outcome. Blood 2006;108(4):1267–79.

68. Loirat C, Noris M, Fremeaux-Bacchi V. Complement and the atypical hemolytic uremic syndrome in children. Pediatr Nephrol 2008;23(11):1957–72.

69. Legendre CM, Licht C, Muus P, et al. Terminal complement inhibitor eculizumab in atypical hemolytic-uremic syndrome. N Engl J Med 2013;368(23):2169–81.

70. Kaplan BS, Meyers KE, Schulman SL. The pathogenesis and treatment of hemolytic uremic syndrome. J Am Soc Nephrol 1998;9(6):1126–33.

71. Stahl AL, Vaziri-Sani F, Heinen S, et al. Factor H dysfunction in patients with atypical hemolytic uremic syndrome contributes to complement deposition on platelets and their activation. Blood 2008;111(11):5307–15.

72. Thompson RA, Winterborn MH. Hypocomplementaemia due to a genetic deficiency of beta 1H globulin. Clin Exp Immunol 1981;46(1):110–9.

73. Warwicker P, Goodship TH, Donne RL, et al. Genetic studies into inherited and sporadic hemolytic uremic syndrome. Kidney Int 1998;53(4):836–44.

74. Dragon-Durey MA, Fremeaux-Bacchi V, Loirat C, et al. Heterozygous and homozygous factor h deficiencies associated with hemolytic uremic syndrome or membranoproliferative glomerulonephritis: report and genetic analysis of 16 cases. J Am Soc Nephrol 2004;15(3):787–95.

75. Seifert PS, Hansson GK. Complement receptors and regulatory proteins in human atherosclerotic lesions. Arteriosclerosi 1989;9(6):802–11.

76. Zuber J, Le Quintrec M, Sberro-Soussan R, et al. New insights into postrenal transplant hemolytic uremic syndrome. Nat Rev Nephrol 2011;7(1):23–35.

77. Loirat C, Niaudet P. The risk of recurrence of hemolytic uremic syndrome after renal transplantation in children. Pediatr Nephrol (Berlin, Germany) 2003;18(11):1095–101.

78. Skerka C, Jozsi M, Zipfel PF, et al. Autoantibodies in haemolytic uraemic syndrome (HUS). Thromb Haemost 2009;101(2):227–32.

79. Waters AM, Pappworth I, Marchbank K, et al. Successful renal transplantation in factor H autoantibody associated HUS with CFHR1 and 3 deficiency and CFH variant G2850T. Am J Transplant 2010;10(1):168–72.

80. Noris M, Brioschi S, Caprioli J, et al. Familial haemolytic uraemic syndrome and an MCP mutation. Lancet (London, England) 2003;362(9395):1542–7.

81. Richards A, Kemp EJ, Liszewski MK, et al. Mutations in human complement regulator, membrane cofactor protein (CD46), predispose to development of familial hemolytic uremic syndrome. Proc Natl Acad Sci U S A 2003;100(22):12966–71.

82. Goicoechea de Jorge E, Harris CL, Esparza-Gordillo J, et al. Gain-of-function mutations in complement factor B are associated with atypical hemolytic uremic syndrome. Proc Natl Acad Sci U S A 2007;104(1):240–5.

83. Fremeaux-Bacchi V, Miller EC, Liszewski MK, et al. Mutations in complement C3 predispose to development of atypical hemolytic uremic syndrome. Blood 2008; 112(13):4948–52.

84. Kavanagh D, Kemp EJ, Mayland E, et al. Mutations in complement factor I predispose to development of atypical hemolytic uremic syndrome. J Am Soc Nephrol 2005;16(7):2150–5.

85. Bienaime F, Dragon-Durey MA, Regnier CH, et al. Mutations in components of complement influence the outcome of factor I-associated atypical hemolytic uremic syndrome. Kidney Int 2010;77(4):339–49.

86. Michael M, Elliott EJ, Craig JC, et al. Interventions for hemolytic uremic syndrome and thrombotic thrombocytopenic purpura: a systematic review of randomized controlled trials. Am J Kidney Dis 2009;53(2):259–72.

87. Ruggenenti P, Noris M, Remuzzi G. Thrombotic microangiopathies. In: Wilcox CS, editor. Therapy in nephrology & hypertension: a companion to Brenner & Rector's the kidney. 3rd edition. Philadelphia: Saunders; 2008. p. 294–312.

88. Ariceta G, Besbas N, Johnson S, et al. Guideline for the investigation and initial therapy of diarrhea-negative hemolytic uremic syndrome. Pediatr Nephrol (Berlin, Germany) 2009;24(4):687–96.

89. Licht C, Weyersberg A, Heinen S, et al. Successful plasma therapy for atypical hemolytic uremic syndrome caused by factor H deficiency owing to a novel mutation in the complement cofactor protein domain 15. Am J Kidney Dis 2005; 45(2):415–21.

90. Zimmerhackl LB, Hofer J, Cortina G, et al. Prophylactic eculizumab after renal transplantation in atypical hemolytic-uremic syndrome. N Engl J Med 2010; 362(18):1746–8.

91. Diamante Chiodini B, Davin JC, Corazza F, et al. Eculizumab in anti-factor h antibodies associated with atypical hemolytic uremic syndrome. Pediatrics 2014; 133(6):e1764–8.

92. Ardissino G, Testa S, Possenti I, et al. Discontinuation of eculizumab maintenance treatment for atypical hemolytic uremic syndrome: a report of 10 cases. Am J Kidney Dis 2014;64(4):633–7.

93. Russo P, Doyon J, Sonsino E, et al. A congenital anomaly of vitamin B12 metabolism: a study of three cases. Hum Pathol 1992;23(5):504–12.

94. Geraghty MT, Perlman EJ, Martin LS, et al. Cobalamin C defect associated with hemolytic-uremic syndrome. J Pediatr 1992;120(6):934–7.

95. Cornec-Le Gall E, Delmas Y, De Parscau L, et al. Adult-onset eculizumab-resistant hemolytic uremic syndrome associated with cobalamin C deficiency. Am J Kidney Dis 2014;63(1):119–23.

96. Delvaeye M, Noris M, De Vriese A, et al. Thrombomodulin mutations in atypical hemolytic-uremic syndrome. N Engl J Med 2009;361(4):345–57.

97. Bu F, Maga T, Meyer NC, et al. Comprehensive genetic analysis of complement and coagulation genes in atypical hemolytic uremic syndrome. J Am Soc Nephrol 2014;25(1):55–64.

98. Ozaltin F, Li B, Rauhauser A, et al. DGKE variants cause a glomerular microangiopathy that mimics membranoproliferative GN. J Am Soc Nephrol 2013;24(3): 377–84.

99. Lemaire M, Fremeaux-Bacchi V, Schaefer F, et al. Recessive mutations in DGKE cause atypical hemolytic-uremic syndrome. Nat Genet 2013;45(5):531–6.

100. Quaggin SE. DGKE and atypical HUS. Nat Genet 2013;45(5):475–6.

101. Moake JL, Byrnes JJ. Thrombotic microangiopathies associated with drugs and bone marrow transplantation. Hematol Oncol Clin North Am 1996;10(2):485–97.

102. Zakarija A, Bennett C. Drug-induced thrombotic microangiopathy. Semin Thromb Hemost 2005;31(6):681–90.

103. Webb RF, Ramirez AM, Hocken AG, et al. Acute intravascular haemolysis due to quinine. N Z Med J 1980;91(651):14–6.

104. Kojouri K, Vesely SK, George JN. Quinine-associated thrombotic thrombocytopenic purpura-hemolytic uremic syndrome: frequency, clinical features, and long-term outcomes. Ann Intern Med 2001;135(12):1047–51.

105. Stroncek DF, Vercellotti GM, Hammerschmidt DE, et al. Characterization of multiple quinine-dependent antibodies in a patient with episodic hemolytic uremic syndrome and immune agranulocytosis. Blood 1992;80(1):241–8.

106. Huynh M, Chee K, Lau DH. Thrombotic thrombocytopenic purpura associated with quetiapine. Ann Pharmacother 2005;39(7–8):1346–8.

107. Saif MW, Xyla V, Makrilia N, et al. Thrombotic microangiopathy associated with gemcitabine: rare but real. Expert Opin Drug Saf 2009;8(3):257–60.

108. Gharpure VS, Devine SM, Holland HK, et al. Thrombotic thrombocytopenic purpura associated with FK506 following bone marrow transplantation. Bone Marrow Transplant 1995;16(5):715–6.

109. Lin CC, King KL, Chao YW, et al. Tacrolimus-associated hemolytic uremic syndrome: a case analysis. J Nephrol 2003;16(4):580–5.

110. Wu DC, Liu JM, Chen YM, et al. Mitomycin-C induced hemolytic uremic syndrome: a case report and literature review. Jpn J Clin Oncol 1997;27(2):115–8.

111. Izzedine H, Isnard-Bagnis C, Launay-Vacher V, et al. Gemcitabine-induced thrombotic microangiopathy: a systematic review. Nephrol Dial Transplant 2006;21(11):3038–45.

112. Saif MW, McGee PJ. Hemolytic-uremic syndrome associated with gemcitabine: a case report and review of literature. JOP 2005;6(4):369–74.

113. Brodowicz T, Breiteneder S, Wiltschke C, et al. Gemcitabine-induced hemolytic uremic syndrome: a case report. J Natl Cancer Inst 1997;89(24):1895–6.

114. Fung MC, Storniolo AM, Nguyen B, et al. A review of hemolytic uremic syndrome in patients treated with gemcitabine therapy. Cancer 1999;85(9):2023–32.

115. Walter RB, Joerger M, Pestalozzi BC. Gemcitabine-associated hemolytic-uremic syndrome. Am J Kidney Dis 2002;40(4):E16.

116. Barz D, Budde U, Hellstern P. Therapeutic plasma exchange and plasma infusion in thrombotic microvascular syndromes. Thromb Res 2002;107(Suppl 1): S23–7.

117. Gore EM, Jones BS, Marques MB. Is therapeutic plasma exchange indicated for patients with gemcitabine-induced hemolytic uremic syndrome? J Clin Apher 2009;24(5):209–14.

118. Al Ustwani O, Lohr J, Dy G, et al. Eculizumab therapy for gemcitabine induced hemolytic uremic syndrome: case series and concise review. J Gastrointest Oncol 2014;5(1):E30–3.

119. Starck M, Wendtner CM. Use of eculizumab in refractory gemcitabine-induced thrombotic microangiopathy. Br J Haematol 2014;164(6):894–6.

120. Faguer S, Huart A, Fremeaux-Bacchi V, et al. Eculizumab and drug-induced haemolytic-uraemic syndrome. Clin Kidney J 2013;6(5):484–5.

121. Bennett CL, Connors JM, Carwile JM, et al. Thrombotic thrombocytopenic purpura associated with clopidogrel. N Engl J Med 2000;342(24):1773–7.

122. Zakarija A, Kwaan HC, Moake JL, et al. Ticlopidine- and clopidogrel-associated thrombotic thrombocytopenic purpura (TTP): review of clinical, laboratory, epidemiological, and pharmacovigilance findings (1989-2008). Kidney Int Suppl 2009;(112):S20–4.

123. George JN, Li X, McMinn JR, et al. Thrombotic thrombocytopenic purpura-hemolytic uremic syndrome following allogeneic HPC transplantation: a diagnostic dilemma. Transfusion 2004;44(2):294–304.

124. Dervenoulas J, Tsirigotis P, Bollas G, et al. Thrombotic thrombocytopenic purpura/hemolytic uremic syndrome (TTP/HUS): treatment outcome, relapses, prognostic factors. A single-center experience of 48 cases. Ann Hematol 2000;79(2):66–72.

125. Laskin BL, Goebel J, Davies SM, et al. Small vessels, big trouble in the kidneys and beyond: hematopoietic stem cell transplantation-associated thrombotic microangiopathy. Blood 2011;118(6):1452–62.

126. Daly AS, Hasegawa WS, Lipton JH, et al. Transplantation-associated thrombotic microangiopathy is associated with transplantation from unrelated donors, acute graft-versus-host disease and venoocclusive disease of the liver. Transfus Apher Sci 2002;27(1):3–12.

127. Choi CM, Schmaier AH, Snell MR, et al. Thrombotic microangiopathy in haematopoietic stem cell transplantation: diagnosis and treatment. Drugs 2009;69(2):183–98.

128. Jodele S, Licht C, Goebel J, et al. Abnormalities in the alternative pathway of complement in children with hematopoietic stem cell transplant-associated thrombotic microangiopathy. Blood 2013;122(12):2003–7.

129. Laskin BL, Maisel J, Goebel J, et al. Renal arteriolar C4d deposition: a novel characteristic of hematopoietic stem cell transplantation-associated thrombotic microangiopathy. Transplantation 2013;96(2):217–23.

130. Kim SS, Patel M, Yum K, et al. Hematopoietic stem cell transplant-associated thrombotic microangiopathy: review of pharmacologic treatment options. Transfusion 2015;55(2):452–8.

131. Verburgh CA, Vermeij CG, Zijlmans JM, et al. Haemolytic uraemic syndrome following bone marrow transplantation. Case report and review of the literature. Nephrol Dial Transplant 1996;11(7):1332–7.

132. Sarode R, McFarland JG, Flomenberg N, et al. Therapeutic plasma exchange does not appear to be effective in the management of thrombotic thrombocytopenic purpura/hemolytic uremic syndrome following bone marrow transplantation. Bone Marrow Transplant 1995;16(2):271–5.

133. Kennedy GA, Kearey N, Bleakley S, et al. Transplantation-associated thrombotic microangiopathy: effect of concomitant GVHD on efficacy of therapeutic plasma exchange. Bone Marrow Transplant 2010;45(4):699–704.

134. de Fontbrune FS, Galambrun C, Sirvent A, et al. Use of eculizumab in patients with allogeneic stem cell transplant-associated thrombotic microangiopathy: a study from the SFGM-TC. Transplantation 2015;99(9):1953–9.

135. Au WY, Ma ES, Lee TL, et al. Successful treatment of thrombotic microangiopathy after haematopoietic stem cell transplantation with rituximab. Br J Haematol 2007;137(5):475–8.

136. Silva VA, Frei-Lahr D, Brown RA, et al. Plasma exchange and vincristine in the treatment of hemolytic uremic syndrome/thrombotic thrombocytopenic purpura associated with bone marrow transplantation. J Clin Apher 1991;6(1):16–20.

137. Corti P, Uderzo C, Tagliabue A, et al. Defibrotide as a promising treatment for thrombotic thrombocytopenic purpura in patients undergoing bone marrow transplantation. Bone Marrow Transplant 2002;29(6):542–3.

138. Uesawa M, Muroi K, Ozawa K. Plasmapheresis-refractory transplantation-associated thrombotic microangiopathy successfully treated with pravastatin and limaprost alfadex. Ther Apher Dial 2013;17(4):462–3.

139. George JN, Nester CM, McIntosh JJ. Syndromes of thrombotic microangiopathy associated with pregnancy. Hematology Am Soc Hematol Educ Program 2015; 2015:644–8.

140. Sibai BM. Imitators of severe pre-eclampsia/eclampsia. Clin Perinatol 2004; 31(4):835–52, vii–viii.

141. Steingrub JS. Pregnancy-associated severe liver dysfunction. Crit Care Clin 2004;20(4):763–76, xi.

142. American College of Obstetricians and Gynecologists, Task Force on Hypertension in Pregnancy. Hypertension in pregnancy. Report of the American College of Obstetricians and Gynecologists' Task Force on Hypertension in Pregnancy. Obstet Gynecol 2013;122(5):1122–31.

143. Baxter JK, Weinstein L. HELLP syndrome: the state of the art. Obstet Gynecol Surv 2004;59(12):838–45.

144. Leeman L, Fontaine P. Hypertensive disorders of pregnancy. Am Fam Physician 2008;78(1):93–100.

145. Steegers EA, von Dadelszen P, Duvekot JJ, et al. Pre-eclampsia. Lancet (London, England) 2010;376(9741):631–44.

146. Le Thi Thuong D, Tieulie N, Costedoat N, et al. The HELLP syndrome in the antiphospholipid syndrome: retrospective study of 16 cases in 15 women. Ann Rheum Dis 2005;64(2):273–8.

147. Geary M. The HELLP syndrome. Br J Obstet Gynaecol 1997;104(8):887–91.

148. Karumanchi SA, Maynard SE, Stillman IE, et al. Preeclampsia: a renal perspective. Kidney Int 2005;67(6):2101–13.

149. Haram K, Svendsen E, Abildgaard U. The HELLP syndrome: clinical issues and management. A review. BMC Pregnancy Childbirth 2009;9:8.

150. Raval DS, Co S, Reid MA, et al. Maternal and neonatal outcome of pregnancies complicated with maternal HELLP syndrome. J Perinatol 1997;17(4):266–9.

151. Martin JN Jr, Perry KG Jr, Blake PG, et al. Better maternal outcomes are achieved with dexamethasone therapy for postpartum HELLP (hemolysis, elevated liver enzymes, and thrombocytopenia) syndrome. Am J Obstet Gynecol 1997;177(5):1011–7.

152. Fonseca JE, Mendez F, Catano C, et al. Dexamethasone treatment does not improve the outcome of women with HELLP syndrome: a double-blind, placebo-controlled, randomized clinical trial. Am J Obstet Gynecol 2005;193(5): 1591–8.

153. Visser W, Wallenburg HC. Temporising management of severe pre-eclampsia with and without the HELLP syndrome. Br J Obstet Gynaecol 1995;102(2): 111–7.

154. Katz L, de Amorim MM, Figueiroa JN, et al. Postpartum dexamethasone for women with hemolysis, elevated liver enzymes, and low platelets (HELLP) syndrome: a double-blind, placebo-controlled, randomized clinical trial. Am J Obstet Gynecol 2008;198(3):283.e1-8.

155. Eser B, Guven M, Unal A, et al. The role of plasma exchange in HELLP syndrome. Clin Appl Thromb Hemost 2005;11(2):211–7.

156. Sullivan CA, Magann EF, Perry KG Jr, et al. The recurrence risk of the syndrome of hemolysis, elevated liver enzymes, and low platelets (HELLP) in subsequent gestations. Am J Obstet Gynecol 1994;171(4):940–3.

157. Bianchi V, Robles R, Alberio L, et al. Von Willebrand factor-cleaving protease (ADAMTS13) in thrombocytopenic disorders: a severely deficient activity is specific for thrombotic thrombocytopenic purpura. Blood 2002;100(2):710–3.

158. Habli M, Eftekhari N, Wiebracht E, et al. Long-term maternal and subsequent pregnancy outcomes 5 years after hemolysis, elevated liver enzymes, and low platelets (HELLP) syndrome. Am J Obstet Gynecol 2009;201(4):385.e1-5.

159. Egerman RS, Sibai BM. Imitators of preeclampsia and eclampsia. Clin Obstet Gynecol 1999;42(3):551–62.

160. Terrell DR, Beebe LA, Vesely SK, et al. The incidence of immune thrombocytopenic purpura in children and adults: a critical review of published reports. Am J Hematol 2010;85(3):174–80.

161. Dashe JS, Ramin SM, Cunningham FG. The long-term consequences of thrombotic microangiopathy (thrombotic thrombocytopenic purpura and hemolytic uremic syndrome) in pregnancy. Obstet Gynecol 1998;91(5 Pt 1):662–8.

162. Gernsheimer T, James AH, Stasi R. How I treat thrombocytopenia in pregnancy. Blood 2013;121(1):38–47.

163. Esplin MS, Branch DW. Diagnosis and management of thrombotic microangiopathies during pregnancy. Clin Obstet Gynecol 1999;42(2):360–7.

164. Vesely SK, Li X, McMinn JR, et al. Pregnancy outcomes after recovery from thrombotic thrombocytopenic purpura-hemolytic uremic syndrome. Transfusion 2004;44(8):1149–58.

165. Jiang Y, McIntosh JJ, Reese JA, et al. Pregnancy outcomes following recovery from acquired thrombotic thrombocytopenic purpura. Blood 2014;123(11): 1674–80.

166. Scully M, Thomas M, Underwood M, et al. Thrombotic thrombocytopenic purpura and pregnancy: presentation, management, and subsequent pregnancy outcomes. Blood 2014;124(2):211–9.

167. Fakhouri F, Roumenina L, Provot F, et al. Pregnancy-associated hemolytic uremic syndrome revisited in the era of complement gene mutations. J Am Soc Nephrol 2010;21(5):859–67.

168. Mandala EM, Gkiouzepas S, Kasimatis E, et al. Pregnancy-associated atypical hemolytic uremic syndrome (aHUS), treated with eculizumab. Blood 2014; 124(21):5019.

169. Kelly RJ, Hochsmann B, Szer J, et al. Eculizumab in pregnant patients with paroxysmal nocturnal hemoglobinuria. N Engl J Med 2015;373(11):1032–9.

170. Jwayyed SM, Blanda M, Kubina M. Acute fatty liver of pregnancy. J Emerg Med 1999;17(4):673–7.

171. Bacq Y. Acute fatty liver of pregnancy. Semin Perinatol 1998;22(2):134–40.

172. Sibai BM. Imitators of severe preeclampsia. Obstet Gynecol 2007;109(4): 956–66.

173. Ko HH, Yoshida E. Acute fatty liver of pregnancy. Can J Gastroenterol 2006; 20(1):25–30.

174. Kaplan MM. Acute fatty liver of pregnancy. N Engl J Med 1985;313(6):367–70.

175. Ranjan V, Smith NC. Acute fatty liver of pregnancy. J Obstet Gynaecol 1997; 17(3):285–6.

176. Tersteeg C, Schiviz A, De Meyer SF, et al. Potential for recombinant ADAMTS13 as an effective therapy for acquired thrombotic thrombocytopenic purpura. Arterioscler Thromb Vasc Biol 2015;35(11):2336–42.

177. Plaimauer B, Kremer Hovinga JA, Juno C, et al. Recombinant ADAMTS13 normalizes von Willebrand factor-cleaving activity in plasma of acquired TTP patients by overriding inhibitory antibodies. J Thromb Haemost 2011;9(5):936–44.

178. Abstracts of the 62nd Annual Meeting of the Scientific and Standardization Committee of the International Society on Thrombosis and Haemostasis May 25-28, 2016. J Thromb Haemost 2016;14(Suppl 1):1–168.

179. Veyradier A. Von Willebrand factor–a new target for TTP treatment? N Engl J Med 2016;374(6):583–5.
180. Peyvandi F, Scully M, Kremer Hovinga JA, et al. Caplacizumab for acquired thrombotic thrombocytopenic purpura. N Engl J Med 2016;374(6):511–22.
181. Patriquin CJ, Thomas MR, Dutt T, et al. Bortezomib in the treatment of refractory thrombotic thrombocytopenic purpura. Br J Haematol 2016;173(5):779–85.
182. Shortt J, Oh DH, Opat SS. ADAMTS13 antibody depletion by bortezomib in thrombotic thrombocytopenic purpura. N Engl J Med 2013;368(1):90–2.
183. Yates S, Matevosyan K, Rutherford C, et al. Bortezomib for chronic relapsing thrombotic thrombocytopenic purpura: a case report. Transfusion 2014;54(8): 2064–7.

Unusual Anemias

Molly Maddock Daughety, MD[a],
Thomas G. DeLoughery, MD, MACP, FAWM[a,b],*

KEYWORDS

- Thalassemia • Aplastic anemia • Paroxysmal nocturnal hemoglobinuria
- Spur cell anemia • Burns • Drug induced

KEY POINTS

- Thalassemia can have a variable presentation ranging from mild microcytosis to transfusion-dependent anemia.
- Paroxysmal nocturnal hemoglobinuria should be considered in any patient with hemolysis, especially if complicated by thrombosis.
- Diverse processes can lead to acquired hemolytic anemias.

A variety of processes lead to anemia, and this review discusses causes beyond the classic conditions often considered (**Box 1**). This report reviews thalassemia, rare nutritional anemias, paroxysmal nocturnal hemoglobinuria, bone marrow failure syndromes, and unusual types of hemolysis.

THALASSEMIA

Although not frequently seen in North America, thalassemias are the most common hemoglobin defect in the world.[1] Thalassemias are diseases of hemoglobin synthesis and are subclassified by the hemoglobin chain involved—most often the α or β chain. Each chromosome 16 carries 2 copies of the gene encoding the α globin chain ($\alpha\alpha/\alpha\alpha$). When any of these genes is mutated, the result is α thalassemia, of which, 4 varieties exist: α thalassemia minor-1 (1 gene affected; α-/$\alpha\alpha$), α thalassemia minor-2 (2 genes affected; α-/α- or $\alpha\alpha$/-), hemoglobin H disease (3 genes affected; α-/–) and hemoglobin Bart's (4 genes affected; –/–). Patients with 1 mutation are considered *silent carriers*, whereas those with 2 mutations are considered to have the α thalassemia trait, which

Both authors report no conflict of interest.
[a] Division of Hematology/Medical Oncology, Department of Medicine, Oregon Health Sciences University, 3181 Southwest Sam Jackson Park Road, Portland, OR 97201-3098, USA; [b] Division of Hematology/Medical Oncology, Department of Medicine, Knight Cancer Institute, Oregon Health and Science University, MC L586, 3181 Southwest Sam Jackson Park Road, Portland, OR 97239, USA
* Corresponding author. Division of Hematology/Medical Oncology, Department of Medicine, Knight Cancer Institute, Oregon Health and Science University, MC L586, 3181 Southwest Sam Jackson Park Road, Portland, OR 97239, USA.
E-mail address: delought@ohsu.edu

Med Clin N Am 101 (2017) 417–429
http://dx.doi.org/10.1016/j.mcna.2016.09.011
0025-7125/17/© 2016 Elsevier Inc. All rights reserved.

Box 1
Less common anemias

Thalassemia
    Clinical clues to diagnosis: microcytosis with normal iron stores, positive family history
    Diagnostic tests: hemoglobin electrophoresis, DNA sequencing
    Treatment: Severe, stem cell transplant, transfusions, iron chelation

Copper deficiency
    Clinical clues to diagnosis: neutropenia, normal platelet counts, sensory neurologic defects
    Diagnostic tests: copper level, ceruloplasmin
    Treatment: copper supplementation

Paroxysmal nocturnal hemoglobinuria
    Clinical clues to diagnosis: Coombs negative hemolysis, thrombosis, pancytopenia
    Diagnostic tests: high-sensitivity flow cytometry
    Treatment: complement C5 inhibitor eculizumab

Aplastic anemia
    Clinical clues to diagnosis: pancytopenia
    Diagnostic tests: bone marrow biopsy and aspirate
    Treatment: stem cell transplant or immunosuppression

Pure red cell aplasia
    Clinical clues to diagnosis: severe anemia with markedly reduce reticulocyte count
    Diagnostic tests: bone marrow biopsy and aspirate
    Treatment: CSA

Microangiopathic hemolytic anemias
    Clinical clues to diagnosis: schistocytes, high low-density lipoprotein level, thrombocytopenia
    Diagnostic tests: blood smear, review of history/examination for severe hypertension, recent mitral valve repair, presence of VAD
    Treatment: treatment of primary cause (eg, reducing blood pressure)

Clostridium sepsis
    Clinical clues to diagnosis: fevers, severe hemolysis
    Diagnostic tests: spherocytes and ghost cells on blood smear
    Treatment: treatment of infection

Spur cell anemia
    Clinical clues to diagnosis: severe hemolysis in the setting of ESLD
    Diagnostic tests: blood smear showing spur cells
    Treatment: liver transplant

Wilson disease
    Clinical clues to diagnosis: Coomb negative hemolysis in the setting of liver disease
    Diagnostic tests: serum copper and ceruloplasmin level, presence of bite cells, and spherocytes in blood smear
    Treatment: copper chelation, liver transplant

Burns
    Clinical clues to diagnosis: history
    Diagnostic tests: spherocytes, fragmented red cells
    Treatment: supportive care

---

typically manifests with mild microcytosis without anemia. Hemoglobin H disease is characterized by pronounced hemolytic anemia, splenomegaly, and complications related to iron overload. Hemoglobin Bart's is the complete failure to produce an α globin chain, resulting in hydrops fetalis and death in utero or soon after birth.

The geographic locations in which α thalassemias are most common are Africa, the Mediterranean, and Southeast Asia.[2] Interestingly, the more severe phenotypes (hemoglobin H disease and hemoglobin Bart's) are typically seen only in the Mediterranean and Southeast Asia.[3] The molecular explanation is that there are 2 forms of α thalassemia minor-2: the *trans* form (α-/α-), which involves 1 mutation on each chromosome 16, and the *cis* form ($\alpha\alpha$/-), which involves 2 mutations on the same chromosome 16. In Africa, the predominate genotype of α thalassemia minor-2 is trans, whereas in the Mediterranean and Southeast Asia, the *cis* configuration is more common. This finding becomes important during reproduction, as inheritance of the *cis* mutation makes the offspring much more likely to acquire clinically significant disease.

Each chromosome 11 carries 1 copy of the gene encoding the β globin chain (β/β), so patients with β thalassemia can be either heterozygous (β thalassemia minor; β/β^T) or homozygous (β thalassemia major; β^T/β^T). Occasionally, patients are homozygous for β chain mutations but still have some residual β globin chain synthesis resulting in an intermediate phenotype (β thalassemia intermedia). The classic presentation of patients with β thalassemia minor is a mild microcytic anemia (hemoglobin ~10–12 g/dL). β thalassemia major presents soon after birth with severe transfusion-dependent anemia. As the name implies, the phenotype of β thalassemia intermedia can range in presentation from moderate anemia to severe, transfusion-dependent anemia.

Also common in Southeast Asia is hemoglobin E disease in which the mutation (glutamic acid to glycine at position 26) reduced β-chain mRNA production, so the phenotype is that of a thalassemic microcytic anemia. Patients who are heterozygous for hemoglobin E (β/β^E) exhibit microcytosis and target cells but tend to be asymptomatic, whereas those who are homozygotes (β^E/β^E) have mild anemia and mild splenomegaly. Of note, patients who are compound heterozygotes for β-thalassemia and hemoglobin E disease (β^T/β^E) tend to manifest a severe thalassemia phenotype resulting in transfusion-dependent anemia.

The amount of reduction in mean corpuscular volume (MCV) can be a clue to etiology, as only rarely does the anemia of inflammation lower the value to less than 70 fL, narrowing the remaining differential diagnosis to iron deficiency anemia and inherited hemoglobinopathies. Specific diagnosis of thalassemias requires the combination of iron studies, hemoglobin electrophoresis, and occasionally DNA testing.

Alpha thalassemia trait (α-/α- or $\alpha\alpha$/-) is electrophoretically silent, and the diagnosis is typically made based on microcytosis with mild or no anemia and normal iron stores.[2] However, definitive diagnosis can be made with DNA analysis. Patients with hemoglobin H disease will have a tetramer of β chains on electrophoresis along with severe microcytosis, hemolysis, and splenomegaly.

Beta thalassemia minor (β/β^T) presents with hemoglobin ranging 10 to 12 g/dL and MCV ranging from 65 to 75 fL typically, as well as increased production of δ globin chains called *hemoglobin A2* (Hgb A2). Hemoglobin electrophoresis in β thalassemia minor shows an increased Hgb A2 fraction. The previous concern that concurrent iron deficiency may blunt the increase in Hgb A2 is not seen in most patients.[4] The hemoglobin electrophoresis for β thalassemia intermedia and major also shows elevated Hgb A2 fraction, but these patients can be distinguished from β thalassemia minor based on their degree of anemia and transfusion dependence.

For most patients with either α or β thalassemia minor, they require no specific therapy. However, if a patient is considering child bearing, the partner should be screened for thalassemia by checking MCV, and if less than 75 fL, then more specific genetic testing should be considered. Thalassemia major appears soon after birth when the production of fetal hemoglobin declines, leading to the onset of severe anemia.

For children born with severe forms of thalassemia, chronic transfusions are necessary to allow normal growth and development.[1] However, without aggressive, concurrent iron chelation therapy, endocrine failure ensues, and many patients will die in the second or third decade of life from complications related to iron overload. Aggressive iron chelation can prevent or delay these complications, but compliance is essential. If available, stem cell transplantation is the best treatment option, minimizing complications associated with lifelong transfusions and chelation therapy.

Treatment of patients with β thalassemia intermedia and hemoglobin H disease is more challenging because of the variety of phenotypic presentations. For patients who require transfusions, iron chelation is essential, as these patients have increased iron absorption, and iron overload can occur even in those with minimal transfusion requirements.

For patients with milder forms of thalassemia who require no treatment, iron supplementation should still be avoided unless clearly iron deficient. All patients with thalassemia should be offered genetic counseling because of their increased risk of having children with thalassemia.

COPPER DEFICIENCY

Copper deficiency is an increasingly recognized cause of anemia and has a unique clinical presentation that warrants mention.[5] Copper—like iron—is absorbed in the duodenum. In the systemic circulation, copper is transported by ceruloplasmin and serves as a cofactor for many oxidoreductases and mono-oxygenases, so deficiency seems to affect a variety of cellular functions.

The hematologic presentation is a severe anemia with variable red cell indices—most often macrocytosis, but occasionally microcytosis occurs.[6] Copper deficiency anemia is accompanied by a severe neutropenia, but unlike many causes of pancytopenia, thrombocytopenia is rare, and a normal platelet count is a clue to the diagnosis.[7] The bone marrow biopsy can mimic myelodysplasia (MDS) with vacuolization of red and white cell precursors and ringed sideroblasts, and copper deficiency should be ruled out before the diagnosis of MDS is made.[7]

Most patients with copper deficiency anemia will have a co-occurring myelopathy, which is another important diagnostic clue.[6] Patients can exhibit gait abnormalities and limb paresthesias, and spinal MRI may show dorsal column defects.

The most frequent cause of copper deficiency is upper gastrointestinal track surgery—most commonly bariatric surgery.[8] Excessive zinc intake can also lead to copper deficiency.[9] Zinc and copper share the same transporter, so if zinc overwhelms the receptor, copper cannot be absorbed. Ironically, patients who ingest "copper" pennies can be copper deficient, as currently pennies are 97.5% zinc. Other causes of copper deficiency include malabsorptive states like celiac disease and iron replacement therapy, as iron also competes with copper for the transporter. Finally, up to 20% of cases are idiopathic.

Detecting low serum copper levels makes the diagnosis. Decreased levels of ceruloplasmin are uniformly seen and have the advantage of more rapid turnaround time than copper levels in many laboratories. The treatment is oral elemental copper supplementation of around 2 to 4 mg/d, but some patients may require more aggressive replacement.[8,10] Removal of zinc and iron supplements is crucial. The hematologic response to therapy is usually rapid, but the neurologic deficits may persist, highlighting the importance of early diagnosis.

PAROXYSMAL NOCTURNAL HEMOGLOBINURIA

Paroxysmal nocturnal hemoglobinuria (PNH) is a complement-mediated hemolytic anemia characterized by bouts of hemolysis and a propensity for thrombosis. The severity of hemolysis can range from well-compensated and episodic to transfusion-dependent anemia. Severe thrombophilia is often observed, making thromboembolism the leading cause of morbidity and mortality in these patients.[11–13] Both venous and arterial thrombosis can occur, but PNH seems to have a predilection for visceral vein thrombosis. Thus, patients who present with unexplained portal or hepatic vein thrombosis should be screened for PNH. The cause of the hypercoagulable state is multifactorial and complex, but complement-mediated platelet activation has been most strongly implicated.[14]

The molecular defect in PNH is a mutation in the phosphatidylinositol glycan complementation group A gene in hematopoietic stem cells, which is responsible for the biosynthesis of glycosylphosphatidylinositol (GPI)-linked proteins. Among these GPI-linked proteins are complement-regulatory proteins CD55 and CD59. The deficiency of these regulatory proteins in PNH stem cells increases complement activation, which results in an inflammatory cascade and intravascular hemolysis.

PNH frequently arises in association with disorders of bone marrow failure, particularly aplastic anemia. Mutations in the phosphatidylinositol glycan complementation group A gene can occur in normal individuals who do not go on to have PNH because the abnormal clone does not have a growth advantage compared with the normal hematopoietic stem cells. However, if there is a concurrent bone marrow failure syndrome, the PNH clone may have a relative growth advantage, leading to expansion of the abnormal clone and the clinical syndrome of PNH.[15]

Traditionally, the diagnosis of PNH was based on in vitro demonstrations of increased sensitivity of red blood cells to complement-mediated lysis. Currently, flow cytometry is used to detect severe deficiency of GPI-anchored proteins in at least 2 cell lines (ie, lack of CD55 or CD59 on erythrocytes, or lack of CD16 or CD24 on granulocytes).[16] The most sensitive flow cytometric technique is fluorescein-labeled proaerolysin, which labels GPI anchors and allows detection of small clones. Patients with PNH should also be screened for bone marrow failure syndromes with bone marrow analysis and cytogenetic testing, as these frequently co-occur.

The mainstay of treatment for PNH is eculizumab, a humanized monoclonal antibody that specifically binds complement protein C5 and inhibits the terminal portion of the complement cascade. By blocking C5, eculizumab inhibits many of the proinflammatory, hemolytic, and prothrombotic effects responsible for the adverse clinical outcomes in PNH.[17] In studies, eculizumab has been shown to reduce hemolysis and improve anemia, fatigue, and quality of life in these patients.[18] Additionally, eculizumab reduces thrombotic events in PNH. In an aggregate review of 3 major trials examining the rates of thromboembolism in patients with PNH, the event rate in the group treated with eculizumab was 1.07 events per 100 patient-years compared with 7.37 events per 100 patient-years (P <.001) in the group not on eculizumab treatment (relative reduction, 85%; absolute reduction, 6.3 thromboembolism events/100 patient-years).[19]

APLASTIC ANEMIA

Aplastic anemia (AA) is defined as pancytopenia in the setting of hypocellular bone marrow in the absence of an abnormal bone marrow infiltration or fibrosis. The age of onset is typically bimodal, with peaks occurring between 10 and 25 years and more than 60 years.[20] AA characteristically manifests with symptoms of trilineage marrow failure: fatigue and pallor from anemia, easy bruising and bleeding from thrombocytopenia, and infections from neutropenia. The complete blood count shows pancytopenia with macrocytosis and low reticulocyte count. Bone marrow biopsy is necessary to make the diagnosis and shows hypocellular marrow. Occasionally, patients can have marrow hot spots of hematopoiesis and may require repeat bone marrow sampling if the rest of the testing suggests aplastic anemia. Several primary bone marrow failure syndromes should be ruled out before initiating treatment. For example, MDS can also present with a hypocellular marrow, so cytogenetic and molecular testing should be performed to rule out this diagnosis. A careful history should be conducted to identify any offending medications or infections that could cause a reversible toxic or postviral aplasia. Additionally, given that AA can be the initial presentation of Fanconi anemia or telomere disease, testing for these etiologies should be performed in younger patients (<40 years) as well.[21,22] Lastly, all patients should be screened for PNH with flow cytometry on peripheral blood to detect deficiency of GPI-anchored proteins. Small PNH clones are identified in up to 50% of AA patients and do not typically change management; however, large PNH clones may predispose patients to hemolysis and increased risk of thrombosis and may necessitate anti-complement therapy. [20]

Severe AA is defined by hypocellular marrow with 2 of 3 of the following: neutrophil count less than 0.5×10^9/L, platelet count less than 20×10^9/L, or reticulocyte count less than 20×10^9/L.[20] Patients are considered to have very severe AA if the neutrophil count is less than 0.2×10^9/L. Patients with severe AA require treatment. The main determinant of mortality and severity of disease in aplastic anemia is the neutrophil count.

Although a detailed mechanism of the pathophysiology is lacking, T cell–mediated inhibition of marrow progenitor growth has been implicated in idiopathic aplastic anemia.[23] Some cases of AA have been attributed to direct drug-induced stem cell toxicity, but even these patients seem to respond to intense immunosuppression, supporting an immune etiology in most patients.[24]

The epidemiology of aplastic anemia has been studied thoroughly by several national and international registries, including the International Aplastic Anemia and Agranulocytosis Study, in attempts to clarify the role certain medicines play in pathogenesis.[25,26] In these studies, it is reported that 17% to 45% of AA cases are related to medication toxicity.[27] The drugs most often implicated are gold salts, penicillamine, nonsteroidal anti-inflammatory agents (indomethacin, diclofenac), ticlopidine, and anticonvulsants (**Box 2**).[24,25,27] When there is a high suspicion of drug-induced AA, therapy consists of removing the offending drug and supporting the patient through the pancytopenia phase. If no improvement is seen after a week, more definitive treatment is required.

Currently, there are 2 mainstays of therapy: (1) hematopoietic stem cell transplantation (HSCT) and (2) immunosuppression therapy (IST). In general, patients younger than 50 years with severe AA should be considered for upfront HSCT if a matched sibling donor (MSD) is immediately available, as cure rates reach up to 75% to 90% in these patients.[20] If an MSD is not readily available, IST is the next step. The outcomes for patients receiving unrelated donor and partial HLA-matched donor stem cell transplants are improving, but this intervention is reserved for patients who first do not respond to immunosuppression.

In patients older than 50 years with severe AA, first-line therapy is IST with horse antithymocyte globulin (ATG) and cyclosporine (CSA).[28] Immunosuppression is effective in many patients with AA, with response rates of up to 75% to 85%.[20] In general, IST has less initial toxicity compared with HSCT but is associated with higher rates of relapse and leukemic transformation. Response to IST may take several months, and most patients do not recover their counts fully, but many can be weaned off transfusions and are able to maintain an absolute neutrophil count high enough to prevent

Box 2
Drugs commonly implicated in leading to aplastic anemia

Acetazolamide

Allopurinol

Amphotericin

Aspirin

Captopril

Carbamazepine

Chlorpheniramine

Chloroquine

Chlorpromazine

Colchicine

Dapsone

Diclofenac

Ethosuximide

Furosemide

Gold

Ibuprofen

Indomethacin

Lithium

Mepacrine

Methicillin

Methyldopa

Naproxen

Nifedipine

Nonsteroidal anti-inflammatory drugs

Penicillamine

Penicillin

Phenylbutazone

Phenothiazine

Phenytoin

Pyrimethamine

Quinacrine

Quinidine

Sulindac

Sulphonamides

Thiouracil

Ticlopidine

Sulphonylurea

infections. Patients who do not respond to IST after 6 months are considered to have refractory AA. If they have an MSD, allogenic stem cell transplant is the next step. If not, then a repeat course of ATG and CSA is given. If this fails, then an alternate donor stem cell transplant can be considered.[29] In the last few years, eltrombopag—a thrombopoietin receptor agonist—has been used to stimulate stem cell maturation and has a 44% response rate in refractory AA.[30] Currently, the use of eltrombopag is reserved for patients with refractory disease, but trials of upfront eltrombopag combined with initial immunosuppressive regimens are underway.[31]

Novel immunosuppressive drugs such as daclizumab, alemtuzumab, high-dose cyclophosphamide, and mycophenolate have been used in refractory AA, but toxicities often outweigh benefit.[20,28]

Good supportive care is imperative in all patients with aplastic anemia. Blood transfusions should be provided to improve symptoms and products limited to leukoreduced blood for all patients (plus, irradiated products for patients undergoing treatment with HSCT or IST). Prophylactic platelet transfusions are recommended for patients receiving treatment if platelet counts are less than $10,000 \times 10^9$/L. Severely neutropenic patients with counts less than 0.5×10^9/L should receive prophylactic antibiotics, antifungal medications, and antiviral medications in accordance with local policies, although routine prophylaxis against *Pneumocystis jiroveci* is not necessary.[20]

PURE RED CELL APLASIA

Pure red cell aplasia (PRCA) is a rare bone marrow disorder in which the red cell line is selectively suppressed.[32,33] Patients present with severe anemia and very low reticulocyte counts (<0.5%). Bone marrow biopsy finds loss of the erythroid lineage and preservation of other cell lines.

The cause of PRCA is thought to be autoimmune, but viral infections and drug toxicities have also been implicated. As with aplastic anemia, a detailed mechanism of the pathophysiology remains uncertain, but support for autoimmune destruction of red cell precursors is favored based on patient response to immunosuppression and elevated levels of T lymphocytes in the serum of patients with PRCA. Additionally, there is increased incidence of thymoma in these patients, and thymectomy has been therapeutic in some.[34]

Parvovirus B19 is a common viral infection that infects and destroys red cell precursors.[35] In most patients, it causes a mild, transient anemia until the infection clears. However, parvovirus can lead to more serious clinical sequela in 2 groups of patients: patients with congenital hemolytic anemia syndromes and immunosuppressed patients. Patients with congenital hemolytic anemias—sickle cell anemia, for example—require high baseline reticulocyte production to compensate for red cell destruction. Parvovirus infection induces periods of reticulocytopenia, which can lead to profound anemia and the so-called aplastic crisis in sickle cell patients. On the other hand, immunocompromised patients have difficulty clearing the infection, which can cause prolonged anemia.

Many drugs have been imputed as a cause of PRCA, but correlation is perhaps only well established for azathioprine, chlorpropamide, erythropoietin, isoniazid, phenytoin, and valproic acid (**Box 3**).[36,37]

The first clinical clue to PRCA is severe reticulocytopenia (<0.1% or <10,000/μL). Diagnosis is based on bone marrow examination, which shows severe and selective loss of erythroid precursors. Patients should be screened for thymoma with chest computed tomography or MRI and peripheral blood sent for flow cytometry to look

Box 3
Drugs implicated in pure red cell aplasia
Allopurinol
Ampicillin
Azathioprine
Carbamazepine
Cephalothin
Chloroquine
Chlorpropamide
Dapsone/Pyrimethamine
Erythropoietin
Fenbufen
Fenoprofen
Gold
Halothane
Isoniazid
Mepacrine
Methyldopa
Penicillamine
Penicillin
Phenobarbital
Phenytoin
Procainamide
Rifampin
Salicylazosulfapyridine
Sulfasalazine
Sulfathiazole
Tolbutamide
Trimethoprim-sulfamethoxazole
Valproic acid

for an increased T lymphocyte population, especially of large granular lymphocytes.[33] Active parvovirus infection can be detected on bone marrow stains and serum polymerase chain reaction.

There is no standard treatment for PRCA. Any suspect drug should be discontinued with marrow recovery expected in a few weeks. A course of prednisone is often effective, but many patients cannot be weaned. Increasingly, CSA is effective in both induction and maintenance and is now considered first-line therapy for PRCA.[33] Cyclophosphamide alone or in combination with CSA is also used with reported benefit in some. Alemtuzumab, ATG, and rituximab are options for patients who do not respond to CSA or cyclophosphamide but with mixed results. Rituximab may be effective for erythropoietin-related PRCA.[38] Finally, in patients with viral PRCA, immunoglobulin infusions with antiparvovirus antibodies have been effective in clearing the infection and correcting the anemia.[39]

ACQUIRED HEMOLYTIC ANEMIAS

Microangiopathic hemolytic anemias (MAHA) are a group of disorders characterized by destruction of circulating erythrocytes in the setting of intravascular disease and red blood cell fragmentation.[40] MAHA is commonly associated with thrombotic micro-angiopathies such as hemolytic uremic syndrome, disseminated intravascular coagulation, and thrombotic thrombocytopenic purpura, in which fibrin and platelet aggregates deposit in small vessels resulting in microvascular thrombi and intravascular hemolysis. However, there are many other disease states in which MAHA has been observed. These will be reviewed below.

MAHA has been associated with several cardiovascular diseases. MAHA occurs in patients with malignant hypertension via disruption of the endothelial wall, resulting in severe hemolysis as erythrocytes transverse damaged glomeruli.[41] Fortunately, the disease reverses rapidly with appropriate blood pressure control. Cardiac valvulopathies can induce MAHA, most commonly after mitral valve repair. When small perivalvular leaks occur around the mitral annulus, a regurgitant jet develops, which creates shearing stress and leads to red cell destruction.[42] Although some patients are treated conservatively with afterload reduction, definitive therapy requires additional surgery or percutaneous valve repair.[21,42]

MAHA is a well-recognized complication of ventricular assist devices (VADs). The high shearing forces that occur within VADs can damage erythrocytes. However, the magnitude of the shear force needed to disrupt erythrocytes is markedly higher (about 15 times) than the force required to unfold von Willebrand protein and 3 times higher than the force required to activate platelets.[43] Nonetheless, VADs cause a low, baseline level of hemolysis, which increases dramatically if in-pump thrombosis occurs. These patients typically present with classic signs of hemolysis (dark urine, high low-density lipoprotein levels, low hemoglobin levels), device alarms, decompensated heart failure, and cardiogenic shock in severe cases.[44] Diagnosis is typically made by echocardiography. Therapy is anticoagulation, and medical stabilization until surgical pump exchange can be performed.

In addition to vascular events, MAHA can be toxin mediated. For example, infection with *Clostridium perfringens* can lead to hemolysis by directly damaging red cell membranes.[45] The bacteria secrete α-toxin with phospholipase activity, which dissolves red cell membranes and causes subsequent leakage of hemoglobin out of the cell. In some cases, this is so severe that the measured hemoglobin may equal the hematocrit level. Additionally, an empty red cell "ghost" may be seen on the blood smear. The clinical course is often fatal with a greater than 80% mortality rate.[45]

End-stage liver disease can cause a specific type of hemolysis known as *spur cell anemia*.[46] Alterations in lipid metabolism in end-stage liver disease lead to cholesterol crystal deposition in the red cell membrane,[47] which leads to both deformed red cells—spur cells—and expedited removal by the spleen. In addition to the classic findings of hemolysis, patients with spur cell anemia have laboratory abnormalities associated with severe liver disease, such as elevated international normalized ratios and total bilirubin (average of 9.5 mg/dL).[46] Spur cell anemia is associated with an ominous prognosis with an average survival of 1.9 months. Treatment options are limited to liver transplantation versus supportive care.

Wilson disease—an inherited disorder of copper metabolism characterized by cooper accumulation resulting in end organ damage—can present initially with episodic hemolysis. Erythrocyte destruction in Wilson disease is likely caused by direct oxidative damage of copper on hemoglobin.[48] The peripheral blood smear typically shows spherocytes and "bite cells." Luckily, hemolysis is often transient.

Finally, severe burns can cause hemolysis owing to direct damage to red cells.[49] The intense heat damages the red cell membrane, leading to instability and destruction. Peripheral blood smear is notable for spherocytes and fragmentation of red cells. Treatment is supportive care.

SUMMARY

In this global age, it is vital for physicians to keep unusual anemias in the clinical differential diagnosis regardless of their practice location. This review serves not only to remind clinicians of these more rare types of anemias, but also to provide a clinical framework to recognize and diagnose these various types of anemias and ultimately promote more appropriate and timely therapeutic interventions.

REFERENCES

1. Martin A, Thompson AA. Thalassemias. Pediatr Clin North Am 2013;60(6): 1383–91.
2. Piel FB, Weatherall DJ. The alpha-thalassemias. N Engl J Med 2014;371(20): 1908–16.
3. Ryan K, Bain BJ, Worthington D, et al. Significant haemoglobinopathies: guidelines for screening and diagnosis. Br J Haematol 2010;149(1):35–49.
4. Passarello C, Giambona A, Cannata M, et al. Iron deficiency does not compromise the diagnosis of high HbA(2) beta thalassemia trait. Haematologica 2012; 97(3):472–3.
5. Lazarchick J. Update on anemia and neutropenia in copper deficiency. Curr Opin Hematol 2012;19(1):58–60.
6. Jaiser SR, Winston GP. Copper deficiency myelopathy. J Neurol 2010;257(6): 869–81.
7. Gassmann M, Muckenthaler MU. Adaptation of iron requirement to hypoxic conditions at high altitude. J Appl Physiol (1985) 2015;119(12):1432–40.
8. Levi M, Rosselli M, Simonetti M, et al. Epidemiology of iron deficiency anaemia in four European countries: a population-based study in primary care. Eur J Haematol 2016. [Epub ahead of print].
9. Duncan A, Yacoubian C, Watson N, et al. The risk of copper deficiency in patients prescribed zinc supplements. J Clin Pathol 2015;68(9):723–5.
10. Halfdanarson TR, Kumar N, Li CY, et al. Hematological manifestations of copper deficiency: a retrospective review. Eur J Haematol 2008;80(6):523–31.
11. Matei D, Brenner B, Marder VJ. Acquired thrombophilic syndromes. Blood Rev 2001;15:31–48.
12. Ray JG, Burows RF, Ginsberg JS, et al. Paroxysmal nocturnal hemoglobinuria and the risk of venous thrombosis: review and recommendations for management of the pregnant and nonpregnant patient. Haemostasis 2000;30:103–17 [Review; 66 refs].
13. Socie G, Mary JY, de Gramont A, et al. Paroxysmal nocturnal haemoglobinuria: long-term follow-up and prognostic factors. French Society of Haematology. Lancet 1996;348:573–7 [see comments].
14. Gralnick HR, Vail M, McKeown LP, et al. Activated platelets in paroxysmal nocturnal haemoglobinuria. Liver 1995;91:697–702.
15. Parker C, Omine M, Richards S, et al. Diagnosis and management of paroxysmal nocturnal hemoglobinuria. Blood 2005;106(12):3699–709.

16. Preis M, Lowrey CH. Laboratory tests for paroxysmal nocturnal hemoglobinuria. Am J Hematol 2014;89(3):339–41.
17. Devalet B, Mullier F, Chatelain B, et al. Pathophysiology, diagnosis, and treatment of paroxysmal nocturnal hemoglobinuria: a review. Eur J Haematol 2015;95(3):190–8.
18. Hillmen P, Young NS, Schubert J, et al. The complement inhibitor eculizumab in paroxysmal nocturnal hemoglobinuria. N Engl J Med 2006;355(12):1233–43.
19. Hillmen P, Muus P, Duhrsen U, et al. Effect of the complement inhibitor eculizumab on thromboembolism in patients with paroxysmal nocturnal hemoglobinuria. Blood 2007;110(12):4123–8.
20. Marsh JC, Ball SE, Cavenagh J, et al. Guidelines for the diagnosis and management of aplastic anaemia. Br J Haematol 2009;147(1):43–70.
21. Pate GE, Al ZA, Chandavimol M, et al. Percutaneous closure of prosthetic paravalvular leaks: case series and review. Catheter Cardiovasc Interv 2006;68(4):528–33.
22. Scheinberg P, Young NS. How I treat acquired aplastic anemia. Blood 2012;120(6):1185–96.
23. Young NS, Maciejewski J. The pathophysiology of acquired aplastic anemia. N Engl J Med 1997;336(19):1365–72 [Review; 72 refs].
24. Vincent PC. Drug-induced aplastic anaemia and agranulocytosis. Incidence and mechanisms. Drugs 1986;31(1):52–63.
25. Kaufman DW, Kelly JP, Jurgelon JM, et al. Drugs in the aetiology of agranulocytosis and aplastic anaemia. Eur J Haematol Suppl 1996;60:23–30.
26. Wiholm BE, Emanuelsson S. Drug-related blood dyscrasias in a Swedish reporting system, 1985-1994. Eur J Haematol Suppl 1996;60:42–6.
27. Young NS. Acquired aplastic anemia. In: Handin RI, Stossel TP, Lux SE, editors. Blood: principles and practice of hematology. Philadelphia: J.B. Lippincott Co; 1995. p. 293–365.
28. Willis L, Rexwinkle A, Bryan J, et al. Recent developments in drug therapy for aplastic anemia. Ann Pharmacother 2014;48(11):1469–78.
29. Marsh JC, Kulasekararaj AG. Management of the refractory aplastic anemia patient: what are the options? Blood 2013;122(22):3561–7.
30. Olnes MJ, Scheinberg P, Calvo KR, et al. Eltrombopag and improved hematopoiesis in refractory aplastic anemia. N Engl J Med 2012;367(1):11–9.
31. Gill H, Leung GM, Lopes D, et al. The thrombopoietin mimetics eltrombopag and romiplostim in the treatment of refractory aplastic anaemia. Br J Haematol 2016. [Epub ahead of print].
32. Ishii K, Young NS. Anemia of central origin. Semin Hematol 2015;52(4):321–38.
33. Sawada K, Fujishima N, Hirokawa M. Acquired pure red cell aplasia: updated review of treatment. Br J Haematol 2008;142(4):505–14.
34. Fisch P, Handgretinger R, Schaefer HE. Pure red cell aplasia. Br J Haematol 2000;111(4):1010–22.
35. Rogo LD, Mokhtari-Azad T, Kabir MH, et al. Human parvovirus B19: a review. Acta Virol 2014;58(3):199–213.
36. DeLoughery T. Drug-induced immune hematologic disease. Immunol Allergy Clin N Am 1998;18(4):829–31.
37. Smalling R, Foote M, Molineux G, et al. Drug-induced and antibody-mediated pure red cell aplasia: a review of literature and current knowledge. Biotechnol Annu Rev 2004;10:237–50.
38. Mohd Slim MA, Shaik R. Pure red cell aplasia associated with recombinant erythropoietin: a case report and brief review of the literature. N Z Med J 2013;126(1386):106–10.

39. Sawada K, Hirokawa M, Fujishima N. Diagnosis and management of acquired pure red cell aplasia. Hematol Oncol Clin North Am 2009;23(2):249–59.
40. Hughes DA, Stuart-Smith SE, Bain BJ. How should stainable iron in bone marrow films be assessed? J Clin Pathol 2004;57(10):1038–40.
41. van den Born BJ, Honnebier UP, Koopmans RP, et al. Microangiopathic hemolysis and renal failure in malignant hypertension. Hypertension 2005;45(2):246–51.
42. Spargias K, Chrissoheris M, Halapas A, et al. Percutaneous mitral valve repair using the edge-to-edge technique: first Greek experience. Hellenic J Cardiol 2012; 53(5):343–51.
43. Fraser KH, Zhang T, Taskin ME, et al. A quantitative comparison of mechanical blood damage parameters in rotary ventricular assist devices: shear stress, exposure time and hemolysis index. J Biomech Eng 2012;134(8):081002.
44. Birschmann I, Dittrich M, Eller T, et al. Ambient hemolysis and activation of coagulation is different between HeartMate II and HeartWare left ventricular assist devices. J Heart Lung Transplant 2014;33(1):80–7.
45. van Bunderen CC, Bomers MK, Wesdorp E, et al. Clostridium perfringens septicaemia with massive intravascular haemolysis: a case report and review of the literature. Neth J Med 2010;68(9):343–6.
46. Alexopoulou A, Vasilieva L, Kanellopoulou T, et al. Presence of spur cells as a highly predictive factor of mortality in patients with cirrhosis. J Gastroenterol Hepatol 2014;29(4):830–4.
47. Doll DC, Doll NJ. Spur cell anemia. South Med J 1982;75(10):1205–10.
48. Attri S, Sharma N, Jahagirdar S, et al. Erythrocyte metabolism and antioxidant status of patients with Wilson disease with hemolytic anemia. Pediatr Res 2006; 59(4 Pt 1):593–7.
49. Lawrence C, Atac B. Hematologic changes in massive burn injury. Crit Care Med 1992;20(9):1284–8.

Blood Transfusion Therapy

Lawrence Tim Goodnough, MD[a,b,*], Anil K. Panigrahi, MD, PhD[a,c]

KEYWORDS

- Anemia • Red blood cell transfusion • Clinical decision support
- Restrictive transfusion practices

KEY POINTS

- Transfusion of red blood cells (RBCs) is a balance between providing benefit for patients while avoiding risks of transfusion.
- Randomized, controlled trials of restrictive RBC transfusion practices have shown equivalent patient outcomes compared with liberal transfusion practices, and meta-analyses have shown improved in-hospital mortality, reduced cardiac events, and reduced bacterial infections.
- This body of level 1 evidence has led to substantial, improved blood utilization and reduction of inappropriate blood transfusions with implementation of clinical decision support via electronic medical records, along with accompanying educational initiatives.

INTRODUCTION

Blood transfusion therapy is frequently used in the supportive care for treatment of anemia. The transfusion of red blood cells (RBC) is a balance between the benefits of maintaining oxygen delivery and the inherent risks from blood transfusion. The signs and symptoms of anemia vary based on the acuity of the anemia, compensatory change in blood volume, and the compensatory change in cardiac output from the patient's cardiovascular system. Chronic anemia is generally well tolerated due to compensatory expansion of intravascular plasma volume, increased cardiac output, vasodilatation, increased blood flow due to decreased viscosity, and not least, increased RBC 2,3 diphosphoglycerate, with a right shift of the oxygen dissociation curve, so that oxygen is unloaded to the peripheral tissues more readily. Symptoms of anemia are often nonspecific and can include fatigue, pallor, dizziness, headaches, vertigo, tinnitus, dyspnea, and inactivity. Fatigue particularly has been associated with poor quality of life.[1]

[a] Department of Pathology, Stanford University, Stanford, CA, USA; [b] Department of Medicine, Stanford University, Stanford, CA, USA; [c] Department of Anesthesiology, Stanford University, Stanford, CA, USA
* Corresponding author. Department of Pathology, Stanford University, 300 Pasteur Drive, Room H-1402, Stanford, CA 94305-5626.
E-mail address: ltgoodno@stanford.edu

Med Clin N Am 101 (2017) 431–447
http://dx.doi.org/10.1016/j.mcna.2016.09.012
0025-7125/17/© 2016 Elsevier Inc. All rights reserved.

The traditional therapy for chronic, medically related anemia has been RBC transfusions. However, transfusion therapy has been identified as one of the most overused (and inappropriate) therapeutic interventions by national accreditation (Joint Commission) and medical societies, such as the American Board of Internal Medicine,[2] the American Medical Association, the American Society of Hematology (ASH), and the American Association of Blood Banks (AABB; http://www.choosingwisely.org/doctor-patient-lists/american-society-of-hematology/). Recommendations have been published by several medical societies for RBC transfusion therapy in adult[3] and pediatric[4] patients.

The authors have previously reviewed blood transfusion practices,[3,5,6] and herein they provide an updated review of RBC therapy in adult and pediatric patients. The article summarizes current blood risks and indications for RBC transfusion. Important, alternative therapies for management of anemia, such as iron therapy and erythropoietic stimulating agents (ESAs), are outside the scope of this review, but have been published elsewhere.[7,8] Where possible, the article provides evidence-based guidelines for best transfusion practices.

RISKS OF BLOOD TRANSFUSION

Transfusion-transmitted infections prompted concern by patients and health care providers since the 1980s, with the recognition of transfusion transmission of human immunodeficiency virus (HIV) and hepatitis C virus (HCV).[9] These risks have decreased substantially, and responses to emerging pathogens transmitted by blood transfusion have been rapid (**Fig. 1**).[10] Nevertheless, emerging threats of blood-transmissible pathogens is always a concern, the most recent example of which is the Zika virus, in which potential blood donors who are acutely ill and viremic may be asymptomatic and not be deferred during donor screening.[11] For this reason, an experimental nucleic acid test (NAT) was implemented for universal donor testing by end of November 2016. Between 2007 and 2011, transfusion-related acute lung injury (TRALI) caused the highest percentage (43%) of fatalities reported to the US Food and Drug Administration (FDA), followed by hemolytic transfusion reactions (23%) caused by non-ABO- (13%) or ABO- (10%) incompatible blood transfusions.[12]

Increasing evidence suggests that a far greater number of patients now have adverse clinical outcomes (increased morbidity and mortality) associated with unnecessary blood transfusions.[13–15] **Table 1** lists risks that include not only known transmissible pathogens for infectious disease, transfusion reactions, TRALI, errors in blood administration, and circulatory overload but also potential, as yet undefined risks such as immunomodulation (eg, perioperative infection or tumor progression), unknown or emerging risks (such as the new variant Creutzfeldt-Jakob disease and Zika virus),[10,16] and potential risks associated with storage lesions from blood transfusions.[17,18]

Awareness of blood risks and costs[19] has led providers to develop institution-based initiatives in Patient Blood Management, including the adoption of recommendations that limit the use of blood transfusion.[3] Patient Blood Management encompasses an evidence-based approach that is multidisciplinary (transfusion medicine specialists, surgeons, anesthesiologists, and critical care specialists) and multiprofessional (physicians, nurses, pump technologists, and pharmacists).[20] Preventative strategies are emphasized to identify, evaluate, and manage anemia in medical[6] and surgical[21] patients, use of pharmacologic interventions,[7,8] and the avoidance of unnecessary diagnostic testing to minimize iatrogenic blood loss[22]; and to establish clinical practice recommendations for blood transfusions.[3] For anemic patients being evaluated for

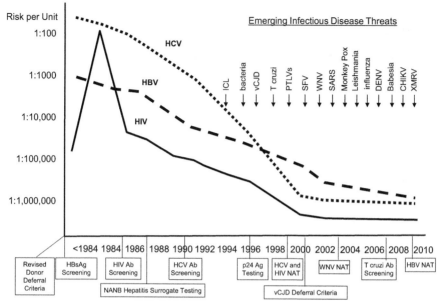

Fig. 1. Risks of major transfusion-transmissible viruses linked to interventions, and accelerating rate of EIDs of concern to blood safety. Evolution of the risks of transmission by blood transfusion for HIV, HBV, and HCV. Major interventions to reduce risks are indicated below the time line on the x-axis. Emerging infectious disease threats over the past 20 years are indicated above in the top right quadrant of the figure. Ab, antibody; Ag, antigen; CHIKV, Chikungunya virus; DENV, dengue virus; HBsAg, hepatitis B surface antigen; ICL, idiopathic CD4+ T lymphocytopenia; PTLV, posttransplant lymphoproliferative disease; SARS, severe acute respiratory syndrome; SFV, simian foamy virus; vCJD, variant Creutzfeldt-Jakob disease; WNV, West Nile virus; XMRV, xenotropic murine leukemia virus-related virus. (*From* Perkins HA, Busch MP. Transfusion-associated infections: 50 years of relentless challenges and remarkable progress. Transfusion 2010;50:2092; with permission.)

elective procedures with the potential for blood loss, counseling on the risks of blood transfusion should be provided and steps taken to further characterize and treat anemia before surgery,[21,23] because preoperative anemia is associated with increased morbidity,[24] mortality,[25,26] and hospital length of stay.[27]

INDICATIONS FOR RED BLOOD CELL TRANSFUSION THERAPY
Pediatric Patients

A single randomized, prospective multicenter trial to evaluate a hemoglobin (Hb) "trigger" in children was published in 2007.[28] In this study, more than 600 children admitted to the pediatric intensive care units (ICU) were randomized to either a restrictive-strategy group where Hb threshold was set at 7 g/dL or a liberal-strategy transfusion group where Hb threshold was set at 9 g/dL. The investigators found that the restrictive strategy resulted in a 44% decrease in the number of packed RBC transfusions without increasing rates of new or progressive multiorgan dysfunction, the primary outcome of the study. Several secondary outcomes, including sepsis, transfusion reactions, nosocomial respiratory infections, catheter-related infections, adverse events, length of stay in the ICU and hospital,

Table 1
Transfusion-associated adverse events

I. Infectious Agents

Transfusion-transmitted disease routinely tested	
Hepatitis B virus (HBV; 1970 [surface antigen]; 1986–1987 [core antibody]; 2009 [nucleic acid])	1:1,000,000
HIV (1985 [antibody]; 2000 [nucleic acid])	1:2,000,000
HCV (1986–1987 [alanine aminotransferase]; 1990 [antibody]; 1999 [nucleic acid])	1:2,000,000
Human T-cell lymphotropic virus (1988 [antibody])	Very rare
West Nile virus (2003 [nucleic acid])	Very rare
Bacteria (in platelets only; 2004)	1:20,000
Trypanosoma cruzi (2007 [antibody])	Very rare
Syphilis	Very rare
Cytomegalovirus (for patients at risk)	Rare
Zika virus	Rare
Transfusion-transmitted disease not currently routinely tested	Very rare or unknown
Hepatitis A virus	
Parvovirus B19	
Dengue fever virus	
Malaria	
Hepatitis E	
Babesia sp	
Plasmodium sp	
Leishmania sp	
Brucella sp	
New variant Creutzfeldt-Jakob disease prions	
Unknown pathogens	

II. Transfusion-associated adverse reactions events

Estimated risk per unit infused	
ABO incompatible blood transfusions	1 in 60,000
Symptoms	40%
Fatalities	1 in 600,000
Delayed serologic reactions	1 in 1600
Delayed hemolytic reactions	1 in 6700
TRALI	1 in 20,000
Graft-versus-host disease	Very rare
Posttransfusion purpura	Very rare
Febrile, nonhemolytic transfusion reactions	
RBCs	1 in 200
Platelets	1 in 5–20
Allergic reactions	1 in 30–100
Transfusion-associated circulatory overload	1 in 12
Anaphylactic reactions (Immunoglobulin A deficiency)	1 in 150,000
Iron overload	Estimated 80–100 U for adults
Transfusion-related immunosuppression	Unestablished
Storage lesions	Unestablished

Adapted from Goodnough LT. Blood management: transfusion medicine comes of age. Lancet 2013;381:1792; with permission.

and mortality were no different between the groups. The investigators recommended a restrictive RBC transfusion strategy in pediatric patients who are stable in the ICU.[28]

In addition, the TOTAL trial involving children aged 6 to 60 months presenting with severe anemia due to malaria or sickle cell disease revealed significant improvements in signs and symptoms of anemia after RBC transfusion to increase Hb concentrations from 3.7 to 7.1 g/dL.[29] Serum lactate levels decreased from 9.1 mmol/L to less than or equal to 3 mmol/L 6 hours after transfusion in 59% of children. Similarly, cerebral tissue oxygen saturation, as measured by near-infrared spectrometry, increased by more than 5% at the completion of transfusion. Furthermore, rates of stupor or coma were reduced by half, whereas respiratory distress decreased by 60%. These findings suggest that tissue perfusion with Hb concentrations of 7 g/dL may be sufficient in this population.

Other randomized trials investigating Hb thresholds have been completed or are underway in neonates.[30–32] The Prematures in Need of Transfusion study[30] suggested that liberal RBC transfusions were beneficial to neurocognitive outcomes of premature infants at 18 to 22 months, in contrast to a randomized clinical trial that showed poorer neurologic outcomes at 7- to 10-year follow-up for those premature infants who were transfused liberally.[31] The Transfusion of Prematures trial is underway to address these conflicting results.[32] In a survey of pediatric centers from Children's Oncology Group, 60% of centers used a transfusion trigger of Hb 8 g/dL, whereas 25% of centers used 7 g/dL.[33]

The notable exception in which liberal RBC transfusions have been found to be superior for improved clinical outcomes is in children with sickle cell anemia, who have overt stroke or abnormal transcranial Doppler ultrasonography and who are managed with chronic blood transfusions to keep the percentage of sickle cell hemoglobin less than 30% and the total Hb level at approximately 10 g/dL.[34,35] Interruption of such aggressive transfusion therapy when children reach the age of 18 to 20 years during transition of care to adult medical services has been described as associated with increased mortality and overt stroke events.[36]

Adult Patients

Symptomatic manifestations in medical anemias generally occur when the Hb is less than two-thirds of normal (ie, <9–10 g/dL), because basal cardiac output increases with anemia and is manifested by symptoms of increased cardiac work.[37] The historical practice was to correct mild to moderate anemia with RBC transfusions in order to treat these signs and symptoms or to transfuse blood prophylactically. The view at that time was reflected in one publication that stated "when the concentration of hemoglobin is less than 8 to 10 g/dL, it is wise to give a blood transfusion before operation."[38]

This readjustment of the transfusion trigger from an Hb of 10 g/dL to a somewhat lower threshold was triggered by concern over blood risks, particularly HIV; accompanied by the realization in populations such as Jehovah's Witness patients, who decline blood transfusions because of religious beliefs, that morbidity and mortality do not increase until the Hb is very low.[39] Data from this population indicate that the critical level of hemodilution, as defined as the point at which oxygen consumption starts to decrease because of insufficient oxygen delivery, occurs at an Hb level of approximately 4 g/dL,[40] which was corroborated in a recent study of RBC transfusions in Ugandan children with SS anemia or malaria.[29]

For anemic patients known to have cardiovascular disease (CVD), perioperative mortality has been reported to be increased significantly, when compared with patients not known to have CVD.[41] Management of anemia and the Hb threshold for RBC therapy should therefore be different for these patients. A post hoc analysis of one study[42] was accompanied by an editorial observing that "survival tended to decrease for patients with pre-existing heart disease in the restrictive transfusion strategy group, suggesting that critically ill patients with heart and vascular disease may benefit from higher Hb."[43] Previously published clinical practice guidelines concluded "the presence of coronary artery disease likely constitutes an important factor in determining a patient's tolerance to low Hb."[44] A retrospective analysis of 79,000 elderly patients (>65 years of age) hospitalized with acute myocardial infarction (MI) in the United States found that blood transfusion in patients whose admission hematocrit values were less than 33% was associated with significantly lower mortalities.[45] A more aggressive use of blood transfusion in the management of anemia in elderly patients with cardiac disease might well be warranted.[6,46]

There are an increasing number of randomized, controlled trials in adults providing level I evidence for blood transfusion practices. A previous systematic review of the literature to year 2000 identified 10 trials.[47] The investigators concluded at that time that the existing evidence supported the use of restrictive transfusion triggers in patients who were free of serious cardiac disease. A Cochrane systematic review of prospective randomized trials to 2012[48] compared "high" versus "low" Hb thresholds of 19 trials involving a total of 6264 patients. The investigators found that (1) "low" Hb thresholds were well tolerated; (2) RBC transfusions were reduced by 34% (confidence interval [CI] 24%–45%) in patients randomized to the "low" Hb cohorts; and (3) the number of RBC transfusions was reduced by 1.2 units (CI 0.5–1.8 units) in the "low" Hb cohorts. A more recent meta-analysis found that a restrictive RBC transfusion strategy aiming to allow an Hb concentration as low as 7 g/dL reduced cardiac events, rebleeding, bacterial infections, and mortality.[15]

There are 7 key randomized, clinical trials in adult patients that compare "restrictive" versus "liberal" RBC transfusion strategies in various clinical settings (**Table 2**). The Transfusion Requirements in Critical Care (TRICC) trial[49] found that intensive care patients could tolerate a restrictive transfusion strategy (Hb range 7–9 g/dL, 8.2 g/dL on average) as well as patients transfused more liberally (Hb range 10–12 g/dL, 10.5 g/dL on average), with no differences in 30-day mortalities. Similarly, in the Transfusion Requirements in Septic Shock trial[50] of lower (<7 g/dL) versus higher (<9 g/dL) Hb thresholds for transfusion in patients with septic shock, equivalent 90-day mortalities (43 vs 45%, respectively) were found for patients in the 2 cohorts. However, a retrospective study of 2393 patients[51] consecutively admitted to the ICU found that an admission hematocrit less than 25%, in the absence of transfusion, was associated with long-term mortality; so that there may be hematocrit levels below which the risk-to-benefit imbalance for transfusion reverses.

The Transfusion Requirements after Cardiac Surgery (TRACS) trial[52] was a large, single-center study of patients randomized to receive either restrictive (hematocrit >24%) or liberal (hematocrit >30%) RBC transfusions postoperatively. Thirty-day all-cause mortality was not different (10% vs 11%, respectively) between the 2 cohorts. The FOCUS trial found that elderly (mean >80 years of age) patients who underwent repair of hip fracture surgery tolerated an Hb trigger without RBC transfusions postoperatively to as low as 8 g/dL (or higher with transfusions, if symptomatic).[53] Subsequently, a single-center prospective study[54] of patients with upper gastrointestinal bleeding demonstrated that patients randomized to a restrictive (Hb <7 g/dL) versus a liberal (Hb <9 g/dL) Hb threshold for blood transfusions had significantly improved outcomes, including mortality at 45 days and rates of rebleeding.

Table 2
Seven key clinical trials in adults of red blood cell transfusion in adults

Clinical Setting (Ref)	Hemoglobin Threshold (g/dL)	Mean Age (y)	Patients Transfused (%)	Deviation from Transfusion Protocol (%)	Mean Hemoglobin (g/dL)[a]	Participation of Eligible Patients (%)
Intensive care[49]	7	57.1	67	1.4	8.5	41
	10	58.1	99	4.3	10.7	
CT surgery[52]	8	58.6	47	1.6	9.1	75
	10	60.7	78	0.0	10.5	
Hip fracture repair[53]	8	81.5	41	9.0	7.9	56
	10	81.8	97	5.6	9.2	
Acute upper GI bleeding[54]	7	NA	49	9.0	7.3	93
	9	NA	86	3.0	8.0	
Symptomatic coronary artery disease[55]	8	74.3	28.3	1.8	7.9	12.2
	10	67.3	NA[b]	9.1	9.3	
Sepsis trial[50]	7	67.0	64	5.9	7.7	82
	9	67.0	99	2.2	9.3	
TITR[56]	7.5	69.9	53.4	30	8–9	98
	9	70.8	92.2	45	9.2–9.8	

Abbreviations: CAD, coronary artery disease; CT, cardiothoracic; TITR, Transfusion Indication Threshold Reduction.
[a] Mean daily hemoglobin.
[b] NA: Not available.
From Goodnough LT, Shah N. Is there a "magic" hemoglobin number? Clinical decision support promoting restrictive blood transfusion practices. Am J Hematol 2015;90:929; with permission.

The MINT trial[55] was a pilot, feasibility study of liberal (Hb $\geq$10 g/dL) versus restrictive (Hb <8 g/dL) transfusion thresholds initiated for a planned enrollment of 200 patients with symptomatic coronary artery disease (acute coronary syndrome or stable angina undergoing cardiac catheterization), but was terminated at the end of 18 months after enrollment of only 110 patients; of eligible screened patients, only 12% were enrolled (see **Table 2**). The primary, composite outcome (death, MI, or revascularization) occurred in 10.9% of the liberal transfusion cohort, compared with 25.9% of the restrictive cohort (P = .054); mortality occurred in 1.8% and 13.0%, respectively (P = .032). In addition, the TITRe2 trial, which focused on postoperative coronary artery bypass graft and valve surgery patients, found no difference in primary outcomes of ischemic events (MI, stroke, bowel infarction, acute kidney injury) or infection (sepsis or wound infection) between restrictive (Hb <7.5 g/dL) and liberal (Hb <9 g/dL) transfusion triggers (35.1% vs 33.0%, P = .30). However, they observed more deaths in the restrictive group as compared with the liberal group (4.2% vs 2.6%, P = .045).[56] Furthermore, a recent meta-analysis stratifying study patients into "context-specific" risk groups based on patient characteristics and clinical setting found increased risk of inadequate oxygen delivery and mortality among patients with CVD undergoing cardiac or vascular surgery as well as elderly patients undergoing orthopedic surgery.[57] These trials[50,55,57] provide evidence that a more liberal transfusion practice to maintain higher Hb thresholds may represent prudent management of high-risk patients who have symptomatic coronary artery disease or are undergoing cardiac surgery.

One of the important limitations of prospectively, randomized clinical trials is that patients who are eligible and who agree to participate in the study may not be particularly reflective of all patients in these clinical settings. Only 41% of the patients who were determined to be eligible for the TRICC trial[49] and 56% of patients eligible for the FOCUS trial[53] were actually enrolled in the studies, leading to concerns over selection bias; did the treating physicians accurately predict which patients would survive the study, and not enroll the others, thereby ensuring that no differences in survival outcomes would be found between treatment groups?

Another limitation is the interpretation of the "transfusion trigger" in these studies. The mean pretransfusion Hb for patients in the "restrictive" red cell transfusion arm of the TRACS trial was 9.1 g/dL (see **Table 2**). Similarly, the mean Hb for patients in the "restrictive" arm of the TRICC trial was 8.5 g/dL; yet many have interpreted this study to advocate that an Hb of 7 g/dL is appropriate for use as the transfusion trigger in critical care patients.

Clinical Practice Guidelines

The number of published clinical practice guidelines for RBC[44,58–75] transfusions attests to the increasing interest and importance of appropriate blood utilization by professional societies and health care institutions (**Table 3**). The selection of a discrete Hb as a "trigger" for RBC transfusion has been controversial.[76] The guidelines generally acknowledge the necessity of considering patient covariables or other patient-specific criteria for making transfusion decisions. Among published guidelines, it is generally agreed that transfusion is not of benefit when the Hb is greater than 10 g/dL, but may be beneficial when the Hb is less than 6 to 7 g/dL.[61–63,66–72]

An editorial[77] summarized the implications of these trials and meta-analyses with a call for a target Hb level for transfusion, stating "it is no longer acceptable to

Table 3
Clinical practice guidelines for red blood cell transfusion

		RBC Transfusion	
Year	Society	Recommendations	Reference
1988	National Institutes of Health Consensus Conference	<7 g/dL (acute)	JAMA 1988;260:2700.[58]
1992	American College of Physicians (ACP)	No number	Ann Int Med 1992;116:393–402.[59]
1996/2006	American Society of Anesthesiologists (ASA)	<6 g/dL (acute) No number	Anesth 1996;84:732–747.[60] Anesth 2006;105:198–208.[61]
1997/1998	Canadian Medical Association (CMA)	No number	Can Med Assoc J 1997;156: S1–24.[44] J Emerg Med 1998;16:129–31.[62]
1998	College of American Pathologists (CAP)	6 g/dL (acute)	Arch Path Lab Med 1998;122:130–8.[63]
2001/2012	British Committee for Standards in Haematology	No number 7–8 g/dL[a]	Br J Haematol 2001;113:24–31.[64] http://www.bcshguidelines. com/documents/BCSH_ Blood_Admin_-_ addendum_August_ 2012.pdf.[65]
2001	Australasian Society of Blood Transfusion	7 g/dL	http://www.nhmrc.health. gov.au.[66]
2007/2011	Society of Thoracic Surgeons (STS) Society of Cardiovascular Anesthesiologists (CVA)	7 g/dL or 8 g/dL[a]	Ann Thorac Surg 2007;83:S27–86.[67] Ann Thorac Surg 2011;91:944–82.[68]
2009	American College of Critical Care Medicine Society of Critical Care Medicine	7 g/dL 7 g/dL	Crit Care Med 2009;37:3124–57.[69] J Trauma 2009;67:1439– 42.[70]
2011	Society for the Advancement of Blood Management	8 g/dL	Trans Med Rev 2011;232– 246.[71]
2012	National Blood Authority, Australia	No number	http://www.nba.gov.au/ guidelines/review.html.[75]
2012	AABB	7–8 g/dL or 8 g/dL[b]	Ann Int Med 2012;157:49–58.[72]
2012	Kidney Disease: Improving Global Outcomes[c]	No number	Kid Int 2012;2:311–316.[73]
2012	National Cancer Center Network (NCCN)	7–9 g/dL	JNCCN 2012;10:628–53.[74]

[a] For patients with acute blood loss.
[b] For patients with symptoms of end-organ ischaemia.
[c] Acute coronary syndrome or cardiac bypass patients.
From Goodnough LT, Levy JH, Murphy MF. Concepts of blood transfusion in adults. Lancet 2013;381:1848; with permission.

recommend that we transfuse using vague approaches such as clinical judgment or in the hope of alleviating symptoms." However, this approach would use transfusion to treat laboratory numbers, rather than patients, and would risk overinterpreting available evidence for a "transfusion trigger" and risk underestimating both the heterogeneity of anemias (eg, acute vs chronic) and the heterogeneity of patients (ie, comorbidities). Given the increasing evidence that shows blood transfusions are poorly effective and possibly harmful, the guiding principle for transfusion therapy should be that "Less is More.". The AABB[78] and the ASH[79] have published recommendations from the American Board of Internal Medicine's *Choosing Wisely* campaign advocating single-unit RBC transfusions for nonbleeding hospitalized patients, which nearly 25 years ago had previously been recommended by the American College of Physicians (ACP).[80] Additional RBC units should be prescribed only after reassessment of the patient between transfusion decisions.

Improving Blood Utilization

Both the pediatric[81] and the adult hospital[82,83] at Stanford Health Care (SHC) have reduced blood use by using computerized physician order entry (POE) process for blood transfusions. The Hb concentration threshold for blood transfusions decreased after clinical effectiveness teams instituted physician education and clinical decision support (CDS) in July 2010, via best practices alerts (BPA) at the time of electronic POE.[82–85] **Fig. 2** shows a subsequent analysis of trends in blood use at SHC. Overall blood component transfusions increased yearly until 2009; after the BPA was implemented in July 2010, however, RBC transfusions have decreased nearly 50% through 2015, over this same interval.[84] Clinical patient outcomes (length of stay, 30-day readmission rate, mortality) showed improvement associated with implementation of CDS for restrictive transfusion practice.

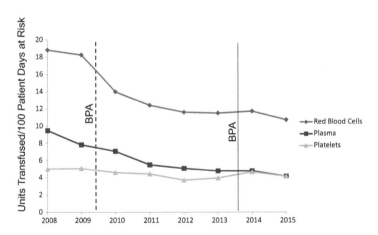

Blood components issued, 2008–2015
---- BPA (best practice alert) for RBC: July 2010
— BPA for plasma: September 2014
Abscissa shows data for end of each year

Fig. 2. Blood components issued to patients at SHC. Transfusion of RBCs per 100 days at risk, decreased by 42% from 2009 through 2015. (*Adapted from* Goodnough LT, Shah N. The next chapter in patient blood management: real-time clinical decision support. Am J Clin Pathol 2014;142:743; with permission.)

Several other institutions have been able to use electronic health records to improve blood utilization, as most recently described by McKinney and colleagues.[86] In another analysis of 21 medical facilities in Kaiser Permanente Northern California and nearly 400,000 inpatients from 2009 to 2013, the incidence of RBC transfusion decreased from 14% to 10.8%, with a decline in pretransfusion Hb levels from 8.1 to 7.6 g/dL; yet 30-day mortality did not change significantly over this same time interval.[87]

Although the improvement in patient outcomes concurrent with reduction in RBC transfusions cannot be proven to be causal, it is reassuring that there was no deleterious effect on patient outcomes after hospital-wide adoption of restrictive transfusion practices.[13] A study monitoring for inappropriate undertransfusion found no evidence that cases of nonadministration of blood were unjustified.[88]

Additional benefits of the restrictive transfusion strategy included a significant improvement in the laboratory budget, with direct cost reductions of $1.6 million annually.[82] Purchase acquisition costs represents a fraction of total costs of blood transfusion that additionally include laboratory testing, reagent costs, nursing time dedicated to transfusion, and monitoring. An activity-based cost summary of blood transfusions estimates that total costs related to transfusion are 3.2 to 4.8 times the purchase costs.[19] Hence, the total transfusion-related savings potentially surpasses $30 million, over a 4-year period. In September 2014, the authors implemented a smart BPA for plasma, triggered when the last recorded international normalized ratio (INR) is less than 1.7 to guide more appropriate plasma transfusion.

This model of concurrent real-time utilization review can be supplemented by peer performance review committees, in which analysis of providers is undertaken for transfusions outside institutional-recommended guidelines. Because up to 30% of RBC transfusions continue to occur in patients whose Hb was greater than 8 g/dL at the authors' institution, peer-performance executive committees can help reduce variability by providers within clinical services that was unchanged by the CDS, and/or help modify the CDS for known clinical exceptions. This process serves as continuous education and feedback, which is seen as vital in the success of utilization programs[89] by augmenting improvements through CDS.

Other programs have been able to use electronic health records to improve blood utilization in a different manner. One center reconfigured their POE system for non-bleeding (excluding procedural units such as operating rooms, cardiac catheterization laboratories) patients to remove single-click ordering for 2-unit RBC transfusions; the provider must select from a drop-down menu if additional RBC units are desired. The proportion of 2-unit RBC transfusions decreased from 47% before to 15% after this intervention.[90] A second center similarly reported a reduction in 2-unit RBC orders (48% to 33%) and an increase in 1-unit RBC transfusions (22% to 48%), before and after, respectively, implementation of a comprehensive education and audit program promoting restrictive transfusion practices.[91] One review concluded that although CDS can improve RBC usage, further data are needed to assess whether CDS can improve plasma and platelet use utilization.[92] The authors have been able to show a 19% reduction in plasma utilization after implementing a smart BPA for plasma orders in the context of a most recent INR result in the patient's electronic medical record (EMR), at the authors' institution.[93]

Additional opportunities to improve blood utilization are in patients undergoing surgical procedures. Because the most important predictor of the need for blood transfusion during perioperative bleeding is the patient's preoperative RBC volume, preadmission testing to include identification and correction of anemia in patients undergoing elective surgical procedures is particularly important.[21] The authors' hospital has initiated a checklist and boarding pass "timeout" before induction of anesthesia, designed to facilitate a conversation between the surgical and anesthesiology teams for individual patients on their anticipated blood loss, cross-matched blood availability, and strategies for managing blood loss anemia; this initiative was based on a strategy described by Atul Gawande using a surgical checklist at his own institution.[94]

SUMMARY

According to the Institute of Medicine, $2.5 trillion was spent on health care, consuming 17.6% of the gross domestic product. In 2009, almost one-third of this health care expenditure was estimated to be wasteful. Transfusion therapy has been identified as one of the most overused (and inappropriate) therapeutic interventions. Reducing this waste helps improve patient outcomes by reducing unnecessary blood donor exposures. The increased adoption of EMRs and features such as CDS allows the practice of prospective, real-time monitoring of transfusion therapy in an automated fashion at the critical time of POE.

Future measures include providing the prescriber with evidence-based and practical RBC ordering options,[95] and distributing the CDS burden to personnel with the highest knowledge base to make decisions. Long term, these users will be engaged for further education or refinement of CDS for continuous quality improvement.[96]

REFERENCES

1. Straus DJ, Testa MA, Sarokhan BJ, et al. Quality-of-life and health benefits of early treatment of mild anemia: a randomized trial of epoetin alfa in patients receiving chemotherapy for hematologic malignancies. Cancer 2006;107:1909–17.
2. Bulger J, Nickel W, Messler J, et al. Choosing wisely in adult hospital medicine: five opportunities for improved healthcare value. J Hosp Med 2013;8:486–92.
3. Goodnough LT, Levy JH, Murphy MF. Concepts of blood transfusion in adults. Lancet 2013;381:1845–54.
4. Roseff SD, Luban NL, Manno CS. Guidelines for assessing appropriateness of pediatric transfusion. Transfusion 2002;42:1398–413.
5. Shah N, Andrews J, Goodnough LT. Transfusions for anemia in adult and pediatric patients with malignancies. Blood Rev 2015;29:291–9.
6. Goodnough LT, Schrier SL. Evaluation and management of anemia in the elderly. Am J Hematol 2014;89:88–96.
7. Goodnough LT, Shander A. Current status of pharmacologic therapies in patient blood management. Anesth Analg 2013;116:15–34.
8. Spahn DR, Goodnough LT. Alternatives to blood transfusion. Lancet 2013;381: 1855–65.
9. Perkins HA, Busch MP. Transfusion-associated infections: 50 years of relentless challenges and remarkable progress. Transfusion 2010;50:2080–99.
10. Goodnough LT. Blood management: transfusion medicine comes of age. Lancet 2013;381:1791–2.
11. Fauci AS, Morens DM. Zika virus in the Americas–yet another arbovirus threat. N Engl J Med 2016;374:601–4.
12. US Food and Drug Administration Center for Biologics Evaluation and Research. Fatalities reported to FDA following blood collection and transfusion. Annual summary for fiscal year 2011. Available at: http://www.fda.gov/downloads/ BiologicsBloodVaccines/SafetyAvailability/ReportaProblem/TransfusionDonation Fatalities/UCM300764.pdf. Accessed June 9, 2016.

13. Goodnough LT, Murphy MF. Do liberal blood transfusions cause more harm than good? BMJ 2014;349:g6897.

14. Brunskill SJ, Millette SL, Shokoohi A, et al. Red blood cell transfusion for people undergoing hip fracture surgery. Cochrane Database Syst Rev 2015;(4):CD009699.

15. Salpeter SR, Buckley JS, Chatterjee S. Impact of more restrictive blood transfusion strategies on clinical outcomes: a meta-analysis and systematic review. Am J Med 2014;127:124–31.e3.

16. Bloch EM, Simon MS, Shaz BH. Emerging infections and blood safety in the 21st century. Ann Intern Med 2016. [Epub ahead of print].

17. Wang D, Sun J, Solomon SB, et al. Transfusion of older stored blood and risk of death: a meta-analysis. Transfusion 2012;52:1184–95.

18. Steiner ME, Triulzi DJ, Assmann SF, et al. Randomized trial results: red cell storage is not associated with a significant difference in multiple-organ dysfunction score or mortality in transfused cardiac surgery patients. Transfusion 2014;54:15A.

19. Shander A, Hofmann A, Ozawa S, et al. Activity-based costs of blood transfusions in surgical patients at four hospitals. Transfusion 2010;50:753–65.

20. Goodnough LT, Shander A. Patient blood management. Anesthesiology 2012;116:1367–76.

21. Goodnough LT, Maniatis A, Earnshaw P, et al. Detection, evaluation, and management of preoperative anaemia in the elective orthopaedic surgical patient: NATA guidelines. Br J Anaesth 2011;106:13–22.

22. Salisbury AC, Reid KJ, Alexander KP, et al. Diagnostic blood loss from phlebotomy and hospital-acquired anemia during acute myocardial infarction. Arch Intern Med 2011;171:1646–53.

23. Guinn NR, Guercio JR, Hopkins TJ, et al. How do we develop and implement a preoperative anemia clinic designed to improve perioperative outcomes and reduce cost? Transfusion 2016;56:297–303.

24. Jans Ø, Jorgensen C, Kehlet H, et al. Role of preoperative anemia for risk of transfusion and postoperative morbidity in fast-track hip and knee arthroplasty. Transfusion 2014;54:717–26.

25. Wu WC, Schifftner TL, Henderson WG, et al. Preoperative hematocrit levels and postoperative outcomes in older patients undergoing noncardiac surgery. JAMA 2007;297:2481–8.

26. Beattie WS, Karkouti K, Wijeysundera DN, et al. Risk associated with preoperative anemia in noncardiac surgery: a single-center cohort study. Anesthesiology 2009;110:574–81.

27. Gruson KI, Aharonoff GB, Egol KA, et al. The relationship between admission hemoglobin level and outcome after hip fracture. J Orthop Trauma 2002;16:39–44.

28. Lacroix J, Hebert PC, Hutchison JS, et al. Transfusion strategies for patients in pediatric intensive care units. N Engl J Med 2007;356:1609–19.

29. Dhabangi A, Ainomugisha B, Cserti-Gazdewich C, et al. Effect of transfusion of red blood cells with longer vs shorter storage duration on elevated blood lactate levels in children with severe anemia: the total randomized clinical trial. JAMA 2015;314:2514–23.

30. Kirpalani H, Whyte RK, Andersen C, et al. The Premature Infants in Need of Transfusion (PINT) study: a randomized, controlled trial of a restrictive (low) versus liberal (high) transfusion threshold for extremely low birth weight infants. J Pediatr 2006;149:301–7.

31. Bell EF, Strauss RG, Widness JA, et al. Randomized trial of liberal versus restrictive guidelines for red blood cell transfusion in preterm infants. Pediatrics 2005; 115:1685–91.

32. Kirpalani H, Bell E, D'Angio C, et al. Transfusion of Prematures (TOP) trial: does a liberal red blood cell transfusion strategy improve neurological-intact survival of extremely-low-birth-weight infants as compared to a restricitve strategy? Available at: http://www.nichd.nih.gov/about/Documents/TOP_Protocol.pdf. Accessed June 9, 2016.

33. Bercovitz RS, Quinones RR. A survey of transfusion practices in pediatric hematopoietic stem cell transplant patients. J Pediatr Hematol Oncol 2013;35: e60–3.

34. Adams RJ, McKie VC, Hsu L, et al. Prevention of a first stroke by transfusions in children with sickle cell anemia and abnormal results on transcranial Doppler ultrasonography. N Engl J Med 1998;339:5–11.

35. Adams RJ, Brambilla D. Discontinuing prophylactic transfusions used to prevent stroke in sickle cell disease. N Engl J Med 2005;353:2769–78.

36. McLaughlin JF, Ballas SK. High mortality among children with sickle cell anemia and overt stroke who discontinue blood transfusion after transition to an adult program. Transfusion 2016;56:1014–21.

37. Finch CA, Lenfant C. Oxygen transport in man. N Engl J Med 1972;286:407–15.

38. Adams RC, Lundy JS. Anesthesia in cases of poor surgical risk: some suggestions for decreasing the risk. Surg Gynecol Obstet 1941;71:1011–4.

39. Carson JL, Noveck H, Berlin JA, et al. Mortality and morbidity in patients with very low postoperative Hb levels who decline blood transfusion. Transfusion 2002;42: 812–8.

40. van Woerkens EC, Trouwborst A, van Lanschot JJ. Profound hemodilution: what is the critical level of hemodilution at which oxygen delivery-dependent oxygen consumption starts in an anesthetized human? Anesth Analg 1992;75:818–21.

41. Carson JL, Duff A, Poses RM, et al. Effect of anaemia and cardiovascular disease on surgical mortality and morbidity. Lancet 1996;348:1055–60.

42. Hebert PC, Yetisir E, Martin C, et al. Is a low transfusion threshold safe in critically ill patients with cardiovascular diseases? Crit Care Med 2001;29:227–34.

43. Parrillo JE. Journal supplements, anemia management, and evidence-based critical care medicine. Crit Care Med 2001;29(Supplement):S139–40.

44. Expert Working Group. Guidelines for red blood cell and plasma transfusion for adults and children. Can Med Assoc J 1997;156(Suppl 11):S1–24.

45. Wu WC, Rathore SS, Wang Y, et al. Blood transfusion in elderly patients with acute myocardial infarction. N Engl J Med 2001;345:1230–6.

46. Goodnough LT, Bach RG. Anemia, transfusion, and mortality. N Engl J Med 2001; 345:1272–4.

47. Carson JL, Hill S, Carless P, et al. Transfusion triggers: a systematic review of the literature. Transfus Med Rev 2002;16:187–99.

48. Carson JL, Carless PA, Hebert PC. Transfusion thresholds and other strategies for guiding allogeneic red blood cell transfusion. Cochrane Database Syst Rev 2012;(4):CD002042.

49. Hebert PC, Wells G, Blajchman MA, et al. A multicenter, randomized, controlled clinical trial of transfusion requirements in critical care. Transfusion Requirements in Critical Care Investigators, Canadian Critical Care Trials Group. N Engl J Med 1999;340:409–17.

50. Holst LB, Haase N, Wetterslev J, et al. Lower versus higher hemoglobin threshold for transfusion in septic shock. N Engl J Med 2014;371:1381–91.

51. Mudumbai SC, Cronkite R, Hu KU, et al. Association of admission hematocrit with 6-month and 1-year mortality in intensive care unit patients. Transfusion 2011;51: 2148–59.
52. Hajjar LA, Vincent JL, Galas FR, et al. Transfusion requirements after cardiac surgery: the TRACS randomized controlled trial. JAMA 2010;304:1559–67.
53. Carson JL, Terrin ML, Noveck H, et al. Liberal or restrictive transfusion in high-risk patients after hip surgery. N Engl J Med 2011;365:2453–62.
54. Villanueva C, Colomo A, Bosch A, et al. Transfusion strategies for acute upper gastrointestinal bleeding. N Engl J Med 2013;368:11–21.
55. Carson JL, Brooks MM, Abbott JD, et al. Liberal versus restrictive transfusion thresholds for patients with symptomatic coronary artery disease. Am Heart J 2013;165:964–71.e1.
56. Murphy GJ, Pike K, Rogers CA, et al. Liberal or restrictive transfusion after cardiac surgery. N Engl J Med 2015;372:997–1008.
57. Hovaguimian F, Myles PS. Restrictive versus liberal transfusion strategy in the perioperative and acute care settings: A context-specific systematic review and meta-analysis of randomized controlled trials. Anesthesiology 2016;125(1): 46–61.
58. Consensus Conference. Perioperative red blood cell transfusion. JAMA 1988; 260:2700–3.
59. Welch HG, Meehan KR, Goodnough LT. Prudent strategies for elective red blood cell transfusion. Ann Intern Med 1992;116:393–402.
60. Practice Guidelines for blood component therapy: a report by the American Society of Anesthesiologists Task Force on Blood Component Therapy. Anesthesiology 1996;84:732–47.
61. Practice guidelines for perioperative blood transfusion and adjuvant therapies: an updated report by the American Society of Anesthesiologists Task Force on Perioperative Blood Transfusion and Adjuvant Therapies. Anesthesiology 2006; 105:198–208.
62. Innes G. Guidelines for red blood cells and plasma transfusion for adults and children: an emergency physician's overview of the 1997 Canadian blood transfusion guidelines. Part 1: red blood cell transfusion. Canadian Medical Association Expert Working Group. J Emerg Med 1998;16:129–31.
63. Simon TL, Alverson DC, AuBuchon J, et al. Practice parameter for the use of red blood cell transfusions: developed by the Red Blood Cell Administration Practice Guideline Development Task Force of the College of American Pathologists. Arch Pathol Lab Med 1998;122:130–8.
64. Murphy MF, Wallington TB, Kelsey P, et al. Guidelines for the clinical use of red cell transfusions. Br J Haematol 2001;113:24–31.
65. British Committee for Standards in Haematology (BCSH) Guideline on the Administration of blood components. Available at: http://www.bcshguidelines.com/documents/BCSH_Blood_Admin_-_addendum_August_2012.pdf. Accessed June 9, 2016.
66. Australasian Society of Blood Transfusion. Clinical Practice Guidelines: Appropriate use of red blood cells. Available at: http://www.nhmrc.gov.au/_files_nhmrc/publications/attachments/cp78.pdf. Accessed June 9, 2016.
67. Society of Thoracic Surgeons Blood Conservation Guideline Task Force, Ferraris VA, Ferraris SP, et al. Perioperative blood transfusion and blood conservation in cardiac surgery: the Society of Thoracic Surgeons and The Society of Cardiovascular Anesthesiologists clinical practice guideline. Ann Thorac Surg 2007;83:S27–86.

68. Society of Thoracic Surgeons Blood Conservation Guideline Task Force, Ferraris VA, Brown JR, et al. 2011 Update to the Society of Thoracic Surgeons and the Society of Cardiovascular Anesthesiologists blood conservation clinical practice guidelines. Ann Thorac Surg 2011;91:944–82.

69. Napolitano LM, Kurek S, Luchette FA, et al. Clinical practice guideline: red blood cell transfusion in adult trauma and critical care. Crit Care Med 2009;37:3124–57.

70. Napolitano LM, Kurek S, Luchette FA, et al. Clinical practice guideline: red blood cell transfusion in adult trauma and critical care. J Trauma 2009;67:1439–42.

71. Shander A, Fink A, Javidroozi M, et al. Appropriateness of allogeneic red blood cell transfusion: the international consensus conference on transfusion outcomes. Transfus Med Rev 2011;25:232–46.e53.

72. Carson JL, Grossman BJ, Kleinman S, et al. Red blood cell transfusion: a clinical practice guideline from the AABB*. Ann Intern Med 2012;157:49–58.

73. Kidney Disease: Improving Global Outcomes (KDIGO) Anemia Work Group. KDIGO Clinical Practice Guideline for anemia in chronic kidney disease. Kidney Int Suppl 2012;2:279–335.

74. Rodgers GM 3rd, Becker PS, Blinder M, et al. Cancer- and chemotherapy-induced anemia. J Natl Compr Canc Netw 2012;10:628–53.

75. National Blood Authority, Australia. Patient blood management guidelines. Available at: https://www.blood.gov.au/pbm-guidelines. Accessed June 9, 2016.

76. Goodnough LT, Shah N. Is there a "magic" hemoglobin number? Clinical decision support promoting restrictive blood transfusion practices. Am J Hematol 2015;90:927–33.

77. Carson JL, Hebert PC. Should we universally adopt a restrictive approach to blood transfusion? It's all about the number. Am J Med 2014;127:103–4.

78. Callum JL, Waters JH, Shaz BH, et al. The AABB recommendations for the Choosing Wisely campaign of the American Board of Internal Medicine. Transfusion 2014;54:2344–52.

79. Hicks LK, Bering H, Carson KR, et al. The ASH choosing wisely campaign: five hematologic tests and treatments to question. Blood 2013;122:3879–83.

80. Audet AM, Goodnough LT, Parvin CA. Evaluating the appropriateness of red blood cell transfusions: the limitations of retrospective medical record reviews. Int J Qual Health Care 1996;8:41–9.

81. Adams ES, Longhurst CA, Pageler N, et al. Computerized physician order entry with decision support decreases blood transfusions in children. Pediatrics 2011;127:e1112–9.

82. Goodnough LT, Shieh L, Hadhazy E, et al. Improved blood utilization using real-time clinical decision support. Transfusion 2014;54:1358–65.

83. Goodnough LT, Maggio P, Hadhazy E, et al. Restrictive blood transfusion practices are associated with improved patient outcomes. Transfusion 2014;54:2753–9.

84. Goodnough LT, Shah N. The next chapter in patient blood management: real-time clinical decision support. Am J Clin Pathol 2014;142:741–7.

85. Tim Goodnough L, Andrew Baker S, Shah N. How I use clinical decision support to improve blood cell utilization. Transfusion 2016;56(10):2406–11.

86. McKinney ZJ, Peters JM, Gorlin JB, et al. Improving red blood cell orders, utilization, and management with point-of-care clinical decision support. Transfusion 2015;55:2086–94.

87. Roubinian NH, Escobar GJ, Liu V, et al. Trends in red blood cell transfusion and 30-day mortality among hospitalized patients. Transfusion 2014;54:2678–86.

88. Hibbs S, Miles D, Staves J, et al. Is undertransfusion a problem in modern clinical practice? Transfusion 2015;55:906–10.

89. Yeh DD. A clinician's perspective on laboratory utilization management. Clin Chim Acta 2014;427:145–50.
90. Yerrabothala S, Desrosiers KP, Szczepiorkowski ZM, et al. Significant reduction in red blood cell transfusions in a general hospital after successful implementation of a restrictive transfusion policy supported by prospective computerized order auditing. Transfusion 2014;54:2640–5.
91. Oliver JC, Griffin RL, Hannon T, et al. The success of our patient blood management program depended on an institution-wide change in transfusion practices. Transfusion 2014;54:2617–24.
92. Hibbs SP, Nielsen ND, Brunskill S, et al. The impact of electronic decision support on transfusion practice: A systematic review. Transfus Med Rev 2015;29:14–23.
93. Shah NK, Shepard J, Hadhazy E, et al. Decreasing Inappropriate Plasma (FFP) Transfusion with Real-time Clinical Decision Support (CDS). Transfusion 2015; 55:107A.
94. Notable & Quotable: Atul Gawande. The Wall Street Journal; 12/12/2014. Available at: http://www.wsj.com/articles/notable-quotable-atul-gawande-1418425543?tesla=y&mod=djemITP_h&mg=reno64-wsj. Accessed June 9, 2016.
95. McWilliams B, Triulzi DJ, Waters JH, et al. Trends in RBC ordering and use after implementing adaptive alerts in the electronic computerized physician order entry system. Am J Clin Pathol 2014;141:534–41.
96. Berwick DM. Continuous improvement as an ideal in health care. N Engl J Med 1989;320:53–6.

Index

Note: Page numbers of article titles are in **boldface** type.

Med Clin N Am 101 (2017) 449–463
http://dx.doi.org/10.1016/S0025-7125(17)30010-X
0025-7125/17

medical.theclinics.com

Moving?

Make sure your subscription moves with you!

To notify us of your new address, find your **Clinics Account Number** (located on your mailing label above your name), and contact customer service at:

Email: journalscustomerservice-usa@elsevier.com

800-654-2452 (subscribers in the U.S. & Canada)
314-447-8871 (subscribers outside of the U.S. & Canada)

Fax number: 314-447-8029

Elsevier Health Sciences Division
Subscription Customer Service
3251 Riverport Lane
Maryland Heights, MO 63043

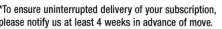
*To ensure uninterrupted delivery of your subscription, please notify us at least 4 weeks in advance of move.

ELSEVIER

Printed and bound by CPI Group (UK) Ltd, Croydon, CR0 4YY

03/10/2024

01040398-0002